'This lucid and accessible book confronts bias against therapies of depth, insight, and relationships – bias that threatens to undermine the credibility of the entire field and that fails those struggling with mental and substance use disorders. In a world facing a crisis in mental health, billions spent on pharmaceuticals, brain research, and treatment limited by insurance entities to crisis intervention, have failed to move the needle on outcomes. The authors offer a perspective reminding us that the rediscovered "social determinants of mental health" not only play a role in causation, but also in treatment. The book summarizes evidence for the effectiveness of long-term therapies and emphasizes the importance of human connection in treatment relationships within which individuals feel heard. Through their market research and focus groups, the authors show that most people want more than they are getting from quick fix, crisis-focused treatment – they want to feel deeply understood, not judged, and to be empowered by self-understanding to take charge of their lives. Kudos to the authors!'

Eric Plakun, *medical director/CEO of the Austen Riggs Center, Stockbridge MA; founding leader, APA Psychotherapy Caucus*

'This landmark book is essential for everyone with an interest in mental health. It illuminates the powerful economic forces that are channeling patients toward the most superficial treatments and clarifies the numerous problems with this approach. To use a medical analogy, the prevailing system resembles treating a patient's fever with aspirin because "evidence" shows the fever usually improves. But unless the cause of the fever can heal on its own, the patient's real problems, those that caused the fever, will persist. Individually and collectively, we can do so much better. This book shows us why and how.'

David D. Clarke, *president, Psychophysiologic Disorders Association and assistant director, Center for Ethics, Oregon Health & Science University, Portland, OR, USA*

'The mental health crises experienced throughout the world are all too evident these days. It is hard to know where to turn for answers. A good place to start is *Advancing Psychotherapy for the Next Generation: Humanizing Mental Health Policy and Practice*. In this edited volume, an ecumenical roster of clinicians, lawyers, MBAs, and physicians argue why we need to promote "therapies that stick" and describe how depth therapy not only makes good financial sense but how they advance our national wellbeing. We are all connected. This book shows us that such connection is both possible and worthwhile.'

Karen G. Foley, *president & CEO, Juvenile Protective Association*

'*Advancing Psychotherapy for the Next Generation: Humanizing Mental Health Policy and Practice* offers a widely encompassing lens for the policies and practices shaping modern psychotherapy. With our society facing a youth mental health crisis and with parity in treatment yet to be achieved, the careful examinations provided by Nancy McWilliams, Farhad Dalal, Pratyusha Tummala-Narra, Susan G. Lazar, Kirk Schneider, Todd Essig, Bill Meyer, Meiram Bendat, and other notable authors, are invaluable.'

Amy Lauren Kennedy, *The Kennedy Forum*

Advancing Psychotherapy for the Next Generation

This book brings together a global community of mental health professionals to offer an impassioned defense of relationship-based depth psychotherapy.

Expressing ideas that are integral to the mission of the Psychotherapy Action Network (PsiAN), the authors demonstrate a shared vision of a world where this therapy is accessible to all communities. They also articulate the difficulties created by the current mental health diagnostic system and differing conceptualizations of mental distress, the shortsightedness of evidence-based care and research, and the depreciation of depth therapy by many stakeholders. The authors thoughtfully elucidate the crucial importance of therapies of depth, insight, and relationship in the repertoire of mental health treatment and speak to the implications of PsiAN's mission both now and in the future.

With a distinguished international group of authors and a clear focus on determining a future direction for psychotherapy, this book is essential reading for all psychotherapists.

Linda L. Michaels is the chair and co-founder of the Psychotherapy Action Network (PsiAN), consulting editor of Psychoanalytic Inquiry, clinical associate faculty of the Chicago Center for Psychoanalysis, and fellow of the Lauder Institute Global MBA program. She is a psychologist with a private practice in Chicago.

Tom Wooldridge is chair in the Department of Psychology at Golden Gate University as well as a psychoanalyst and board-certified, licensed psychologist. He has published several books and numerous journal articles and book chapters on topics such as eating disorders, masculinity, technology, and psychoanalytic treatment. He is on the Scientific Advisory Council of the National Eating Disorders Association, faculty at the Psychoanalytic Institute of Northern California (PINC) and the Northern California Society for Psychoanalytic Psychology (NCSPP), an assistant clinical professor at UCSF's Medical School, and has a private practice in Berkeley, CA.

Nancy Burke is an associate clinical professor, Feinberg School of Medicine of Northwestern University, past president, board member and faculty at the Chicago Center for Psychoanalysis, vice-chair of EMHS-NFP, and secretary of ISPS-US and ABAPsa. She is the originating founder of PsiAN. She maintains a private practice of psychoanalysis, psychotherapy, and consultation in Evanston IL.

Janice R. Muhr is the treasurer and co-founder of the Psychotherapy Action Network (PsiAN) and clinical associate faculty at the Chicago Center for Psychoanalysis. She is a psychologist with a psychotherapy practice in the Chicago area for over 40 years.

Advancing Psychotherapy for the Next Generation

Humanizing Mental Health Policy and Practice

Edited by Linda L. Michaels,
Tom Wooldridge, Nancy Burke
and Janice R. Muhr

Routledge
Taylor & Francis Group
LONDON AND NEW YORK

Designed cover image: Brian P. Bullock, https://bpbullock.com

First published 2023
by Routledge
4 Park Square, Milton Park, Abingdon, Oxon OX14 4RN

and by Routledge
605 Third Avenue, New York, NY 10158

Routledge is an imprint of the Taylor & Francis Group, an informa business

British Library Cataloguing-in-Publication Data
A catalogue record for this book is available from the British Library

Library of Congress Cataloging-in-Publication Data
A catalog record has been requested for this book

ISBN: 9781032351445 (hbk)
ISBN: 9781032351469 (pbk)
ISBN: 9781003325512 (ebk)

DOI: 10.4324/9781003325512

Typeset in Garamond
by codeMantra

To our patients, whose complexity, humanity, and courage set a standard not only for therapists to meet, but for our mental health system to recognize, respect, and embrace as a defining foundation for healing.

To Erika Schmidt and William Meyer, in loving memory.

Contents

Credits List xi
List of Contributors xiii

Introduction 1
TOM WOOLDRIDGE

1 Psychotherapy Action Network: Seeing beyond the crossroads 8
NANCY BURKE, LINDA L. MICHAELS AND JANICE R. MUHR

SECTION I
The social, political, and economic context **17**

2 CBF: Cognitive behavioral fallacies 19
FARHAD DALAL

3 The cost-effectiveness of psychodynamic therapy: The obstacles, the law, and a landmark lawsuit 38
SUSAN G. LAZAR

4 In name only? Mental health parity or illusory reform 57
MEIRAM BENDAT

5 The exclusion of psychoanalysis in academic and organized U.S. psychology: On voodooism, witch-hunts, and the legion of followers 78
OKSANA YAKUSHKO

6 The psycho-politics of evidence-based practice and the assault on our mental health and mental health care 100
ALLAN SCHOLOM

SECTION II
Therapies of depth, insight, and relationship 119

7 Relational healing in psychotherapy: Reaching beyond the research 121
ENRICO GNAULATI

8 Two perspectives of mental distress 135
JOHN THOR CORNELIUS

9 Diagnosis and its discontents: Reflections on our current dilemma 162
NANCY MCWILLIAMS

10 Toward a science of the heart: Romanticism and the revival of psychology 182
KIRK SCHNEIDER

SECTION III
Implications and future actions 209

11 Going beneath the surface: What people want from therapy 211
SANTIAGO DELBOY AND LINDA L. MICHAELS

12 Mirror and window: What each reveals 240
TODD ESSIG

13 Psychoanalytic applications in a diverse society 254
PRATYUSHA TUMMALA-NARRA

14 The rights of children 274
ERIKA SCHMIDT

15 Long-term treatment in the rearview mirror 290
WILLIAM S. MEYER

Stepping toward the future: PsiAN's vision 298
LINDA L. MICHAELS, JANICE R. MUHR AND NANCY BURKE

Index 303

Credits List

The editors and contributors also gratefully acknowledge the permission provided to republish the following material:

Farhad Dalal (2021) CBF: Cognitive Behavioral Fallacies, *Psychoanalytic Inquiry*, 41:8, 580–592, DOI: 10.1080/07351690.2021.1983399, © Melvin Bornstein, Joseph Lichtenberg, Donald Silver, reprinted by permission of Taylor & Francis Ltd., http://www.tandfonline.com on behalf of Melvin Bornstein, Joseph Lichtenberg, Donald Silver.

Susan G. Lazar (2021) The Cost-Effectiveness of Psychodynamic Therapy: The Obstacles, the Law, and a Landmark Lawsuit, *Psychoanalytic Inquiry*, 41:8, 624–637, DOI: 10.1080/07351690.2021.1983404, © Melvin Bornstein, Joseph Lichtenberg, Donald Silver, reprinted by permission of Taylor & Francis Ltd., http://www.tandfonline.com on behalf of Melvin Bornstein, Joseph Lichtenberg, Donald Silver.

Bendat, Meiram. (2012) In Name Only? Mental Health Parity or Illusory Reform, *Psychodynamic Psychiatry*, 42:3, 253–375. Reprinted with permission of Guilford Press.

Oksana Yakushko (2021) The Exclusion of Psychoanalysis in Academic and Organized US Psychology: On Voodooism, Witch-Hunts, and the Legion of Followers, *Psychoanalytic Inquiry*, 41:8, 638–653, DOI: 10.1080/07351690.2021.1983405. © Melvin Bornstein, Joseph Lichtenberg, Donald Silver, reprinted by permission of Taylor & Francis Ltd., http://www.tandfonline.com on behalf of Melvin Bornstein, Joseph Lichtenberg, Donald Silver.

Enrico Gnaulati (2021) Relational Healing in Psychotherapy: Reaching Beyond the Research, *Psychoanalytic Inquiry*, 41:8, 593–602, DOI: 10.1080/07351690.2021.1983403, © Melvin Bornstein, Joseph Lichtenberg, Donald Silver, reprinted by permission of Taylor & Francis Ltd., http://www.tandfonline.com on behalf of Melvin Bornstein, Joseph Lichtenberg, Donald Silver.

John Thor Cornelius (2021) Two Perspectives of Mental Distress, John Thor Cornelius, *Psychoanalytic Inquiry*, 41:8, 654–672, DOI: 10.1080/07351690.2021.1983407, © Melvin Bornstein, Joseph Lichtenberg, Donald Silver, reprinted by permission of Taylor & Francis Ltd., http://www.tandfonline.com on behalf of Melvin Bornstein, Joseph Lichtenberg, Donald Silver.

Nancy McWilliams (2021) Diagnosis and Its Discontents: Reflections on Our Current Dilemma, *Psychoanalytic Inquiry*, 41:8, 565–579, DOI: 10.1080/07351690.2021.19833950, © Melvin Bornstein, Joseph Lichtenberg, Donald Silver, reprinted by permission of Taylor & Francis Ltd., http://www.tandfonline.com on behalf of Melvin Bornstein, Joseph Lichtenberg, Donald Silver.

Schneider, Kirk J. (1998). Toward a science of the heart: Romanticism and the revival of psychology. *American Psychologist*, 53(3), 277–289. Copyright © 1998 by the American Psychological Association. Reproduced with permission.

Tummala-Narra, Pratyusha. (2013). Psychoanalytic applications in a diverse society. *Psychoanalytic Psychology*, 30(3), 471–487, © 2013 by the American Psychological Association. Reproduced with permission.

Long-Term Treatment in the Rearview Mirror by William S. Meyer from *Reflections on Long-Term Relational Psychotherapy and Psychoanalysis*, by Susan A. Lord (eds.) Copyright (© 2019) by Routledge. Reproduced by permission of Taylor & Francis Group.

Contributors

Meiram Bendat is an attorney licensed by the State Bar of California as well as a psychotherapist licensed by the California Board of Behavioral Sciences. With a background in law, clinical psychology, marriage and family therapy, and psychoanalysis, he serves as a consultant to national mental health advocacy organizations and frequently presents on access to treatment and mental health parity. He is a member of the American Psychoanalytic Association Committee on Government Relations and a distinguished Ittleson Consultant to the Group for the Advancement of Psychiatry (GAP). He has lectured at universities around the country, including Yale Medical School, Butler Hospital (Brown University), UCLA, and Antioch University. Dr. Bendat has been interviewed by CBS, National Public Radio, *The New York Times*, *Forbes*, *Psychiatric News,* and other media. In collaboration with the GAP, he authored "In Name Only? Mental Health Parity or Illusory Reform." The article was published in a special issue of the *Journal of Psychodynamic Psychiatry* devoted to the impact of mental health parity and the Affordable Care Act. Along with the National Council for Behavioral Health, he authored two companion pieces on negotiating managed care contracts with an eye toward protecting patient rights. Most recently, along with the Coalition for Psychotherapy Parity, he co-authored *Clinical Necessity Guidelines for Psychotherapy, Insurance Medical Necessity and Utilization Review Protocols and Mental Health Parity.*

Nancy Burke is a psychoanalyst on the faculty of the Chicago Center for Psychoanalysis, of which she is a past president. She is the originating founder of the Psychotherapy Action Network (PsiAN), served previously as a co-chair, and is currently an advisor to PsiAN. She is also an associate clinical professor at the Feinberg School of Medicine of Northwestern University, is past vice-president of ISPS-US, and is on the boards of CCP, Expanded Mental Health Services of Chicago, NFP, and SUSU. Her writing has appeared in *Psychoanalytic Psychology*, the *Psychoanalytic Review*, *JAMA, Gender and Psychoanalysis*, and various literary magazines, and she is the editor of *Gender and Envy* (Routledge). She has presented on the anorexia of language, the domestication of envy, the fear of knowing, and the art of mis-reading Freud, among other topics. She is the recipient of Gradiva, Fish, Fiske, and three Illinois Arts Council awards, and her novel, *Undergrowth,* was published in 2017 by Gibson House Press. She has a private practice in Evanston, IL, devoted to psychoanalysis, psychotherapy, couples/family therapy, and supervision.

John Thor Cornelius is a medical doctor and psychoanalyst who works in Sacramento, California. He trained as a psychiatrist and worked psychiatrically in hospitals, outpatient clinics, and as the medical director of an intensive county program before going on to complete psychoanalytic training at the Psychoanalytic Institute of Northern California. He taught psychoanalysis at the University of California at Davis for many years, is the current president of the Sacramento Psychoanalytic Society, and writes and speaks nationally on the intersection of science and psychoanalysis. In his practice, he prescribes medications, engages in psychoanalytic psychotherapy, and sees people in many forms of distress, including those struggling with trauma and extreme states. Over 98% of his income in 2019 was from direct patient care. He has no financial relationships with mental health drug companies or device manufacturers.

Farhad Dalal is a psychotherapist and group analyst in private practice in Devon, UK. He is a training group analyst and supervisor for the Institute of Group Analysis, London. He also works with organizations. With colleagues, he has recently started delivering a long-term psychodynamic group psychotherapy training in India (which is supported by donations) at groupanalysisindia.com. He has been studying and writing on the themes of psychotherapy, discrimination, equality, and diversity for over 25 years. He has published many papers and four books to date: *Taking the Group Seriously, Race, Colour and the Processes of Racialization, Thought Paralysis: The Virtues of Discrimination.* The content of this paper draws on some of themes from his most recent work *CBT – The Cognitive Behavioural Tsunami: Managerialism, Politics and the Corruptions of Science.* For more information, see his website at *www.dalal.org.uk.*

Santiago Delboy is a psychotherapist in private practice in Chicago. He is a graduate of the Psychoanalytic Psychotherapy Program at the Chicago Center for Psychoanalysis, is currently faculty at the Institute for Clinical Social Work and clinical associate faculty at the Chicago Center for Psychoanalysis, past reflective practice supervisor at The Family Institute at Northwestern University, and serves on the board of Expanded Mental Health Services in Chicago. Prior to becoming a clinician, Santiago spent over a decade in the corporate world, working in marketing research and consumer insights, both in Peru, his home country, and in the US. In his last role, as a consumer insights expert at a global management consulting firm, he focused on market segmentation, branding, and developing marketing and business strategies to drive growth. Santiago earned a Master of Business Administration from The University of Texas at Austin, a Master of Social Work from Loyola University Chicago, and an undergraduate degree in Psychology from Pontificia Universidad Católica del Perú.

Todd Essig is training and supervising psychoanalyst at the William Alanson White Institute, co-chair of APsaA's Covid-19 Advisory Team, and an advisor to PsiAN. Widely known as a pioneer in the innovative uses of mental health technologies, he publishes and lectures widely. He has served on editorial boards for *Contemporary Psychoanalysis* and *JAPA* and recently co-edited along with Gillian Isaacs Russell a special issue of *Psychoanalytic Perspectives* on psychoanalysis and technology. In the aftermath of 9/11, he was board chair for the NY Disaster Counseling Coalition (NYDCC) providing free mental health care to first responders and their families. He writes "Managing Mental Wealth" for *Forbes* where he covers the intersection of technology, psychology, and culture. His practice is in New York City where he treats individuals and couples, almost all of whom (used to) come to his office.

Enrico Gnaulati is a clinical psychologist based in Pasadena, California, and affiliate professor of Psychology at Seattle University. He has published numerous journal and magazine articles, and his work has been featured on *Al Jazeera America*, *China Global Television Network*, *KPCC,* Los Angeles, *KPFK*, Los Angeles, *KPBS*, San Diego, *WBUR*, Boston, *KPFA* Berkeley, *Wisconsin Public Radio*, *Public Radio Tulsa*, and online at the *Atlantic, Salon*, *Psychology Today*, and *Psychotherapy Networker*, as well as reviewed in *Maclean's*, *Pacific Standard*, the *Huffington Post, The Australian, Prevention*, and the *New Yorker*. He is a blogger for *Mad in America,* a nationally recognized reformer of mental health practice and policy, and the author of *Back to Normal: Why Ordinary Childhood Behavior is Mistaken for ADHD, Bipolar Disorder, and Autism Spectrum Disorder* (Beacon Press, 2013) and *Saving Talk Therapy: How Health Insurers, Big Pharma, and Slanted Science are Ruining Good Mental Health Care* (Beacon Press, 2018).

Susan G. Lazar has presented and also published widely on the cost-effectiveness of psychotherapy, including the special place for psychodynamic therapy, in book chapters and articles. Her publications include co-authoring a 1997 *American Journal of Psychiatry* cover article 'The Economic Impact of Psychotherapy: A Review', two edited and co-authored special issues of psychiatric journals including the *Psychoanalytic Inquiry* 1997 supplement *Extended Dynamic Psychotherapy: Making the Case in an Era of Managed Care* as well as the *Psychodynamic Psychiatry* 2014 special issue *Psychotherapy, The Affordable Care Act, and Mental Health Parity: Obstacles to Implementation,* the volume *Psychotherapy Is Worth It: A Comprehensive Review of Its Cost-Effectiveness*, and the 2018 article 'The Place for Psychodynamic Therapy and Obstacles to Its Provision in Psychiatric Clinics of North America'. She chaired the group that formed the Coalition for Psychotherapy Parity and co-authored its document *Clinical Necessity Guidelines for Psychotherapy, Insurance Medical Necessity and Utilization Review Protocols, and Mental Health Parity*, which is available on the website of the Coalition, psychotherapyparity.org. Dr. Lazar served as a consultant to The Mental Health Work Group of The White House Task Force for National Health Care Reform in the Clinton administration and was instrumental in the inclusion of psychotherapy as a medically covered service without arbitrary limitation in the bills considered by Congress at that time. She is a supervising and training analyst at the Washington Baltimore Psychoanalytic Society and clinical professor of Psychiatry at the George Washington University School of Medicine and the Uniformed Services University of the Health Sciences, member and former chair of the Committee on Psychotherapy at the Group for the Advancement of Psychiatry (GAP), member of the American College of Psychiatrists, and distinguished life fellow of the American Psychiatric Association.

Nancy McWilliams teaches at Rutgers University's Graduate School of Applied and Professional Psychology and has a private practice in Lambertville, NJ. She is author of *Psychoanalytic Diagnosis* (1994; rev. ed. 2011), *Psychoanalytic Case Formulation* (1999), and *Psychoanalytic Psychotherapy* (2004), all with Guilford Press. She has edited, co-authored, or contributed to several other books, and is associate editor of both editions of the Psychodynamic Diagnostic Manual (2006; 2nd ed. 2017). A former president of the Division of Psychoanalysis (39) of the American Psychological Association (APA), she is on the editorial board of *Psychoanalytic Psychology* and on the board of directors of the Austen Riggs Center. Dr. McWilliams graduated from the National Psychological Association for Psychoanalysis and is also affiliated with the Center for Psychotherapy and Psychoanalysis of New Jersey. She was featured in three master-therapist videos for the APA and was plenary speaker for their 2015 convention. Dr. McWilliams is an honorary member of the American Psychoanalytic Association, the Moscow Psychoanalytic Society, the Institute for Psychoanalytic Psychotherapy of Turin, Italy, and the Warsaw Scientific Association for Psychodynamic Psychotherapy. Her writings have been translated into twenty languages.

William S. Meyer was director of training for Social Work and associate professor in the Departments of Psychiatry and Ob/Gyn at Duke University Medical Center. He practiced in Duke's high-risk obstetrics clinic and taught and supervised social work interns and 3rd year psychiatry residents at Duke for over 30 years. Additionally, he was on the faculty of the Psychoanalytic Center of the Carolinas, the University of North Carolina, and Smith College. He lectured and published clinical papers on a variety of mental health topics, including the painful history of Psychiatry and the LGBTQ+ community. He was in private practice in Durham, NC.

Linda L. Michaels is a clinical psychologist in private practice in Chicago. She is the chair and co-founder of the Psychotherapy Action Network (PsiAN), a consulting editor of *Psychoanalytic Inquiry*, clinical associate faculty at the Chicago Center for Psychoanalysis, and a fellow of the Lauder Institute Global MBA program. She has published and presented on the value of psychotherapy, the therapeutic relationship and technology, and the public narratives about therapy. She has a former career in marketing, innovation, and strategy, with over 15 years' experience consulting to organizations in the US and Latin America. In addition to her doctorate degree in clinical psychology from the Illinois School of Professional Psychology, Linda is a graduate of the Chicago Psychoanalytic Institute's Psychoanalytic Psychotherapy program. She also has an MBA from Wharton, and a BA from Harvard.

Janice R. Muhr is a clinical psychologist in private practice in Chicago. She is the treasurer and co-founder of the Psychotherapy Action Network (PsiAN) and clinical associate faculty at the Chicago Center for Psychoanalysis. Her 40-some years of clinical practice, following a short career teaching high school English, began in community mental health and has always been informed by it. In addition to her practice with adult individuals and couples, she has consulted in business settings and was clinical adjunct faculty in Northwestern University's Counseling Psychology program for 18 years. She has presented on a wide range of topics which address both systemic and therapeutic responses to the person-in-distress from traumatic life events, and most recently on othering in the field of psychology. In addition to a PhD from Northwestern University, she has an AB and MAT from the University of California, Berkeley.

Erika Schmidt was president of the Chicago Psychoanalytic Institute, a training and supervising adult analyst and child analyst, and faculty member. She was the vice chair of the Psychotherapy Action Network (PsiAN). With a commitment to the provision of mental health services to children who might not otherwise have access, she initiated two programs to provide these services: The Center for Child and Adolescent Psychotherapy at the Chicago Psychoanalytic Institute which offers psychotherapy and on-site therapeutic services in schools and the Chicago chapter of A Home Within which offers pro bono psychotherapy to children in foster care. Her publications were in the areas of child psychotherapy and analysis and the history of psychoanalysis. She was on the editorial board of the *Journal of the American Psychoanalytic Association* and she served as a director-at-large on the Board of Directors of the American Psychoanalytic Association.

Kirk Schneider is a licensed psychologist and leading spokesperson for contemporary existential-humanistic psychology. Dr. Schneider is the current president of the Existential-Humanistic Institute (EHI), council member of the American Psychological Association (APA), past president of the Society for Humanistic Psychology (Division 32) of the APA, recent past editor of the *Journal of Humanistic Psychology*, a member of the Steering Committee of the Psychotherapy Action Network (PsiAN), and an adjunct faculty member at Saybrook University and Teachers College, Columbia University. Dr. Schneider has authored or edited 13 books including *The Spirituality of Awe, The Polarized Mind, Awakening to Awe, The Handbook of Humanistic Psychology, Existential-Humanistic therapy, Existential-Integrative Psychotherapy, The Wiley World Handbook of Existential Therapy,* and *The Depolarizing of America: A Guidebook for Social Healing.* For more information on Dr. Schneider's work, visit https://kirkjschneider.com

Allan Scholom is immediate past president of the Section of Psychoanalyst Practitioners of the Society for Psychoanalysis and Psychoanalytic Psychology of the American Psychological Association, on the faculty and board of the Chicago Center for Psychoanalysis, on the faculty of the Institute for Clinical Social Work, and a founder and member of the Steering Committee of the Psychotherapy Action Network. He has served as president of the Chicago Association for Psychoanalytic Psychology, first vice chairperson of the Chicago Community Mental Health Board, founder and chairperson of the Illinois Coalition of Mental Health Professionals and Consumers, and as a mental health policy advisor to Illinois US Senator Adlai Stevenson, Jr. Dr. Scholom has published and presented widely on the interface between psychoanalysis and politics, primarily regarding mental/health care issues. He has taught classes and led workshops on Psychoanalysis and Politics, the Therapist's Subjectivity, the Clinical Use of Dreams, and Case Conferences. Dr. Scholom is in the private practice of psychotherapy, psychoanalysis, and supervision in Chicago.

Pratyusha Tummala-Narra is a clinical psychologist and the director of Community-Based Education at the Albert and Jessie Danielsen Institute and research professor in the Department of Psychological and Brain Sciences at Boston University. Her research and scholarship focus on immigration, trauma, race, and culturally informed psychoanalytic psychotherapy. Her publications include over 90 peer-reviewed articles and chapters in books. She is also in Independent Practice, and works primarily with survivors of trauma from diverse sociocultural backgrounds. Dr. Tummala-Narra is an associate editor of *Psychoanalytic Dialogues* and the *Asian American Journal of Psychology*. She is the author of *Psychoanalytic Theory and Cultural Competence in Psychotherapy* (2016) and the editor of *Trauma and Racial Minority Immigrants: Turmoil, Uncertainty, and Resistance* (2021), both published by the American Psychological Association Books.

Tom Wooldridge is chair in the Department of Psychology at Golden Gate University as well as a psychoanalyst and board-certified, licensed psychologist. He has published journal articles and book chapters on topics such as eating disorders, masculinity, technology, and psychoanalytic treatment.

His first book, *Understanding Anorexia Nervosa in Males*, was published by Routledge in 2016 and has been praised as "groundbreaking" and a "milestone publication in our field." His second book, *Psychoanalytic Treatment of Eating Disorders: When Words Fail and Bodies Speak*, an edited volume in the Relational Perspectives Book Series, was published by Routledge in 2018, and has been well reviewed. His third book, *Eating Disorders (New Introductions to Contemporary Psychoanalysis),* was released in 2022. In addition, Dr. Wooldridge has been interviewed by numerous media publications including Newsweek, Slate, WebMD, and others for his work. He is on the Scientific Advisory Council of the National Eating Disorders Association, faculty at the Psychoanalytic Institute of Northern California (PINC) and the Northern California Society for Psychoanalytic Psychology (NCSPP), an assistant clinical professor at UCSF's Medical School, and has a private practice in Berkeley, CA.

Oksana Yakushko received her doctoral education in Counseling Psychology and Women and Gender Studies from the University of Missouri. Her initial scholarly work focused on migration, human trafficking, gender, and xenophobia. Recently she has focused on connecting centrality of eugenics among leading American psychologists to propagation of xenophobic, racist, sexist, anti-psychotherapeutic, and anti-psychoanalytic patterns in US psychology. Dr. Yakushko is an author of several books and numerous peer-reviewed articles. She is a professor of clinical psychology at Pacifica Graduate Institute and has a private practice in Santa Barbara, CA. Dr. Yakushko is completing her training in psychoanalysis at the National Training in Psychoanalysis, New York. She is a fellow of the American Psychological Association and has received several awards for her work from several national psychological organizations.

Introduction

Tom Wooldridge

I can still remember the excitement in the air as at the Psychotherapy Action Network (PsiAN) conference held in San Francisco at Golden Gate University in December 2019. As I write this, that was almost exactly one year ago, but it feels like it was in an altogether different world: a time when people came together *in person* without worrying about COVID-19. It was at this event that I first met the three remarkably dedicated women who developed and co-led PsiAN: Nancy Burke, PhD, Linda Michaels, PsyD, MBA, and Janice Muhr, PhD.

Only a year previously I had learned about their vision for PsiAN. Inspired by this, when I discovered they were searching for a location to hold a conference in the Bay Area, I immediately reached out to offer space at Golden Gate University, knowing that we'd have plenty of room after students returned home for the winter holiday. The conference, entitled "Advancing Psychotherapy for the Next Generation: Rehumanizing Mental Health Policy and Practice," was a huge success, drawing attendees from all over the country, each of whom shared a passion for preserving, promulgating, and elaborating dynamically informed, relationship-based treatment.

The present volume attempts to capture the spirit of both this event and its predecessor held in Chicago two years prior. Many of the contributors were, in fact, presenters at one or both of these conferences, whereas others have been involved with PsiAN in other ways. All the authors express, each in his or her own idiosyncratic way, ideas that are integral to the mission of the larger organization. That mission recognizes that while depth-based psychotherapy is alive and well, it is also under attack. Insurance companies are reluctant to cover substantial treatments. Psychology training programs are increasingly constrained to teach manualized, behaviorally oriented treatments. Public policy is similarly biased toward short-term, structured interventions and medications. The shared vision of organizing to "push back" against medicalization, managed care, instrumentalization, and reductionism unites the present group.

In our lead chapter, *Psychotherapy Action Network: Seeing beyond the crossroads,* Nancy Burke, Linda Michaels, and Janice Muhr – founding co-chairs of PsiAN – offer a lovely meditation on many of the issues that animate the work

DOI: 10.4324/9781003325512-1

of the organization and that will be discussed in later chapters in this book. They emphasize the importance of recognizing the environments in which our patients are embedded, including the financial, ideological, and cultural forces that impinge upon them and upon the therapeutic work that occurs (or fails to occur) in our treatments with them. Therapies of depth, insight, and relationship are in the "cross hairs," they insist, and their survival depends upon the strength of our advocacy on their behalf. In this vein, they describe the origins of PsiAN, the principles that form the backbone of its mission, and its three main audiences: policymakers, the general public, and mental health professional organizations. They describe, too, some of the organization's main efforts over the past several years which, as readers will soon see, have been substantial and far-reaching. It is surely a hopeful beginning.

The remainder of this book is divided into three sections, paralleling the conferences' themes. In the first are collected articles exploring the social and political contexts that help to both define and explain the challenges PsiAN faces in accomplishing its mission.

Farhad Dalal, in Chapter 2, *CBF: Cognitive behavioral fallacies*, delivers an impassioned critique of the cognitive behavioral therapy (CBT), including its underlying philosophy and "facile understanding of the human condition," the flawed research protocols that have been used to develop its so-called evidence based, the neoliberal and managerialist political surround in which CBT prospers, and the delivery of CBT in the United Kingdom's health system. He astutely traces the philosophical origins from Jeremy Bentham's utilitarianism, which quantified the notion of happiness and drove psychology toward positivism with its insistence that only what can be observed and measured is real. This fundamentalist ideology, by which psychology today is still gripped, can be described as follows: "Only the countable counts. And that which happens to be countable is MADE TO count. And that which cannot be counted, is simply discounted" (p. 1). This ideology, naturally, led to the ascension of behaviorism, descriptive psychiatry, and research paradigms that are fundamentally tied to the diagnostic categories of the DSM. His critique of these research paradigms is devastating and unveils the vested interests, sleights of hand, and abhorrently compromised standards that characterize much of the so-called "evidence" for CBT.

Susan G. Lazar, in our third chapter, *The cost-effectiveness of psychodynamic therapy: The obstacles, the Law, and a landmark lawsuit,* provides an overview of the research and laws that demand the provision of psychodynamic psychotherapy. In this effort, she describes how psychodynamic psychotherapy has been poorly supported by insurance although the Mental Health Parity Act mandates benefits for mental health care at parity with other health care and that the Affordable Care Act lists mental health care as an Essential Health Benefit. She draws out the consequences of limiting insurance support for psychotherapy upon poorer patients and those with a range of chronic and co-morbid conditions. Finally, Lazar describes 2019 class action lawsuit against United

Behavioral Health for declining to cover research-backed standards for mental health care and of a subsequent California state law mandating sufficient insurance coverage.

Meiram Bendat, in Chapter 4, *In name only? Mental health parity or illusory reform*, describes important insurance and patient protection reforms – the Paul Wellstone and Pete Domenici Mental Health Parity and Addiction Equity Act of 2008 and the Affordable Care Act – that have arisen in the face of inadequate access to mental health resources, stemming in part from discrimination against coverage by private insurers, managed behavioral healthcare organizations, and employers. Yet, as he shows, poor regulatory enforcement and lack of consumer and provider sophistication have led to continued deprivation of mental health and substance abuse treatment by insurers despite these reforms. As a result, whatever gains have been made are negated and the need for further legislative reform is urgent. He proposes a multi-pronged response to this situation.

In Chapter 5, *Exclusion of psychoanalysis in academic and organized U.S. Psychology: On voodooism, witch-hunts and the legion of followers*, Oksana Yakushko turns an eye toward the precarious place of psychoanalysis in American psychology throughout its history. Despite its influence upon the wider culture, psychoanalysis has been marginalized and excluded in academic psychology, with notable consequences including a lack of psychoanalytic ideas in psychology academic training, practice guidelines, grants, and scholarship. Yakushko attempts to understand this exclusion within the historical context of values embraced by American psychology since its inception. After surveying the attitudes toward psychoanalysis of important figures such as William James, John Watson, B.F. Skinner, Albert Ellis, and Martin Seligman, among others, she turns to the socio-historical origins of the attitudes toward psychoanalysis within the academy. Here she cites the influence of the eugenics movement on American psychology, whose assumptions were incompatible with those of psychoanalysis in fundamental ways as well as the organizational dynamics of the American Psychological Association from its inception.

In our sixth chapter, *The psycho-politics of evidence-based practice and the assault on our mental health and mental health care*, Allan Scholom critically examines the notion of evidence-based practice in the context of relevant historical, political, and economic forces. Set against a backdrop of profit-based, market-driven healthcare system in the United States that drives the most expensive, and most poorly ranked, healthcare system in the world, he convincingly casts EBP as a means to curtail services so as to increase the profit of health insurance companies and pharmaceutical industries while also cutting government costs. With a psychoanalytic sensibility, he exposes the mythologies and belief systems that perpetuate a system that supports EBPs and, in the process, cripples our country's mental healthcare system. He emphasizes how CBT fits into the neoliberal paradigm, reducing the costs of health insurance companies and governmental entities while shifting the financial burden to patients and practitioners, and the neoliberal ideology, which values the illusory triumph of individual control over interdependence.

Section II considers the value of therapies of depth, insight, and relationship, with thoughtful explication of their crucial importance in the repertoire of mental health treatment

Enrico Gnaulati, in Chapter 7, *Relational healing in psychotherapy: Reaching beyond the research*, argues for a humanistic revival in the education and training of psychotherapists in an effort to help clinicians-in-training to acquire the relational repertoire, self-expansion, and ethical know-how that is an essential aspect of the clinical profession. It is now a well-known fact that the alliance between therapist and patient is one of the strongest predictors of treatment outcome. In addition, while relatively neglected in the current evidence-based zeitgeist, therapist qualities, such as the capacity for empathic immersion and genuine, authentic care, have long been recognized as essential in the psychodynamic, existential, and humanistic therapeutic traditions. In his chapter, Gnaulati definitionally and descriptively unpacks key aspects of alliance building, therapist empathy, and therapist authenticity and genuineness for pragmatic learning purposes. His effort, it is hoped, will serve clinicians-in-training who are attempting to develop these fundamental capacities and more seasoned clinicians who are revisiting and honing them as well.

Drawing on his real-world experience as a psychiatrist and psychoanalyst, in Chapter 8, *Two perspectives of mental distress*, John Thor Cornelius reflects upon the tension between two perspectives on mental distress: the "broken brain," which understands mental distress from a localized, mechanistic perspective and as caused by discrete mechanical failures of organic brain function, and the "symphonic" perspective, which sees mental distress as a non-local, wholistic, and distributed process spread across the entirety of the mental capacity and as resulting from the impact of tragic life events upon the normally functioning mind. Despite their overlaps, these two perspectives lead to dramatically different ways of relating to, and attempting to ameliorate, suffering. While the "broken brain" perspective has been prominent in recent decades, he highlights questions about its scientific validity and relation to clinical outcomes. The "symphonic" perspective, he suggests, is buttressed by emerging scientific evidence of its theoretical credibility and clinical efficacy.

In Chapter 9, *Diagnosis and its discontents: Reflections on our current dilemma*, Nancy McWilliams reflects on contemporary diagnostic conventions in mental health and their impact on clinical practice, describing the historical evolution from diagnosis that is inferential, dimensional, contextual to descriptive and categorical ways of characterizing mental suffering and the unfortunate consequences for the field entailed by this shift. With a view informed by the history of our field, she highlights the consequences upon diagnosis and treatment of efforts at cost containment, the interests of pharmaceutical companies in mental health, and the sweeping changes in the academic landscape. Finally, McWilliams describes the international project of creating and improving the

Psychodynamic Diagnostic Manual, an effort to restore a clinically useful diagnostic sensibility that values inference, dimensionality, context, and meaning

Kirk Schneider, in Chapter 10, *Toward a science of the heart: Romanticism and the revival of psychology*, begins with the recognition that although emotional, intuitive, and holistic bases for understanding behavior have never been prominent in American psychology as a discipline, now the very existence of such understandings is under threat. His chapter elaborates the reasons for this threat to "romanticism" and spells out the consequences associated with it. With the term *romanticism,* he refers specifically to a lineage of thought that manifests in contemporary psychology in orientations such as existential-humanistic, hermeneutical, narrative, semiotic, cultural, relational, transpersonal, and ecological psychologies (Bevan & Kessel, 1994; Messer et al., 1988; O'Hara, 1994; Sass, 1988; Taylor, 1992; Walsh & Vaughan, 1993). Each of these, in his view, converges with the overarching concern of the human "lifeworld" (Husserl, 1962; Valle & Halling, 1989). Schneider makes an impassioned argument for reclaiming romanticism's legacy, which he sees as important for the future of our discipline. He also, finally, discusses romanticism in contrast to postmodernism, with which he sees a partial compatibility.

Section III, the final section in the book, speaks to the implications of PsiAN's mission and where the movement is headed in the coming years.

Santiago Delboy and Linda Michaels, in Chapter 11, *Going beneath the surface: What people want from therapy*, share the results from their extensive qualitative and quantitative research. They listened deeply to the general public and assessed attitudes, beliefs, biases, motivations, and concerns regarding therapy, therapists, and mental health. Importantly, they found that a sizeable percentage of the public wants what depth therapy has to offer and has an intuitive understanding that their symptoms can be superficial, transitory, and meaningful. People also understand that changing repeating patterns and opening up new choices takes time, and they are willing to make the investment of time, money, and emotion, for they feel both that therapy is a worthy endeavor and they are worthy of its benefits. It is heartening that the public seems receptive to learning more about therapies of depth, insight, and relationship, and their research provides the blueprint for revitalizing these therapies in the mind of the public. Yet much work will need to be done, as the public experiences a dearth of resources and clear information

Todd Essig, in Chapter 12, *Mirror and window: What each reveals*, shares curated excerpts and summaries of articles from his *Forbes* column, written for the general public. He explores topics ranging from some of the troubling trends threatening psychotherapy's future, the need for a stance of activism rather than pessimism in relation to these trends, the rising appeal of artificial intimacy and the deterioration of our relational expectations of others, the media's glamorization of apps to address depression and other mental health problems, the differences between an in-person and online psychotherapeutic process, and the difficulties entailed by returning to in-person treatment during the middle of a pandemic. His reflections offer a thoughtful, pro-active engagement with many of the themes that are the focus of this book.

In Chapter 13, *Psychoanalytic applications to diverse communities*, Pratyusha Tummala-Narra explores ways in which psychoanalysis might be understood through a more inclusive lens in an effort to develop a fuller understanding of racial and cultural diversity across clinical and community applications and focuses on the application of psychoanalytic theory in clinical and community contexts with an eye toward racial and cultural diversity. She proposes an approach to intervention that integrates multiple theoretical perspectives to facilitate engagement with issues of diversity and elaborates how practice with diverse populations may inform psychoanalytic theory. These ideas are illustrated with two case examples that concern the application of psychoanalytic theory to therapeutic work and consultation across sociocultural contexts. The implications of these ideas for minority individuals and communities are discussed.

In Chapter 14, *The rights of children*, Erika Schmidt passionately explores our ambivalence toward children that allows us both to mythologize childhood while at the same time obstructing the legitimate developmental needs of children. She begins with an exploration of our attitudes toward children, focusing on Young-Bruehl's concept of *childism* as a system of thoughts and assumptions akin to sexism and racism that rationalizes harm to children and failure to meet their basic needs, and then turns to two areas in which these prejudices are prominent: immigration, which often spells tragedy for children and their families as forcefully depicted in Luiselli's (2019) book, *Lost Children Archive*, and education, such as when public schools – which often provide not only education but also a larger community as well as meals, health care, and a range of other special services – close to the detriment of children and their families. Her chapter reinforces the need to recognize childism as a part of the social fabric that determines these policies and practices.

In our final chapter, William Meyer revisits his ideas about the value of long-term treatment, for which he is an impassioned advocate especially for those with severe emotional difficulties, with the benefit of experience and hindsight, including the moving clinical case discussed in an earlier paper but from the perspective of several decades later. Here, we can witness his deep and transformative engagement in his clinical work as it unfolds over many years. His chapter reminds us of the benefits to be accrued from pursuing PsiAN's mission. Meyer was involved with the organization before his death in 2021, and this chapter offers readers an opportunity to revisit his thoughtful contributions to the field.

In our epilog, Linda Michaels, Janice Muhr, and Nancy Burke remind us of the essential and vital role for psychotherapies of depth, insight, and relationship and revisit some of the central themes from this special issue, highlighting both the reasons for hope and the threats to the overarching vision expressed here. As they suggest, and as I want to reiterate in this introduction, the ideas discussed by our contributors have real-world import and urgently demand our attention. Our thoughtfulness about these complex issues, efforts toward advocacy in the public and professional spheres, and the important work of community building have the potential to make an enormous difference in the wider world and in the lives of our patients. It is work worth doing.

References

Bevan, W., & Kessel, F. (1994). Plain truths and home cooking: Thoughts on the making and remaking of psychology. *American Psychologist*, *49*, 505–509.

Husserl, E. (1962). *Ideas: General introduction to pure phenomenology*. New York: Collier.

Luiselli, Valeria. (2019). *Lost Children Archive*. New York: Knopf Doubleday Publishing Group.

Messer, S. B., Sass, L. A., & Woolfolk, R. L. (1988). *Hermeneutics and psychological theory: Interpretive perspectives on personality, psychotherapy, and psychopathology*. New Brunswick, NJ: Rutgers University Press.

O'Hara, M. (1994). Relational humanism: Psychology for a pluralistic world. In F. J. Wertz (Ed.), *The humanistic movement: Recovering the person in psychology* (pp. 322–329). Lake Worth, FL: Gardner.

Sass, L. (1988). Humanism, hermeneutics, and the concept of the subject. In S. B. Messer, L. A. Sass, & R. L. Woolfolk, (Eds.), *Hermeneutics and psychological theory: Interpretive perspectives on personality, psychotherapy, and psychopathology* (pp. 222–271). New Brunswick, NJ: Rutgers University Press.

Taylor, E. (1992). William James and the humanistic tradition. *Journal of Humanistic Psychology*, *31*(1), 56–74.

Valle, R., & Halling, S. (1989). *Existential-phenomenological perspectives in psychology: Exploring the breadth of human experience*. New York: Plenum.

Walsh, R., & Vaughan, F. (1993). *Paths beyond ego: The transpersonal vision*. Los Angeles, CA: Tarcher.

1

Psychotherapy Action Network

Seeing beyond the crossroads

Nancy Burke, Linda L. Michaels and Janice R. Muhr

As therapists, we are devoted to the delicate, painstaking work of individual change that happens in the sheltered intimacy of our offices, where we provide opportunities for thinking and feeling before acting, and sometimes instead of acting. Within that protected space and time, the therapy relationship provides both the canvas and the vehicle for healing and growth. At the same time, we cannot confine our vision of our role solely to that therapeutic space, nor can we view our patients' suffering in isolation from their experiences beyond its walls. As we continue to develop our appreciation for the integrity and import of our patients' psychic lives, we do so recognizing the environments in which they are embedded, viewing through their eyes the formative relationships, achievements and, too often, injustices that have shaped them.

In parallel, if our profession and the transformative gifts it yields are to survive, we must embrace acting on behalf of the very work we do in the environments in which we practice. These environments not only influence internal worlds but also play a significant role in determining the very possibility of accessing such intensive therapeutic opportunities. We cannot ignore the financial, ideological and cultural forces that impinge on our work both in establishing a therapeutic process in the first place and in conducting one in which healing from these forces can occur. The world outside has shifted dramatically socially, culturally, economically and politically, and we need to take notice – and action – if we want therapies of depth, insight and relationship to confirm and expand their place of meaning and relevance in helping others navigate that world. In short, psychotherapy is in the crosshairs, and its survival, especially for those who cannot afford to pay out of pocket for treatment or advanced training, will depend upon the skill and strength of our advocacy.

These broader forces simultaneously impact the public, our own professions and policymakers. Marketers play upon the public's fears and fantasies by pathologizing expectable human experiences and downplaying the environmental exigencies that help to explain them. They also promote distorted descriptions and definitions of evidence, creating illusory seals of approval for certain therapeutic protocols, and placing pressure upon practitioners to offer simple and rapid treatments that can produce an easy remission of pain-become-pathology.

DOI: 10.4324/9781003325512-2

The technology industry, with its instant-gratification ideology and free-flowing reserves of investor cash, has sold the idea of well-being as a digitizable commodity available anywhere, anytime, with a swipe of the finger, dehumanizing people and their struggles, and minimizing the impacts of greater societal forces in the process. Insurance companies, responsible to their investors and the quarterly bottom line, will do what they can to discourage the provision of treatments that, at least on the surface and over the short term, appear to be more expensive. Partnerships between insurance companies and technology platforms that are then marketed to employers and the public capitalize on all of these trends simultaneously, increasingly driving a wedge into the therapeutic relationship, if not sidelining it altogether. In addition, while parity for mental health treatment is now the law of the land through the Mental Health Parity and Addiction Equity Act (MHPAEA) of 2008 and the Affordable Care and Patient Protection Act (ACA) of 2010, we continue to see new failures of both the letter and spirit of the law; enforcement has been difficult, and new incursions from insurance companies continue to be experienced by therapists and patients like.

Finally, many therapists no longer feel that their professional organizations represent their work and world views adequately and express disillusionment at many of their initiatives. For example, we highlight psychology's destructive insistence on promoting itself almost exclusively as a hard science, cleaved from its foundation in the human spheres of meaning and experience. Psychology's professional organization has invited insurance company representatives into its inner-circle of practitioners and researchers, offering them a hand in writing treatment guidelines which are later used by those same insurance companies to ration care in the name of "science" (Courtois, & Brown, 2019; See also Dauphin, 2019). It has likewise prioritized randomized controlled trial research over real-world clinical practice, and has developed its training programs accordingly, building a monoculture (Leichsenring et al., 2018) of theory and practice that treats cultural realities almost as an after-thought. Recent graduates from advanced degree programs in many disciplines often report not feeling fully equipped to work with patients and the complex problems with which they can present. And these issues in the mental health professions along with the cultural, technological, legal and financial forces playing out today actively shape law and policy – all of which exercises a determining influence over the broad landscape of mental health treatment, and, intentionally or otherwise, contributes to the marginalization of therapies of depth, insight and relationship.

While many therapists have expressed deep concern about this state of affairs, they have often either withdrawn to practice within a rarified bubble of like-minded colleagues or didn't have the resources to sustain efforts to press for change over the long term. Others challenged specific assaults to psychotherapy in a circumscribed way by marshaling the energy of their individual groups, but without the benefit of more widespread organizational support. And of course, most therapists have been primarily dedicated to the essential task of doing what they do best – of changing the world one person at a time through the revolutionary practice of insight-oriented, relationship-based treatment. Indeed, offering this form of treatment, which upholds the values of development, exploration, tolerance for ambiguity, fantasy, humility, complexity and relatedness, may be our most truly radical act, but it is admittedly hard to operationalize as the basis for organized activism.

Still, only with our concerted active efforts will the general public, policymakers and newer generations of therapists understand and appreciate what depth therapies have to offer. The evidence base for these therapies – over 100 years in the making – is substantial (Shedler, 2010). From meta-analyses of randomized controlled trials to qualitative analyses of therapy process to in-depth case studies, these therapies are shown to be highly effective, both in relieving symptoms and in improving relationships and ongoing deeper patterns of distress (Steinert et al., 2017). These treatments are also a tremendous value: they are relatively inexpensive (when compared to higher levels of care) and they are cost-effective – they reduce and prevent more costly interventions such as hospitalizations, diminish workplace absenteeism and contribute to better physical health outcomes, as offset data show (Lazar, 2010). In addition to being a great value, depth therapies are also an enduring investment; far from a quickly fading quick fix (Westen et al., 2004), the benefits stick with patients over time, and patients continue to improve, months and even years after their last therapy session (de Maat et al., 2009; See also Beutel et al., 2004). Finally, these therapies align with what people want from their treatment experiences (Paris, 2008; Patterson, 2008; Delboy & Michaels, 2021). Extensive qualitative and quantitative market research conducted by consumer insights professionals on behalf of PsiAN clearly demonstrates that many in the general public desire therapies that help them change and grow, make different choices in their lives and address the roots of their concerns. They see therapy as a worthwhile undertaking, an investment in themselves and their future. (The complete discussion of this research can be found in Chapter 11, "Going beneath the surface: What people want from therapy – PsiAN's original research," by Santiago Delboy and Linda Michaels.)

Recognition of the value of therapies of depth, insight and relationship has been as extensive as its history, and yet this recognition has been marginalized along with the treatments themselves, indicating the need for intensified advocacy. To be sure, some of the prior and continuing advocacy efforts have been significant. Both the American Psychoanalytic Association and the Society for Psychoanalysis and Psychoanalytic Psychology (previously, Division 39 of the American Psychological Association) have, in recent years, provided strong and consistent voices aimed at fending off efforts to marginalize relationship-based psychotherapy in professional organizations, with insurers and with the public. The National Association for the Advancement of Psychoanalysis labored for decades so that psychoanalysis could achieve statute recognition in New York State. David against Goliath, the National Coalition of Mental Health

Professionals and Consumers and the Illinois Coalition of Mental Health Professionals and Consumers pushed back hard against the pressures toward capitation models, managed care and short-term treatments stemming from the rise of HMOs that swept the healthcare world during the 1980s. Yet, with the exception of the NCMHPC, most of the advocacy for in-depth treatments had represented the exertion of isolated groups – psychoanalysts, psychologists, social workers or practitioners in specific states – on their own behalf, without the backing of the wide variety of professionals who see depth-oriented psychodynamic, humanistic and other forms of open-ended treatment as their life-giving vocation.

Clearly, there was a need to stand on the shoulders of these giant efforts, to integrate the relatively isolated endeavors of these individuals and groups into a chorus loud enough to get the mental health world – and beyond – to listen. Such an opportunity came in 2017, when the Chicago School of Professional Psychology offered the space to hold a conference, "Advancing Psychotherapy for the Next Generation: Rehumanizing Mental Health Policy and Practice," and the Chicago Center for Psychoanalysis agreed to sponsor it. Without much lead time, a conference committee led by one of us (Nancy Burke) came together. Soon enough, an impressive group of presenters were speaking about the value of, assaults to and avenues for activism on behalf of psychotherapy to a rapt audience over the course of an enlightening, exasperating and exhilarating weekend. Many of the attendees were hearing about the multiple challenges to their work for the first time. Between that Saturday evening and the next Sunday morning, thanks to the energy in the room and the conference's vision to channel it, PsiAN was born. Janice Muhr and Linda Michaels signed on immediately, and, for the next five years, this trio of colleagues from Chicago led PsiAN – an advocacy organization devoted to protecting psychotherapy for the next generation and beyond, especially for those who need it most.

Several principles emerged from that conference which formed the backbone of PsiAN's mission. First, it was clear that PsiAN needed to be a unifying organization, a big tent that welcomed practitioners with an array of practice orientations. If we couldn't set aside theoretical differences, we would get nowhere in our efforts to secure the right to practice and to convey the essential contributions of depth work. We also needed to create a meeting place where those from all corners – even the outskirts – of the field were welcome; thus, we opened our arms to individuals regardless of theoretical orientation in terms of how they practice or theorize. Finally, it was imperative that PsiAN be explicitly interdisciplinary, unfettered by the artificial professional boundaries that foster the illusion that significant differences exist between the psychologists, social workers, psychiatrists, art therapists, marriage and family therapists and counselors who often collaborate extensively and study side by side in peer consultation groups, institutes and continuing education events. We founding co-chairs of PsiAN, psychologists all by license, have been struck by the power of traditional professional groups to isolate therapists from each other, to the detriment of all of us. Indeed, only by uniting, speaking with a common voice about shared concerns, do we have the power to confront the multitude of forces swirling outside our offices.

An additional belief guiding the creation of PsiAN's organizational structure is that our three main audiences – the general public, policymakers and mental health professional organizations – are interlocking, and that activism in all of these spheres at once offers our best hope of creating lasting change. PsiAN's Committees reflect this dedication to a multi-faceted effort. Our Communications Committee aims to reach the general public, informed by PsiAN's extensive qualitative and quantitative research into public experiences, expectations, preconceptions, associations, biases, behaviors and desires regarding psychotherapy. We are working to educate and inform, correct the record of mis-representations of how therapy works and present compelling accounts of its power to change lives. The Children's Committee works to change patterns in the provision of services to this most vulnerable group, aiming to speak out to students, policymakers, attorneys, pediatricians, parents and school-based professionals about the importance of relationally based interventions that focus on providing needed support and opportunities for children and their families. The Education Committee aims to support students at all levels in their efforts to develop therapeutic capacities and interests, to challenge biases against therapies of depth, insight and relationship in graduate training and accreditation and to support the visibility and identity formation of early career practitioners, with special attention to clearing paths toward places of significance in the field for people from marginalized groups or with fewer financial resources. Our Insurance Committee stepped up to take a strong stand to protect parity and teletherapy during the pandemic. Our Developing Professionals Committee sponsors a mentoring program for undergraduates. Most recently, we have brought the Psychoanalytic Collaboratory, a process group model for project incubation with a seven-year track record that has supported numerous clinicians in developing projects to serve the community, under our umbrella as the Community Collaboratory at PsiAN to form the core of our efforts to expand dynamic perspectives and practice into community work, within and beyond the office.

We crafted our committee structure to respond to the fact that psychotherapy is embedded within overlapping circles of professional practice, psychological theory, healthcare systems and economic and social forces. Each circle is crafted by assumptions about what matters: how power and resources should be managed and distributed, how we understand our place within our environment and, ultimately, what it is to be human. In the US, therapies of depth, insight and relationship were imported into and grew up within a culture in which pragmatism, efficiency and the commodification of human functioning were common features. Some of the unfortunate consequences of these factors include prisons (where people of color are over-represented, see U.S. Department of Justice, 2016) serving as a predominant provider of mental health service (Montross, 2020), and partnerships between insurance companies and large corporations that focus on measuring employee wellness in the name of mental healthcare (McRobbie, 2019). In addition, there are diagnostic systems that stigmatize members of marginalized groups disproportionately (Bell, Jackson & Bell, 2015), treatment for veterans that often leads to re-traumatization instead of rehabilitation (Steenkamp, Litz & Marmar, 2020) and a surge of apps and even bots that promise the eradication of difficult feelings, and of internal life itself.

We view advocacy for therapies of depth, insight and relationship as advocacy for social justice, and believe that our movement offers an alternative set of values that can, potentially, provide needed correctives to these essentializing trends. We aim not merely to protect the accessibility and provision of a specific form of treatment that can heal our patients one by one, but to support a view of human possibility that can act as a wellspring of insight and influence regarding broader cultural forces. In pressing for the availability of depth psychotherapies for those who need them most, we are working toward the creation of a world in which the subjectivity of each of us is honored. To serve in this role, however, depth therapies also must look inward, take stock of their legacies and embrace this necessary form of self-reflection with even greater urgency. As it stands, people with means and privilege are far more likely than people without to receive psychological services that treat them as subjects rather than objects. While broader cultural forces have had a determinative role in rationing these treatments, psychoanalytic organizations and institutes have often fostered an insular elitism, restricting training programs to the well-heeled, in which one aspect of their privilege is their ability to complete advanced training with little to no exposure to the world of human suffering beyond their social boundaries. Similarly, we as depth therapists must work to face the extent to which we've operated as if social context, systemic inequities and other daily manifestations of dehumanization play a relatively small role in a healing therapeutic process, until recently giving them little attention in our theory-building and in the therapy relationship itself. To recalibrate our core beliefs in light of a heightened sensitivity to cultural factors is to amplify our capacity to appreciate not only the limits, but the integrity and power of the workings of our internal worlds.

Just as artists and other activists-from-the-margins are often most effective in challenging systems that have marginalized core aspects of humanity, it is we practitioners of this often-marginalized art of emotional healing who, in finding ways to bear the unbearable with our patients, are well prepared to build bridges to understanding and connection, and to give credibility to those whose suffering must be heard. The tools of our trade – the cultivation of listening, the development of vocabularies for understanding and transcending our fears and their effects and the appreciation that our most sacred tenets are provisional – are a most effective means to creating understanding and connection. If we apply these tools in equal measure to our patients and to our own guiding concepts and assumptions, we will likely be of greater service in both the clinical and social arenas.

If we need a test case to illuminate the crucial juncture at which our mental health systems, like our other social systems, find themselves, we need look no further than to the mental health pandemic that has been sparked by the COVID-19 viral one. Isolation, helplessness and instability on many fronts, framed and exacerbated by social inequity, have, not surprisingly, given rise to deep distress on a massive scale. Such a historical moment might have created insight on the part of the mental health community, leading its members, who are experiencing the same stressors and effects as our patients, to challenge the illusion of distress-as-diagnosable-illness, and to recognize depression, anxiety and even psychosis, as human problems, even understandable reactions to external circumstances. Instead, we saw institutionalized racism at work in terms of which groups were most likely to suffer the tragic effects of the virus, correlated with those who were far less able to access support for their emotional well-being in a time of crisis. We likewise witnessed a tsunami of money-making start-ups emerging in the surge of this devastation (Landi, 2020), offering putative technological shortcuts to emotional well-being, amplified by the enthusiasm of insurance companies that saw an opportunity to provide ever cheaper interventions under the guise of increasing access.

Nevertheless, these are also times of great promise, offering opportunities to re-envision the mental health landscape, to promote effective care and real equity and to motivate our colleagues to work with us toward that end as never before. Our national crises have raised awareness of the impacts of social upheaval and have energized an empowered and activist citizenry devoted to defending our vision of a world in which empathy guides action. By drawing therapists, generally a reclusive bunch, out of their consulting rooms and into the world, such advocacy and action cannot help but reinforce appreciation of and support for efforts to recognize the effects of traumas upon psyches and cultures, and the urgent need to remediate them. We are hoping to provide a home for these advocates that is large enough to hold practitioners and non-practitioners alike. It is our belief that in so doing, therapies of depth, insight and relationship will be valued on a widespread basis for their vital role in protecting and acknowledging personal, interpersonal and cultural embodied experience in ways that algorithmic, one-size-fits-all, symptom-focused treatments simply cannot.

On our journey toward the formation of a robust, multi-faceted advocacy organization, we cannot have found better guidance than that offered by our Advisors and Steering Committee members, several of whom are represented in this book. Our fervent wish is that, inspired by their insights, you find an aspect of our advocacy that activates you, draws you into our PsiAN family and empowers you to do the work that needs to be done to assure that therapies of depth, insight and relationship can be available to those who need them most. To achieve the paradigm shifts we desire, to restore the value of therapies of depth, insight and relationship in the minds of the public, policymakers and our own professions, we will need many voices, many experiences and many perspectives. PsiAN has already seen growth and progress beyond our wildest dreams, testifying to the power of our mission and the promise of our vision. We eagerly look toward a future in which the therapies that offer powerful benefits that stick (Michaels, 2020) are respected as evidence that counts, valued as the worthy endeavors they are for so many and accessible by all who desire healing and seek life-giving transformation. Welcome to our big tent.

References

Bell, C. C., Jackson, W. M., & Bell, B. H. (2015). Misdiagnosis of African-Americans with psychiatric issues–part II. *Journal of the National Medical Association, 107*(3), 35–41.

Beutel, M. E., Rasting, M., Stuhr, U., Rüger, B. & Leuzinger-Bohleber, M. (2004). Assessing the Impact of Psychoanalysis and Long-term Psychoanalytic Therapies on Health Care Utilization and Costs. *Psychotherapy Research, 14*, 146–160. https://doi.org/10.1093/ptr/kph014.

Courtois, C. & Brown, L. (2019). Guideline Orthodoxy and Resulting Limitations of the American Psychological Association's Clinical Practice Guideline for the Treatment of PTSD in Adults. *Psychotherapy, 56* (3), 329–339.

Dauphin, V. B. (2020). A Critique of the American Psychological Association Clinical Practice Guideline for the Treatment of Posttraumatic Stress Disorder (PTSD) in Adults. *Psychoanalytic Psychology, 37* (2), 117–127. https://doi.org/10.1037/pap0000253.

de Maat, S., de Jonghe, F., Schoevers, R. & Dekker, J. (2009). The Effectiveness of Long-term Psychoanalytic Therapy: A Systematic Review of Empirical Studies. *Harvard Review of Psychiatry, 17*, 1–23. https://doi.org/10.1080/10673220902742476.

Delboy, S. & Michaels, L. (2021). Going Beneath the Surface: What People Want from Therapy. *Psychoanalytic Inquiry, 41* (8), 603–623. https://doi.org/10.1080/07351690.2021.1992232

Landi, H. (2020, July 06). Digital behavioral health startups scored $588M in funding amid COVID-19 pandemic. FierceHealthcare.com. Retrieved February 09, 2021, from https://www.fiercehealthcare.com/tech/funding-for-digital-behavioral-health-startups-surged-amid-covid-19-pandemic.

Lazar S. G., ed. (2010). *Psychotherapy Is Worth It: A Comprehensive Review of Its Cost-Effectiveness.* Arlington, VA: American Psychiatric Association Publishing.

Leichsenring, F., Abbass, A., Hilsenroth, M., Luyten, P., Munder, T., Rabung, S. & Steinert, C. (2018). "Gold Standards," Plurality and Monocultures: The Need for Diversity in Psychotherapy. *Frontiers in Psychiatry, 9*, 159. https://www.frontiersin.org/articles/10.3389/fpsyt.2018.00159/full.

McRobbie, L. (2019, August 19). Offering mental health apps as part of corporate wellness programs can be risky. Strategy-Business.com. Retrieved February 09, 2021, from https://www.strategy-business.com/blog/Offering-mental-health-apps-as-part-of-corporate-wellness-programs-can-be-risky.

Michaels, L. (2020, March 24). Why depth therapy is more enduring than a quick fix of CBT. Aeon. Retrieved February 09, 2021, from https://aeon.co/essays/why-depth-therapy-is-more-enduring-than-a-quick-fix-of-cbt.

Montross, C. (2020). *Waiting for An Echo: The Madness of American Incarceration.* New York: Penguin Press.
Paris, J. (2008). Clinical Trials of Treatment for Personality Disorders. *Psychiatric Clinics of North America, 31*, 517–526. https://doi.org/10.1016/j.psc.2008.03.013.
Patterson, T. L. (2008). Adjunctive Psychosocial Therapies for the Treatment of Schizophrenia. *Schizophrenia Research, 100*, 108–199. https://doi.org/10.1016/j.schres.2007.12.468.
Shedler, J. (2010). The Efficacy of Psychodynamic Psychotherapy. *American Psychologist, 65*, (2), 98–109. https://doi.org/10.1037/a0018378. See also Fonagy, P and Moran, G (1993) Selecting Single Case Research Designs for Clinicians in Miller, N.E., Luborsky, L., Barber, J.P., Docherty, J.P. (eds) *Psychodynamic Treatment Research.*
Steinert, C., Munder, T., Rabung, S., Hoyer, J. & Leichsenring, F. (2017). Psychodynamic Therapy: As Efficacious as Other Empirically Supported Treatments? A Meta-analysis Testing Equivalence of Outcomes. *American Journal of Psychiatry, 174*, (10), 943–953. https://doi.org/10.1176/appi.ajp.2017.17010057.
Steenkamp, M., Litz, B. & Marmar, C. (2020). First-line Psychotherapies for Military-related PTSD. *JAMA, 323* (7), 656–657. https://doi.org/10.1001/jama.2019.20825.
U.S. Department of Justice. (2016). "Prisoners in 2015." NCJ 250229 (Bureau of Justice Statistics Bulletin). https://www.bjs.gov/content/pub/pdf/p15.pdf.
Westen, D., Novotny, C. M. & Thompson-Brenner, H. (2004). The Empirical Status of Empirically Supported Psychotherapies: Assumptions, Findings, and Reporting in Controlled Clinical Trials. *Psychological Bulletin, 130*, 631–663. https://doi.org/10.1037/0033-2909.130.4.631.

Section 1

The social, political, and economic context

2

CBF: Cognitive behavioral fallacies

Farhad Dalal

Introduction

Cognitive behavioral therapy (CBT) has become a global success story because it presents itself as the only therapy that has scientific empirical evidence proving its effectiveness. But as soon as one starts looking into it, one discovers that the so-called science of CBT is not just bad science – which can be excused as sloppy science – but corrupt science. Corrupt, because bad science is being knowingly promoted as good science.

Although what follows is primarily about the rise and rise of CBT in Great Britain, it also serves as a cautionary tale for situations in the USA, mainland Europe and elsewhere.

The entire CBT edifice is deeply problematic, from the shabby research protocols that it utilizes, to its philosophy, to its facile understanding of the human condition, to the way that CBT is delivered in the UK.

I should say that my argument is not with CBT per se. It is a way of working that no doubt suits some practitioners and some of those who come for treatment. It's just not my cup of tea. If it stayed in its neck of the woods I would have no problem with it – live and let live I'd say.

But over the last decades, CBT has colonized the entire field of so-called mental-health. Indeed the very term "mental-health" is at the heart of how this colonization process has taken place: this being the medicalization of human suffering.

One of the triggers for this critique of CBT (Dalal, 2018) was an experience we had on arriving at a conference on the Science of Happiness. Delegates were greeted by people holding placards saying "Get Free Hugs Here." During the conference we learnt that the Science of Happiness had discovered that happy people tended to have more physical contact than others. This insight was "reverse-engineered" to decree that one could make oneself happier by hugging others – even strangers.

This was akin to noticing that when dogs were happy they wagged their tails, and then presuming that if one taught distressed dogs to wag their tails, they would become happy.

But there is another thing here. I find myself hugging those who are significant to my emotional life, and when I do, it is an expression of my feelings

DOI: 10.4324/9781003325512-4

toward them; I am not *using them* to enhance my sense of wellbeing. It is in this way that hugs become instrumentalized, stripped of all meaning and reduced to a skill to be mastered, a skill to be taught by CBT.

This gives you a first glimpse into the mind-set that is CBT.

Philosophy: Jeremy Bentham

In the UK, the Cognitive Behavioral Tsunami was triggered in 2004 when the clinical psychologist David Clark met the economist Richard Layard whose specialty was the study of unemployment. They realized that by joining forces each could help further the interests of the other – Layard's Utilitarian Happiness agenda and his interest in unemployment, and Clark's wish to advance the fortunes of CBT and the profession of clinical psychology.

As is well known, the Happiness agenda was initiated in the 18th C. by the philosopher Jeremy Bentham. He thought that intention of government policies should not only focus on the economy, but also deliberately try to increase the happiness level of its citizens.

Now although Bentham's philosophy gave a central place to the wellbeing of the citizen, it did so in ways that drove psychology into the arms of the positivists, and set the stage for the later arrival of hyper-rationality. It all hinges on the word "increasing." One can only speak of *increasing* happiness if it is construed of as a quantity. But how to measure an intangible subjective state? The answer that Bentham came up with was "utility," which is why his philosophy has come to be known as "utilitarianism." Utility was (allegedly) a measure of the amount of happiness any action would generate in a person. However, in practice it was not possible to calculate utility values.

So the notion of happiness languished for some 200 years, until the arrival of the American psychologist Martin Seligman (1972), who claimed to have discovered the Science of Happiness. Early in his career he conducted experiments in which he delivered electric shocks to dogs in situations that they could not escape from. Eventually the dogs lost all hope and lay down on the floor even while being shocked. His great finding was this: that when these dogs were put in new situations – *where there was the possibility of escape* – they did not try to do so. They had truly given up. The dogs were now deemed to have "*learnt* helplessness." Seligman supposed that depression was a form of learnt helplessness. Depression was being stuck in a state of *imagined* helplessness despite a change of circumstances. In this way, *depression became construed of as the opposite of happiness.* In 2005, Layard published his best seller *Happiness*, the thesis of which was condensed into a short but powerful manifesto, "The Depression Report: A New Deal for Anxiety and Depression Disorders" (Bell et al., 2006).

> for some people it seems impossible *to be positive* without some physical help. Until fifty years ago there was no effective treatment for *mental illness*. (Layard, 2005, p. 9)

Almost all the difficulties with the Happiness/CBT theses are encapsulated in the linkage between these two sentences. The subject of the first sentence is "positivity," and that of the second sentence "mental illness." If you cannot be positive, it is because you are suffering from a mental disorder; the treatment for which turns out to be CBT.

To be out of work is undoubtedly depressing. But the report reversed this to claim to say that the unemployed are unable to work *because* they are suffering from mental illnesses like depression and anxiety. This was said to cost the economy over 12 billion pounds a year in unemployment, disability benefits and lost tax revenue. But an investment of just 0.6 billion pounds a year in a CBT service would cure the unemployed anxious and depressed in 12–24 sessions. Cured, they would be employed, which would result in the benefits bill going down and the tax income going up. For every 60 pence invested, the treasury and country as a whole would get back £12 within a year. A stock broker's wet dream.

In effect, CBT was being sold as a money-making venture. It was on the basis of the economic promises made in that report that the government of the day poured eye watering sums of money into CBT. It was the economic argument that had won the day.

Philosophy: Immanuel Kant

Before going any further, it is helpful to recall the basis of the powerful distinction between "cause" and "reason" in Kant's philosophy as it will be critical to the argument that follows.

Kant thought the material world to be broadly mechanistic and predictable as it consisted of interacting inanimate "things." Its functioning (effects) could be explained (and determined) by prior "causes."

In contrast, the human realm is unpredictable. The human capacity to think allows them *to decide* how to respond to events that impinge on them. And so unlike billiard balls, their actions cannot be understood or determined by prior causes. To understand human life, one looks for "reasons" rather than "causes," because humans live in a world of meaning. Further, Kant thought it unethical to treat humans as though they were mechanisms, as things, because to do so was to dehumanize them. But modernity – and specifically CBT – has paid little heed to Kant's critical distinction between cause and reason, between things and persons, and come to view humans as deterministic mechanisms.

Philosophy: The Vienna Circle

Things took a further turn for the worse in the 1930s when the Vienna Circle of philosophy took a hold of rationality and positivism. According to "ordinary" positivism, if some claim cannot be empirically tested, then one has to remain agnostic about whether the claim is true or false. The existence of God being one such example. The Vienna Circle cranked up positivism into Logical Positivism. They went one step further to say that if something could not be observed and measured, then there was no evidence that it existed, *therefore it did not exist*. They declared that all statements about such matters were "nonsense." Therefore, all intangibles which could not be directly observed and measured, including inner psychological life and ethics, ended up in the dustbin called nonsense. It is this fundamentalist ideology that has led to the fetishization of measurement that our world is in the grip of today. Enlightenment rationality had been usurped and distorted into a form of hyper-rationality, according to which

> Only the countable counts
> And that *which happens to be countable* is MADE TO count
> And that which cannot be counted, is simply discounted.

This belief then allows all kinds of bizarre things to take place, one of which is that the psychotherapies which cannot be tested in accordance with hyper-rationalist protocols are by definition ineffective. But before pursuing that topic further, I turn to the story of the Neem tree which exposes the vested interests embedded within hyper-rationalism and the ideological excesses that flow out of it.

The Neem tree

For over 2,000 years, components of the Neem tree have been used by farmers in India as pesticide. In 1992, an American agricultural company called "Grace" patented a version of the pesticide. Now, Indian farmers' continued use of Neem tree as pesticide put them in breach of international law. The protest that followed counted for nothing in the eyes of the patent courts, because in patent law, a challenge to the novelty claim of the patent could only be allowed if it could be demonstrated that the prior knowledge had previously appeared *in a printed publication*, preferably in a "scientific" journal. In other words, the legal system required *documentation*, something tangible as "evidence." As this was folk knowledge, there was obviously no such documentation. On this basis, the courts declared that *there was no evidence.*

The actual lived self-evident fact, that farmers had been using the Neem tree for millennia, was declared anecdotal and dismissed. In this hyper-rationalist world, it is the presence or absence of documentation that is the ultimate arbiter of truth and reality. The point to be underlined is this: that *the idea of evidence itself is up for grabs.* What counts as legitimate evidence is determined by the ruling definition of evidence. This ruling definition also has the effect of *ruling out* other kinds of evidence, even though it is also objective in that it is visibly there for all to see. This is the kind of fundamentalist hyper-rationalist reality that we find ourselves beleaguered by.

Data has become God. Reality is what the numbers decree it to be, and so numbers becoming more real than the reality they are allegedly measuring. Anything not measurable simply does not exist.

It was on this sort of basis that psychoanalysis was dismissed as nonsense. This opened the door to the first challenger for the psychological throne, Behaviorism, whose progenitor Watson declared himself a Logical Positivist, saying:

> [readers of this book will] find no discussion of consciousness and no reference to terms such as sensation, perception... will... and the like. These terms are in good repute but I have found that I can get along without them... I frankly do not know what they mean. (Watson, 1919, p. xii)

Some decades after Watson, the psychoanalyst Aaron Beck made the remarkable discovery that humans were more complicated than Watsonian mechanisms, in that they actually had minds that contributed to *how* they responded to inputs and stimuli. However, like the economists, Beck thought that humans were primarily rational, calculative beings and that their emotional difficulties were caused by logical errors in a rational thinking process. In this moment, CBT was born, a treatment that set out to correct logical errors.

Psychiatry and clinical psychology

Before I get to CBT treatment, I need to say something about CBT's bedfellow, the profession of psychiatry, without which CBT could not have prospered.

In the early part of the 20th C., psychiatry was embarrassed by the fact that there was no consistency or reliability to the diagnoses conducted by psychiatrists:

> A patient identified as a textbook hysteric by one psychiatrist might easily be classified as a hypochondriac depressive by another. (Spiegel, 2005, p. 57)

The psychiatrist called Spitzer took it upon himself to improve the fortunes of psychiatry, by re-defining it as an empirical evidence-based science.

He managed this extraordinary feat by focusing only on observable symptoms. On this basis, the *Diagnostic and Statistical Manual of Mental Disorders* (DSM, 1980) was transformed into the prodigious diagnostic instrument that it is today. Descriptive psychiatry declared itself to be an objective science because it dealt in visible and tangible. The reliability problem had been solved. So they said.

The status and reliability of the DSM is important, because *all* CBT research is hitched onto one of the diagnostic categories found in the DSM. So if the DSM is found to be problematic, then all research based upon it turns to dust.

Spitzer's DSM-III listed 265 "mental disorders," each allegedly discrete and differentiated from the others by virtue of the list of observable symptoms. The new diagnostic process is a pick and mix process. If a person has five out of a list of nine observable symptoms for depression – then they are diagnosed has having the mental disorder called clinical depression.

> During the production of the DSM-IV the American Psychiatric Association… {undertook} a broad reliability study, and although the research phase of the project was completed, the findings were never published. {when asked why,} The director of the project, Jim Thompson said that *the APA ran out of money* (Spiegel, 2005, p. 63, italics added).

This is hard to believe given that the American Psychiatric Association had just made many millions of dollars out of the sale of over 800,000 copies of the DSM-III. It seems pretty obvious that the real reason for not publishing the research was that its findings would have shown that the reliability problem had not been solved. In effect, the bad news was buried.

But then in the 1990s, another major study claiming that the DSM-III had solved the reliability problem was published (Williams et al., 1992). But when researchers Kutchins and Kirk (1997) looked closely into the data, they found that the statistics actually showed the opposite to be the case: not only had reliability *not improved* since the 1950s, "in some cases {they} were {actually} worse." Here by the way are two of the corruptions of science that are habitually practiced today. If the research results are negative then an attempt is made to spin the results and write up the study in a way that it makes it look like the results were positive, and if that is not possible, then the research is buried and never gets to see the light of day.

Meanwhile, the profession of clinical psychology also had little standing in the scientific medical community as they too dealt in intangibles like thoughts and feelings. To compete with the medics, they too had to find a way to redefine themselves and their work as scientific and positivist. CBT, an allegedly evidence-based treatment, made for the perfect entry ticket for them as it fitted the positivist paradigm. It is for this reason that the profession of clinical psychology embraced and fostered CBT. In this way, the fate of CBT became linked to that of the profession of clinical psychology, with the result that both came to prosper.

I should add some correctives here. Not every psychiatrist is signed up to the medicalized view of human distress – for example, those that belong to the movement called critical psychiatry. And not all clinical psychologists are signed up to the cognitivist world view – for instance, the Midlands Psychology Group. But both are marginal to, and marginalized by, the medicalized, hyper-rationalist, cognitivist ethos that has come to rule within both disciplines.

Neoliberalism and managerialism

One cannot make sense of the success of CBT without stepping back and looking at the bigger political picture – specifically neoliberalism and managerialism.

Neoliberalism started to flourish during the time of Regan and Thatcher; today it has become a taken for granted orthodoxy. Its ethos is perfectly captured by the title of Milton Friedman's (1970) article published in 1970 in the *New York Times Magazine*: "The Social Responsibility of Business is to Increase its Profits."

In this new world order, in the pursuit of profit, humans become "human resources" and human labor becomes commodified. The principles of mass production and the conveyor belt are brought to bear on all areas of working life, including that of psychotherapy. All in the name of efficiency. In the UK, from the 1980s on, public services have been cut, industries have collapsed, jobs and livelihoods have been lost, distress and despair have become the norm. There has been a dramatic increase in homelessness and unemployment. What has taken place is nothing other than social carnage, and all in the name of efficiency.

But now, the suffering of the dispossessed is recast as being due to a mental illness, and as having nothing to do with the social conditions that have produced the suffering in the first place. In a final ironic twist of the knife, the state offers the suffering the panacea of CBT to help them get over their mental illnesses.

I will now turn my attention more directly to CBT itself.

Human nature according to CBT

Recall that in Bentham's time, the idea of being able to measure utility – the level of happiness – remained exactly that: simply an idea.

Fast forward several 100 years to a very excited Lord Layard. He is excited because science is deemed to have shown that happiness has a physiological correlate; therefore, it is "real," and a proper subject of study by that self-same science.

> Scientific breakthroughs... have transformed the way we think about happiness. Until recently, if people said they were happy, sceptics would hold that this was just a subjective statement... But now we know that what people say about how they feel corresponds closely to the actual levels of activity in different parts of the brain, which can be measured *in standard scientific ways* ... psychology and brain science are beginning to give us the tools to arrive at *precise answers*. (Layard, 2005, pp. 12, 13)
>
> Happiness is feeling good, and misery is feeling bad... that feeling can now be measured by asking people or by monitoring their brains. (Layard, 2005, p. 6, italics added).

But each and every one of these statements is either exaggeration or untruth. All we can do with the help of brain scans is to notice a *correlation* between an experience and electrical activity in a particular part of the brain. Correlation is not measurement – nor is there anything precise about it. Nor is it particularly surprising to discover that there are neurological and physiological correlates to one's emotional and mental life. Humans are bodies after all, and brains are a part of the body. What would be mysterious is if no cerebral activity were visible in tandem with lived experience.

CBT treatment

Let me turn now to CBT treatment itself.

John and Martin were both unexpectedly made redundant at the same time. A few weeks later John was out there looking for jobs, while Martin had slipped into a state of lassitude. What's going on? CBT's explanation begins with the premise that events produce emotional responses in people. "If an event automatically gave rise to an emotion… it would follow that the same event would have to result in the same emotion for anyone who experienced that event… [therefore] there must be something else… CBT says that this 'something else' is cognition" (Westbrook et al., 2008, p. 3).

This then is one of the fallacies residing at the root of CBT's belief system: the bizarre idea that an event should evoke the *same* emotion in all people…

Pretty much every CBT book, technical or self-help, contains this kind of picture:

Event → Cognition → Emotion

First, the event, then cognition, then the emotional response.

The focus of CBT treatment is "Cognition" – the habituated way of thinking that *maintains* the problem, the thing that keeps it going. Change the cognition, change the emotion. CBT makes a powerful dichotomy between cause and maintenance. CBT texts portray psychoanalysis as endlessly and fruitlessly looking for the *causes* of difficulties in the past, while CBT focuses on the ways that the difficulties are being *maintained* in the present. CBT texts tend to parody psychoanalysis in this kind of way:

> if you want to put out a fire then you had better tackle what keeps it going – heat, fuel, oxygen etc. – rather than look for the match that started the fire. (Westbrook et al., 2008, p. 40)

Layard and Clark say

> It is not 'necessary to know what caused the cancer – you cure it by cutting it out… Similarly, infections are often cured with antibiotics, *without knowing their causes*. (Layard & Clark, 2014, p. 109)

In proceeding in this way, they decontextualize suffering and strip it of all meaning, the *reason* for the suffering. Recall Kant. The CBT ethos makes it a virtue of having nothing to do with meaning. CBT says that unlike John, Martin is suffering because of a logical malfunction in his cognition.

His cognition is habituated to experiencing events in a negative light, and it is this that is creating a sense of helplessness in him. CBT will teach Martin how to change what he thinks. Once he has learnt how to do this, he can rationally *choose* to think optimistically which will change his *feelings* of lassitude and depression. The key word here is control.

> Human beings have largely *conquered* nature, but they have still to *conquer* themselves. (Layard, 2005, p. 9)
>
> The inner life... determine[s] how we react to life... So how can we gain control over our inner life? (Layard, 2005, p. 184)

But first, Martin will be tested at his local CBT clinic to see if he really is suffering from the mental disorder called depression. You might expect these tests to be fearfully complex and sophisticated, as they are able to look deep into the mind.

Patient Health Questionnaire 9

Over the last two weeks, how often have you been bothered by any of the following problems?

> Not at all (0), several days (1), More than half the days (2), Nearly every day (3).
>
> Little interest or pleasure in doing things Feeling down, depressed, or hopeless
>
> Trouble falling or staying asleep, or sleeping too much Feeling tired or having little energy
>
> Poor appetite or overeating
>
> Feeling bad about yourself – or that you are a failure or have let yourself or your family down Trouble concentrating on things, such as reading the newspaper or watching television
>
> Moving or speaking so slowly that other people could have noticed? Or the opposite – being so fidgety or restless that you have been moving around a lot more than usual
>
> Thoughts that you would be better off dead or of hurting yourself in some way

If the total score comes to more than ten, then Martin is diagnosed as suffering from the mental disorder depression. Martin will be given this "test" after each and every session. If his score drops below ten, he will be deemed to have recovered from his mental illness (Patient Health Questionnaire 9, n.d.).

It is by the device of calling questionnaires like this "instruments" and giving subjective experiences a number that it is made to appear that subjective experiences are being scientifically measured in objective ways.

As for the treatment itself, Martin and the practitioner will agree the symptoms the treatment will target for modification. Note the word symptom. If during treatment Martin falls into the error of ruminating about his childhood relationship to his father, this will not be allowed because rumination does not feature in the manual.

The treatment itself consists of catching hold of core beliefs, schemas and "Negative Automatic Thoughts" (for example, "no one likes me"). The idea is to demonstrate rationally and *empirically* to the patient that their cognitions are distorted, and then for the patient to practice replacing negative thoughts with positive ones. The rational patient will now choose to have different thoughts, and this will change how they feel.

Once the patient has learnt to replace distorted thoughts with objective thoughts that correspond with reality, then the patient will feel "happier" and no longer be depressed.

That's it. That's second-wave CBT treatment in its entirety.

But if it turns out that Martin has not recovered from depression despite having gone through CBT treatment, then by definition, this cannot have anything to do with the nature of the treatment itself, because the research has shown that CBT works. So the problem must lie elsewhere. One possibility is that Martin is "CBT-Resistant"; another is that Martin is suffering from a powerful form of depression known as "treatment-resistant depression." The problem is the disease or the person. The treatment itself is fine.

Even so, these sorts of CBT treatments do work to some degree. If someone is helped to leave their flat for the first time in many years and buy a pint of milk, that is a great thing and to be celebrated. No irony intended. For some, this is enough and it is all they need. But for many others, not only is this thin hyper-rationalist gruel, it misses the point entirely in relation to the existential complexities that most people struggle with.

But the thing is that these sorts of successes are insufficient to privilege CBT over the other therapies. Because counselors and therapists of all kinds of persuasions habitually help patients manage these sorts of tasks at least as well as CBT practitioners.

I will now turn my attention to the systems that support and deliver CBT from research to delivery.

CBT research

Borders and boundaries are a means of differentiation. If on one side of the border is acceptable empirical science, then everything on the other side is unacceptable. However, the unacceptable can be made acceptable by the simple device of moving the border. As Ben Goldacre (2012) and others have shown, this is exactly what has happened in psychological and pharmacological research. Over the last few decades, the borders have been consistently moved in directions that have lowered standards to dismally low levels; that which was previously problematic is now the new normal.

For example, the regulators have agreed that all it need take is two clinical trials to demonstrate statistical significance for a treatment to be licensed. However,

> there is no limit to the number of trials that can be conducted in search of these two significant trials. (Kirsch, 2011, p. 195)

Negative trials are either hidden or written up as positive. It turns out that even when the regulatory agencies come to know about the existence of large numbers of negative trials, they discard them.

> All they require are two positive trials to give the green light for public use. The FDA in the US has publicly defended... [this] dubious approval process. (Davies, 2014, p. 71)

CBT tests fully formed treatment packages. The packages themselves are never put to any kind of test, scientific or otherwise. They are articles of faith. In effect, the manual is written before any testing has begun. And strangely, almost every piece of CBT research seems to find that these manualized treatments are efficacious.

Here is a prediction. A new treatment that I have just devised but am yet to test will be found to be efficacious. It is called *Arbitrary Cognitive Therapy* (ArCoT) for the mental illness *Repeated Conflict Disorder* (RCD) – those who repeatedly get into arguments with others (a disorder that has yet to be recognized by the DSM).

The outcomes are bound to be positive for at least two reasons: first, investigator allegiance (Westen et al., 2004, p. 640). It has been empirically found that when investigators are invested in the form of treatment they are testing, the outcomes are almost always positive. Second, it has been empirically demonstrated that patients who think that they are receiving something, anything, do better than those *who know* that they are not receiving anything (Kirsch, 2011). Both are true of CBT research: it habitually tests its treatments against doing nothing, and because those being tested know that they are in treatment, more of them will say that they feel better than those who know that they received nothing. That's a scientific fact.

A dramatic instance of both, negative findings being written up as positive and negative findings buried, was brought to light by a group of researchers, Turner et al. (2008), who tracked all registered clinical trials for all the antidepressants that were launched between 1987 and 2004 (Turner et al., 2008). There were 74 of them. Thirty-eight of the trials concluded that the treatment being tested worked, and 36 found that the treatment did not. Thirty-seven of the 38 trials with positive results were published, while only 3 out of the 36 negative trials were published. Of the remaining 33 trials with negative outcomes, 22 were buried. And most astonishingly, the remaining 11 negative trials were written up in ways that made it seem that the trial was a success. Consequently, when medics looked to the published "research" to help make an informed decision, they found 48 trials apparently demonstrating the efficacy of antidepressants, set against 3 that did not.

Another instance of run-of-the-mill statistical spin is found in a run-of-the-mill CBT study published in 2012 in the prestigious four-star journal, *The Lancet* (Wiles et al., 2013). The abstract claims:

> CBT provided in addition to usual care including antidepressant medication is an *effective treatment* that reduces depressive symptoms. (p. 375)

The abstract also states

> 46% of those who received CBT had improved, reporting at least a 50% reduction in symptoms of depression, compared to 22% [in the control group]. (p. 375)

The first thing to notice is the unusual way that the numbers are mentioned – one number for the treatment group and another for the control group – rather than the statistical amalgam of the two that is the norm. This is to cover up the fact that the treatment was found to be helpful to just 23% of those tested (46 minus 22). And notice, the treatment does not cure; all it manages is *to reduce symptoms by 50%*. Further, the use of the number 50% makes it seem that the measure is objective. But it is not. All that is taking place is that people are being asked is to answer questions like: on a scale of 1–5, how depressed are you feeling? Despite the answer being delivered as a number, it is clear that it is subjective. The answer 5 is no less subjective than the answer "very very depressed." It is in this way – the presence of numbers – that it is made to appear that subjective human experiences are being objectively measured. We are witnessing hyper-rationality at work.

When all this is taken into account, the "results" of this study actually ought to be announced in this way:

> About two out of ten people came to feel somewhat better because of having received CBT; however, although feeling better, they are still depressed, only less depressed. By the way, *eight out of ten people receiving this treatment will not be helped.* And that's a scientific fact.

It is astonishing to me that such shabby pieces of research are being regularly accepted by high-status peer-reviewed journals. The only way to explain it is to say that this sort of chicanery is commonplace and become part of the acceptable norm.

The culmination of this kind of sleight-of-hand-research in prestigious scientific journals has meant that it is now become incontrovertible established scientific "fact" that CBT is unquestionably an entirely effective therapy. For example, the website of the prestigious (Scientific) Royal College of Psychiatrists informs us that:

> CBT has been shown to help with many different types of problems. These include: anxiety, depression, panic, phobias (including agoraphobia and social phobia), stress, bulimia, obsessive compulsive disorder, post-traumatic stress disorder, bipolar disorder and psychosis. CBT may also help if you have difficulties with anger, a low opinion of yourself or physical health problems, like pain or fatigue. (http://www.rcpsych.ac.uk/expertadvice/treatments/cbt.aspx)

Research findings are habitually amplified by a variety of other techniques, one of which is to cite results in the form of *relative* changes rather than *absolute* ones. The difference between the two is crucial. For example, I could say that I have increased my chances of winning the lottery by 100% because I bought two tickets instead of my usual one. This is the *relative* increase – relative to the starting condition of one ticket. But all I have actually done is increase my chances of winning from 1 out of 14 million to 2 out of 14 million. This is the *absolute* increase.

> Which of the two is more meaningful?
> Which of the two looks more impressive?
> Which of the two is used by CBT researchers?

It is on this sort of basis that the abstract of a third-wave CBT treatment called mindfulness-based cognitive therapy (MBCT) has claimed that it helps 50% of folk prone to depression, from relapsing (Teasdale et al., 2000). However, the 50% turns out to be a vast exaggeration. In the body of their paper, the researchers own calculations show that the treatment reduces the chances of relapsing is 39%. What happens next is interesting. Part way through the paper, the 39% is re-written in words as "almost a half." A paragraph or two later the term "almost" disappears, and the claim is further amplified to say a "half." And a while later, they move back to numerals to say that the treatment has been shown to help 50% of those who receive the treatment. Notice the sleight of hand, from numbers to words to words to numbers again. It is by device that 39% is transmuted into 50%.

And indeed, it is this vastly exaggerated claim that we find on the MBCT website:

> The UK National Institute for Clinical Excellence (NICE) has recently endorsed MBCT as an effective treatment for *prevention* of relapse... The evidence from two randomized clinical trials of MBCT indicates that it

> reduces rates of relapse by 50% among patients who suffer from recurrent depression. (MBCT, n.d.)

Notice also the further exaggeration: from "reduction in likelihood" to "prevention."

But there is even more. It turns out that the 39% is the *relative* change. The *absolute* figure turns out to be 25%. Further, the 25% only applies to a very narrow subset: people who have previously suffered and recovered from depression *on at least three occasions*. It then also turned out that the chances of those who had suffered and survived *two or fewer* previous episodes of depression had actually increased following MBCT treatment. This was the case in both studies that tested for the efficacy of MBCT treatment; demonstrating that for this population MBCT is iatrogenic. But, according to the researcher's statistical calculations, this finding was of no consequence despite it being replicated, as it was not "statistically significant." So, no problem.

It is always helpful to reverse the findings: *MBCT will be of no help to seven or eight out of ten people*. This is the case for even for this very narrow grouping of those who have suffered and recovered from depression on at least three previous occasions.

When this cherry-picked category is done away with and one looks at the efficacy for *entire* treatment group that was tested, it turns out that this treatment was shown to help a mere 14% of them, no different to the placebo effect (See details in Dalal, 2018).

Another empirically validated highly respected third-wave treatment is dialectical behavior therapy (DBT). Within 10 years of its introduction, over 25 data-driven scientific papers were published in support of the treatment. However, it turns out that each and every one of these publications drew on data from the original study, and most astonishingly, they were almost all written by the members of the original treatment team. The sample size in the original study was miniscule – 24 in the DBT group and 22 in the control group. Scheel concluded

> All positive published outcome findings are from a single study… [and] rest on no more than 24 DBT subjects… all remaining positive findings are based on 13 or fewer DBT subjects, and all process and most follow-up conclusions are based on seven or fewer DBT subjects. (Scheel, 2000, p. 68)

This is an incredibly small number of persons on which to make predictions and generalizations about humanity at large.

Correlations of this kind in psychological research are mostly meaningless. The researcher Meehl calls this the *crud factor* of psychological science, because everything will and does correlate to everything else to a small but meaningless degree. For example, Jean Twenge et al. (2018) released a study, covered widely in the press, linking screen use to youth suicides. However, another scholar with access to the same dataset noted in an interview that the magnitude of effect is about the same as for eating potatoes on suicide (Ferguson, 2019).

NICE soup

In the UK, once the research is published, the public body called NICE (The National Institute for Health and Care Excellence) is tasked with examining evidence and issuing impartial advice for the treatment all kinds of medical conditions.

But in the field of psychology, the whole process is biased in all kinds of ways. To begin with membership of the committees examining the evidence is made up mostly of clinical psychologists committed to the manualized therapies. The cognitivists advise the legislators, and the legislators based on this advice create policies that decree that the treatments to be provided are those favored by the cognitivists. This is tantamount to poachers writing rules of good practice for gamekeepers, rules that favor the poachers.

It is also the case that NICE will only take account of a very narrow kind of research: one which "tests" a specific manualized treatment for a specific mental disorder from the DSM. It takes no account of other forms of empirical research, for example, research that compares the outcome of two treatments for one mental disorder or naturalistic studies in clinics. It does not even trouble itself to refute them. As far as NICE is concerned, Westen and Shedler's research efforts do not exist, as it does not fit their research template.

The only way that therapies that do not fit the manualized paradigm can put themselves forward to be considered by NICE is by manualizing themselves. In doing so, they effectively distort themselves to such a degree that they become something other than they once were.

For example, I have decided on an experimental protocol to distinguish that which is edible from that which is not. To this end I have decided that only those substances that I am able to pick up with chopsticks will count as food. So according to this "protocol," soup could never count as food because my chopsticks cannot grasp it. Your form of verification, which is your experience (you did ingest it, you enjoyed its taste, you felt nourished, your hunger was assuaged, you did not die), has no legitimacy in my protocol and so I take no account of it.

Within this paradigm, the form of psychotherapy that I and many others practice is soup. In order to enter the paradigm, I have to find a way to *lumpify* my practice so that it is able to be grasped by positivist chopsticks. However, in becoming lumpified, the soup is *no longer soup*. Today, this is what many schools of psychotherapy (including psychoanalysis) are trying to do, lumpify their practice, so that it can be picked up by NICE's positivist chopsticks and be counted as legitimate practice.

Increasing Access to Psychological Therapies (IAPT)

Once NICE has issued its advice, in the UK, the public body called IAPT is given the responsibility for the delivery of *NICE–compliant* treatments to the general public. IAPT is given a number of targets – how many are seen, how long do they spend on the waiting list, how severe are the difficulties, whether the treatment is completed or not, whether the person has recovered and so on. Payments are allocated to each of the targets.

In order to make it seem that IAPT is meeting its targets, it habitually uses two strategies: one of which is to deliver an impoverished service and the other is to cook its statistical books.

The managerialists who are in charge of public bodies have become masters at spinning a reduction in service as an enhancement of that service. For example, face-to-face meetings between patient and practitioner are being replaced with telephone contact. This reduction in service is reframed as an enhancement, by saying that change is for the convenience of the patient as it saves them making an unnecessary journey. Because NICE-compliant therapies only require practitioners to be able to follow manualized instructions, highly trained psychotherapists are thought to be unnecessary, and so they are replaced with lower paid practitioners called psychological wellbeing practitioners (PWP). They are trained for one year in the art of delivering manualized CBT therapies.

One target that IAPT services have to meet has to do with throughput: 75% of those referred to IAPT should be seen within 6 weeks of referral, and 95% should be seen within 18 weeks.

To be able to stay on target, the service is cut back in two ways – reducing the duration of the session to 45 or even 30 minutes, and reducing the number of sessions from 20 to 12 to 6 to 4. One anonymous PWP revealed the following malpractice:

> In the service in which I work, all assessments are marked as 'assessment and treatment' [which makes it look like more people have been treated than is the case]... When I discussed this concern with management, I was told that 'NHS England have told us to do it this way' which would indicate either that the service is wilfully lying or the NHS England are actually aware of this and are allowing the data to be manipulated. (Serioussham, 2016)

But even this is not enough to make the numbers sing the song the data is required to sing. IAPT has developed a bizarre view of what "completed treatment" means. *If a person attends just two sessions* and then does not return for whatever reason – including death – it is counted as a *completed treatment*, which makes the outcome measures look more positive than it actually is.

Another regular scam is to shift patients that are not improving in CBT treatment onto a non-IAPT list, or to mark down the contact as an "assessment" rather than as a failed treatment. Either way, the data will show the service as having met two targets: the accessing services target and the waiting list time target. The non-IAPT data is not "measured" and so disappears from view, making the recovery statistic look better than it actually is.

Another anonymous practitioner said that they were being put through official trainings that taught them how to encourage patients to reconsider their answers on questionnaires to say that they had improved more than they thought they had.

> Oh, you're much better now aren't you – I'm sure that's a six... I think you've been doing much better this week, don't you think that's a two? (Griffiths & Steen, 2013, p. 28)

Official policy dictates that when someone who had previously been declared "recovered" from their "mental illness" following CBT "relapses" and returns to the service, official policy requires them to be seen by another practitioner, not the original one. In this way, what is actually a follow-up treatment is made to look like a new "treatment episode." In other words, the data will show two people have been seen once, rather than one person twice; the data will also show two recoveries rather than one failure.

Conclusions

The cognitivist delusion is exactly that: the delusion that modern humans are primarily cognitive, rational-decision-making beings. The delusion continues: thoughts are not only separable from emotions, they also precede them and are able to control them. Mental life is the controller of emotional life. Irrational thoughts produce problematic emotional states. CBT treatments correct faulty thinking after which emotional life falls into line and the person is in recovery. This is readily achievable in anything between 6 and 20 sessions. Here endeth the delusion.

But that is not the end of the delusion, nor is it its beginning. I have been arguing that the reason that the delusion is able to flourish within psychology is because it is shared by the corrupt scientific systems and managerialist structures that surround and sustain it. It is quite extraordinary that so many of the great and the good – governments and policy makers – have been gullible enough to swallow the CBT fabulation in its entirety, and then, intoxicated by its heady hyper-rationalist promises, they have fostered the cognitivist delusion and in doing so nurtured the corruptions of science.

References

American Psychiatric Association. (1980). *Diagnostic and statistical manual of mental disorders* (3rd ed.). Author.

Bell, S., Knapp, M., Layard, P., Meacher, M., Priebe, S., Thornicroft, G., Turnberg, L., & Wright, B. (2006). *The depression report: A new deal for anxiety and depression disorders.* Mental Health Policy Group, Centre for Economic Performance, London School of Economics.

Dalal, F. (2018). *CBT: The cognitive behavioural tsunami – Managerialism, politics & the corruptions of science.* Routledge.

Davies, J. (2014). *Cracked: Why psychiatry is doing more harm than good.* Icon Books.

Ferguson, C. (2019, March). Embrace the unknown. *The Psychologist.* https://thepsychologist.bps.org.uk/volume-32/march-2019/embrace-unknown

Friedman, M. (1970, September 13). The social responsibility of business is to increase its profits. *The New York Times.*

Goldacre, B. (2012). *Bad pharma: How medicine is broken and how we can fix it.* Fourth Estate.

Griffiths, S., & Steen, S. (2013). Improving Access to Psychological Therapies (IAPT) Programme: Scrutinising IAPT costestimates to support effective commissioning. *The Journal of Psychological Therapies in Primary Care, 2,* 142–156.

Kirsch, I. (2011). Antidepressants and the placebo response. In Rapley, M., Moncrieff, J., & Dillon, J. (Eds.), *De-medicalizing misery: Psychiatry, psychology and the human condition* (pp. 189–196). Palgrave.

Kutchins, H., & Kirk, S. (1997). *Making us crazy – DSM: The psychiatric bible and the creation of mental disorders.* FreePress.

Layard, R. (2005). *Happiness.* Penguin.

Layard, R., & Clark, D. (2014). *Thrive: The power of evidence-based psychological therapies.* Allen Lane.

MBCT. (n.d.). *Mindfulness-based cognitive therapy: Does it work?* Retrieved May 2017 http://mbct.com/about/does-mbct-work/

Patient Health Questionnaire 9. (n.d.). https://patient.info/doctor/patient-health-questionnaire-phq-9

Scheel, K. R. (2000). The empirical basis of dialectical behavior therapy: Summary, critique and implications. *Clinical Psychology: Science and Practice,* 7(1), 68–86. https://doi.org/10.1093/clipsy.7.1.68

Seligman, M. E. P. (1972). Learned helplessness. *Annual Review of Medicine, 23*(1), 407–412. https://doi.org/10.1146/ annurev.me.23.020172.002203

Serioussham. (2016). IAPT waiting list targets. Available at www.clinpsy.org.uk/forum/viewtopic.php?p=180855

Spiegel, A. (2005, January 3). The dictionary of disorder: How one man revolutionized psychiatry. *The New Yorker.* www.newyorker.com/magazine/2005/01/03/the-dictionary-of-disorder.

Teasdale, J. D., Segal, Z. V., Williams, M. G., Ridgeway, V. A., Soulsby, J. M., & Lau, M. A. (2000). Prevention of relapse/ recurrence in major depression by mindfulness-based cognitive therapy. *Journal of Consulting and Clinical Psychology,* 68(4), 615–623. https://doi.org/10.1037/0022-006X.68.4.615

Turner, E., Matthews, A., Linardatos, E., Tell, R., & Rosenthal, R. (2008). Selective publication of antidepressant trials and its influence on apparent efficacy. *The New England Journal of Medicine, 358*(3), 252–260. https://doi.org/10. 1056/NEJMsa065779

Twenge, J. M., Joiner, T. E., Megan, L. R., & Martin, G. M. (2018). Increases in depressive symptoms, suicide-related outcomes, and suicide rates among U.S. adolescents after 2010 and links to increased new media screen time. *Clinical Psychological Science, 6*(1), 3–17.

Watson, J. B. (1919). *Psychology from the standpoint of a behaviorist.* Lippincott.

Westbrook, D., Kennerley, H., & Kirk, J. (2008). *An introduction to cognitive behavioural therapy: Skills and applications.* Sage.

Westen, D., Novotny, C. M., & Thompson-Brenner, H. (2004). The empirical status of empirically supported psychotherapies: Assumptions, findings, and reporting in controlled clinical trials. *Psychological Bulletin, 130*(4), 631–663. https:// doi.org/10.1037/0033–2909.130.4.631

Wiles, N., Thomas, L., Ridgway, L., Turner, N., Campbell, J., Garland, A., Hollinghurst, S., Jerrom, B., Kessler, D., Kuyken, W., Morrison, J., Turner, K., Williams, C., Peters, T., & Lewis, G. (2013). Cognitive behavioural therapy as an adjunct to pharmacotherapy for primary care-based patients with treatment resistant depression: Results of the CoBalT randomised controlled trial. *The Lancet, 381*, 375–384. https:// doi.org/10.1016/S0140-6736(12)61552-9

Williams, J. B., Gibbon, M., First, M. B., Spitzer, R. L., Davies, M., Borus, J., Howes, M. J., Kane, J., Pope, H. G., & Rounsaville, B. (1992). The structured clinical interview for DSM-III-R. *Archives of General Psychiatry, 49*(8), 630–636. https://doi. org/10.1001/archpsyc.1992.01820080038006

3

The cost-effectiveness of psychodynamic therapy

The obstacles, the law, and a landmark lawsuit

Susan G. Lazar

Insurance reimbursement and the law

Psychotherapy, especially psychoanalysis and dynamic psychotherapy, has in recent decades been poorly supported by insurance benefits. This longstanding trend may have begun very slowly and haltingly to improve. A notable milestone in this progress is The Mental Health Parity and Addiction Equity Act (MHPAEA) 2008, the first sweeping national legal mandate for parity for mental health care benefits. The Affordable Care and Patient Protection Act of 2010 (ACA) also strengthened mental health parity and named mental health care as an Essential Health Benefit including psychotherapy as one component.

Despite these important steps, many problems with establishing parity remain. These are most recently being addressed by successful litigation against insurance companies evading parity by utilizing inappropriate treatment limitations and proprietary insurance company "medical necessity" guidelines, mandating improvements in longstanding poor insurance support for mental health. To protect patients, clinicians and advocates need to become familiar with the parity law and specific ways it is evaded by inappropriate treatment limitations and proprietary insurance company "medical necessity" guidelines that are not consistent with professional standards.

Stigma, not expressed toward physical illness, has historically been intense toward the mentally ill, including by association, toward mental health treatment providers and the treatments that help patients, especially toward psychotherapy. Accordingly, one frequent and widespread misconception about psychotherapy would describe it as an "unnecessary indulgence" used by the affluent or the "worried well." Among policy makers, the concept of "price elasticity" reflects the notion that psychotherapy is often accessed unnecessarily and self-indulgently and seeks to require whatever patient copayment for psychotherapy is needed to reduce its use to the same level as other insurance supported health care. Besides higher copays for psychotherapy, coverage exclusions, and dubious "medical necessity" standards are a deliberate increase in patients' cost burden employed to correct an assumed "moral hazard" (unnecessary use of treatment) (Frank & McGuire, 2000).

DOI: 10.4324/9781003325512-5

Since MHPAEA made illegal higher copays and discriminatory reimbursement schedules for mental health services, private insurance companies resorted to indirect means to limit reimbursement and to evade the language of the parity mandate. Such protocols have included "medical reviews" triggered by an arbitrary number of psychotherapy sessions conducted on treatments exceeding a preset, "outlier" session cap (e.g., above 20 or more visits in a given period) that more frequently than not judge continuing treatment "not medically necessary."

Several decades of research counter the belief that psychotherapy is an "unneeded expense." The Rand Health Experiment found that even when psychotherapy is free, 4% of an insured population access it for an average length of care of 11 sessions (Manning et al., 1986). In fact, a higher cost burden for outpatient psychiatric care turns away very ill patients who simply forego treatment (Landerman et al., 1994; Simon et al., 1996). Furthermore, increasing the cost burden for outpatient treatment for seriously ill patients, especially those in lower socioeconomic circumstances, decreases that treatment and increases overall expenses in emergency care and hospitalization by more than is saved in outpatient costs (Ravesteijn et al., 2017).

Insurers very commonly overlook a robust research base documenting the efficacy, effectiveness, and cost-effectiveness especially of psychodynamic therapies (Lazar, 2010, 2018; Lazar & Yeomans, 2014) Despite the claim that their internal insurance medical necessity guidelines adhere to professional mental health care provider guidelines, "standard practice" and "expert opinion" (more commonly informing guidelines for other health care) those for mental health and for psychotherapy in particular are often "cherry-picked" to emphasize brief treatments. Insurance medical necessity guidelines have more often than not excluded the indications for the provision of intensive and extended, especially psychodynamic, psychotherapy. Insufficient treatment due to suboptimal insurance support for mental health services, including psychotherapy, leads to increased morbidity, disability, and greatly expanded overall health care expenses compared to patients without psychiatric illness. The increased medical expenses of those with mental illness are over and above the costs of their psychiatric care and include increased medical expenses, more primary care visits, higher outpatient charges, and longer hospital stays (Deykin et al., 2001; Luber et al., 2000; Melek & Norris, 2008).

Insurance providers prefer to reimburse for lower cost medication treatment, despite findings that psychotherapy augments the effect of medication (the reverse effect is unclear) and often has a higher effect size. Psychotherapy is preferred by 75% of patients (McHugh et al., 2013), has lower dropout rates than medication alone protocols, and obviously lacks the side effects of medication treatment (Levy et al., 2014). A new retrospective study of patients with first-episode mild-to-moderate major depressive disorder found that those treated with brief dynamic psychotherapy alone maintained 72% remission at five years without further treatment compared to those treated with antidepressant medication alone, 47% of whom sustained remission at five years. Of note, those with severe personality disorders and patients with substance abuse were excluded from the cohort studied (Rosso et al., 2019).

"Evidence-based" research protocols of brief cognitive-behavioral psychotherapy

The common claim that short-term cognitive-behavioral therapy (CBT) is the most evidence-based psychotherapy is based on a large body of randomized controlled trials yielding statistically significant improvement in symptoms. These findings provide the rationale supporting insurance companies' preference for reimbursing short-term CBT treatments. However, a different conclusion comes from a meta-analysis of 23 randomized controlled trials using reliable rating methods for a total of 2,751 patients that examined studies of psychodynamic and other treatments established as efficacious, including CBT. The meta-analysis showed an equivalence of psychodynamic therapy to comparison conditions, including CBT, for target symptoms at posttreatment and its equivalence to treatments established in efficacy (Steinertet al., 2017). Leichsenring and Steinert (2017) also dispute the oft-claimed "gold-standard" status of CBT with their analysis of its research corpus and a finding of frequent publication bias, small effect size, weak empirical tests used in many trials, the influence of researcher allegiance on studies, and several meta-analyses revealing its limited efficacy. In addition, a frequent response and remission rates of 50% or less for depression and anxiety in such trials leaves a large percentage of patients with insufficient improvement. The authors also cite the finding that only 7% of CBT randomized controlled trials for anxiety and depression were of high quality (Cuijpers et al., 2016).

Drilling down further into issues of study design, brief, manualized CBT trials are, in fact, generally conducted with subjects with a sole diagnosis under investigation and are not typical of most psychiatric patients who have more complicated conditions and frequent comorbidity. In fact, the aforementioned study comparing the superiority of a brief course of psychodynamic psychotherapy for depressed patients with medication treatment alone is noteworthy for the fact that the patient cohort was narrowly focused on patients with one particular diagnosis and without certain common chronic disorders and who, arguably, could therefore sustain significant recovery after brief treatment alone. The much touted ostensible superiority of brief manualized cognitive-behavioral psychotherapy is also based on studies of patients with a single diagnosis; they are patients who are atypical of most psychiatric patients who have comorbidity with several diagnoses and who turn out to need a more extended course of therapy.

Enduring clinical improvement is not indicated by statistically significant improvement in symptom rating scales. Reviews of manualized brief treatments for depressive and anxiety disorders have found only short-lived benefits with half of patient cohorts seeking further treatment within 6–12 months (Westen et al., 2004). Most of these patients require more therapy to achieve remission and 75% did not recover without it (Driessen et al., 2014). According to Shedler (2015), brief "'evidence-based' therapies are ineffective for most people most of the time" (p. 48). In short, study design flaws and publication bias undermine claims of efficacy (Cuijpers et al., 2010; Leichsenring & Steinert, 2017; Shedler, 2018; Wampold et al., 2011) and thus the design and conclusions of such studies also undermine their potential relevance to most patients' clinical needs and appropriateness in shaping policy or insurance coverage protocols.

The cost-effectiveness of extended psychotherapy for the patients who need more

A claim that a treatment should be covered by insurance should provide evidence for its effectiveness. "*Cost-effectiveness*" does not mean "effectiveness" (in real-world conditions) or "efficacy" (as found in research outcomes) but the financial cost of a treatment related to outcome measures of effectiveness (Cellini & Kee, 2010). "Cost-effective" does not mean "cheap" but what society is willing to pay for measurable positive outcomes – the impact per dollar spent.

A high percentage of the psychiatrically ill are never diagnosed and a majority of those who receive inadequate treatment (Wang, Berglund et al., 2005; Wang, Lane et al., 2005).

More medical conditions and higher medical costs are incurred by patients with chronic, complex, and/or recurrent psychiatric illness who can be treated with psychotherapy with better mental health and overall health outcomes. In ignoring these facts, insurance companies privilege their own short-term cost-saving goals that minimize reimbursement, evade the mandate for mental health parity, and subvert the provision of thorough treatment that would yield better health outcomes and cost-savings in the budgets of other parties on whom subsequent health expenses and increased disability will fall.

Some psychiatric patients improve with brief treatment, but important groups are very costly to society if inadequately treated. These patients need more intensive and/or extended psychotherapy than most insurance companies are willing to support. There are also research data on the provision of adequate care for these patients for recovery and subsequent savings from decreased medical expenses and improved productivity, which constitute the more stringent metric of "cost-offset." It must be said, however, that insisting on a future cost savings in overall medical and other expenses as a condition for supporting mental health care would be an immoral standard in comparison to physical health care in which reimbursed treatments are frequently effective, often life-saving, and also very expensive.

Several diagnostic groups of patients with chronic, debilitating personality disorders, chronic, complex disorders, such as severe longstanding depression and anxiety, and multiple chronic psychiatric disorders need an intensive and longer duration of psychotherapy and often do better with a psychodynamic approach (Leichsenring & Rabung, 2008, 2011; Shedler, 2010). Among the most seriously ill, they are frequently not adequately treated with psychotherapy due to arbitrary limits on reimbursement for psychotherapy by insurance companies (Bendat, 2014).

Both longer duration and higher frequency of psychotherapy have independent positive effects for the more severely and chronically ill and together contribute to the most positive treatment outcomes (Rudolf et al., 1994; Sandell et al., 2000; Grande et al., 2006; Leichsenring & Rabung, 2008, 2011; Huber et al., 2012). The cost-effectiveness of extended intensive psychotherapy for those patients who need it often includes a cost offset from decreased sick leave, decreased medical costs, and decreased hospital costs (Bateman & Fonagy, 1999, 2003, 2008; Clarkin et al., 2007; Dossmann et al., 1997; Duehrssen, 1962; J. F. Clarkin et al., 2001; Hall et al., 2001; Heinzel et al., 1996; Keller et al., 1998).

The lifetime prevalence of *personality disorders* is between 9.1% and 13.5% (Casey & Tyrer, 1986; Maier et al., 1992; Reich et al., 1989; Zimmerman & Coryell, 1990; Lenzenweger, 2008) affecting 30 million Americans of all social classes, races, and ethnicities. These patients have maladaptive, inflexible, and deeply ingrained patterns of thinking, feeling, and impaired relationships. Their sense of interpersonal relatedness is commonly distorted by immature "mentalization" or ways of understanding their own minds, those of others, and their relationships with other people. They also are very costly to society, often unemployed for long periods, with more drug problems, suicide attempts, interpersonal difficulties (Gabbard, 2000; Linehan & Heard, 1999; Pilkonis et al., 1999; Reich et al., 1989), criminal behavior, divorce, child abuse, heavy use of mental and general health care (Skodol et al., 2005), and are among the most chronically impaired psychiatric patients.

Randomized controlled trials of different psychotherapeutic approaches find that dialectical behavior therapy (DBT), CBT, psychodynamic, and other specialized treatments for personality disorders are all effective and lead to reduced symptomatology, improved functioning, and decreased hospitalization. (Bateman, 2012; Bateman & Fonagy, 2009; Cristea et al., 2017; Hadjipavlou & Ogrodniczuk, 2010; Leichsenring et al., 2013; Leichsenring, Leweke et al., 2015; Leichsenring, Luyten et al., 2015; Leuzinger-Bohleber et al., 2019; Linehan et al., 1991; McMain et al., 2012)

Of note, the impaired interpersonal relationships of patients with personality disorders constitute a larger increased risk factor for mortality than smoking, obesity, alcoholism, and hypertension (Holt-Lunstad et al., 2010). Thus, it is of the utmost significance that while psychotherapy of different approaches improves symptoms, studies indicate that long-term psychodynamic treatments are significantly superior in improving maladaptive interpersonal relationships (Huber et al., 2012; Leichsenring & Rabung, 2008, 2011; Levy et al., 2014, 2006; Mullin et al., 2016; Shedler, 2010). Shedler (2010) also emphasized that compared to patients treated with other psychotherapies, patients treated with psychodynamic psychotherapy maintain their therapeutic improvement better and continue to improve after treatment ends, the "sleeper effect," an ongoing improvement after the end of therapy also noted by other researchers over several decades (e.g., Sandell et al., 2000).

Patients with *borderline personality disorder* in particular take significantly longer to improve (Fonagy, 2002; Høglend, 1993; Howard et al., 1986; Kopta et al., 1994; K. N. Levy et al., 2010; Seligman, 1995). In fact, the British Health Service National Institute for Health and Care Excellence cautions against brief psychological interventions for borderline personality disorder stating, "*... there is perhaps an even stronger signal that longer treatments with higher doses are of greater benefit. In several studies, significant improvement was only observed after 12 months of active treatment*" (*NICE clinical guideline;* National Institute for Health and Care Excellence [NICE], 2009, p. 207). And, as mentioned above, very specifically for borderline personality disorder, psychodynamic psychotherapy reaches and impacts more positively the intrapsychic elements of the illness, leading to broader personality changes than supportive psychotherapy or DBT for borderline personality disorder (Clarkin et al., 2007; Levy et al., 2006). In fact, there is no evidence that the core psychopathology of unstable relationships, primitive defenses, identity diffusion, and boredom of patients with borderline personality disorder is affected by one year of DBT (Van Den Bosch et al., 2002).

While *depression* is the most common diagnosis made in primary care, primary care physicians still miss the diagnosis 50% of the time (Katon & Sullivan, 1990). One-fifth of all Americans experience a depressive disorder at some point during their lifetimes (Kessler et al., 2003). Extremely costly to society in increased medical costs, suicide-related mortality costs, and disability, a World Health Organization (2008) study found unipolar depressive disorders to be the greatest cause of worldwide disability.

In addition, the 20% of depressed patients who are treatment resistant have even greater health care costs are twice as likely to be hospitalized for depression and for general medical admissions than other depressed patients. The treatment-resistant depressed group has 12% more outpatient visits, 1.4–3 times more psychotropic medications, over 6 times the mean total medical costs, and 19 times greater total depression-related costs (Crown et al., 2002).

One study of chronically depressed patients found a similar pattern of recovery with extended psychodynamic and cognitive-behavior psychotherapy as measured by symptom rating scales (Leuzinger-Bohleber et al., 2019). However, another study of unipolar depression found that both a psychodynamic approach and the greater intensity of a psychoanalytic schedule add benefit. Long-term cognitive-behavioral, psychoanalytic, and psychodynamic therapies do yield similar improvements in depressive symptoms for all three approaches immediately post treatment. And while CBT and psychodynamic therapy also yield similar levels of depressive symptoms at three-year follow-up, patients treated with the more intensive psychoanalytic treatment sustain greater improvement. Both the more intensively psychoanalytically treated group and less intensively treated psychodynamic therapy groups had fewer interpersonal problems than the CBT group at both post-treatment measurement points. The improvement in interpersonal problems was the one detectable superiority of psychodynamic therapy over CBT. However, further documenting the separate impact of treatment intensity, the more intensively psychoanalytically treated group had greater improvement in general distress and interpersonal problems immediately after treatment and in depressive symptoms, in general distress, interpersonal problems, and self-schema than the CBT group at three-year follow-up (Huber et al., 2012).

Certain character traits of depressed patients complicate their treatment course. Perfectionistic patients do poorly in all brief treatments and substantially better in intensive, extended psychoanalytic treatment than in less intensive long-term therapies (Blatt, 1992; Blatt et al., 1995). Another group of depressed patients who do not readily sustain improvement from briefer treatment are those who, although seemingly recovered; nonetheless, still suffer from overlooked residual symptoms that progress to prodromal symptoms of recurrence. Such residual symptoms are a strong prognostic indication of relapse and are among its most consistent predictors. In particular, dysfunctional social and interpersonal patterns are positively correlated with persistent depression, relapse, and poor long-term outcomes.

Since the number and quality of sub-syndromal symptoms are often not specified in treatments judged to be successful, patients no longer judged to be meeting syndromal criteria are often inaccurately assessed as recovered. In addition to residual depressive symptoms, alertness to pre-disposing dysfunctional interpersonal problems is needed to address ongoing character traits that put patients at risk for recurring illness (Fava et al., 2007). Again, studies indicate that psychodynamic treatments have greater efficacy with these traits (Clarkin et al., 2007; Levy et al., 2006; Leichsenring & Rabung, 2008; Shedler, 2010; Huber et al., 2012). In fact, also reinforcing both the importance of intensity of treatment for more complex cases and of a psychodynamic approach, one study found improvement in interpersonal relationships significantly related to the number of psychodynamic psychotherapy sessions and the frequency of use of psychodynamically informed interventions (Mullin et al., 2016). Another study comparing long-term psychodynamic psychotherapy (LTPP) to treatment as usual for treatment-resistant depression found greater improvement in depression and in social adjustment at two-year follow-up in the psychodynamic-therapy–treated group. For those treated with psychodynamic therapy, 30% sustained partial remission and 44% no longer met criteria for major depressive disorder compared to only 4.4% of the control group who sustained improvement and for whom only 10% no longer met criteria for major depression (Fonagy et al., 2015). The first study documenting the impact of LTPP on the brain reveals treatment-specific changes in the limbic system and regulatory regions in the prefrontal cortex associated with improvement in depression after therapy (Buchheim et al. 2012).

Patients diagnosed with both personality disorders and depression are more treatment resistant and have persistent and recurrent depression, more role limitations, and impaired social functioning and health perceptions than patients with major depressive disorder alone. Poor psychosocial functioning compounds the impairments of major depressive disorder and affects the course of the illness (Skodol et al., 2005; Young, 2018).

Patients whose personality disorders remit experience an improvement in social functioning and greater remittance of depression compared to those with major depression and persisting personality disorders who are the group that functions the poorest. Both personality and mood disorders need to be treated in comorbid patients since the course of personality psychopathology influences depressive outcome as well as psychosocial functioning (Markowitz et al., 2007; Skodol et al., 2005). The patients with both depression and comorbid personality disorders also have longer time to remission than those without personality disorders. Borderline and obsessive-compulsive personality disorders at baseline are robust predictors of accelerated relapse after remission from an episode of major depressive disorder, even when controlling for other negative prognostic predictors (Grilo et al., 2010).

In sum, personality disorders are negative prognostic indicators for the course of major depressive disorder. In fact, borderline personality disorder is the *strongest independent predictor of persistence* of major depressive disorder (found in 57% of persistent cases) followed by schizoid and schizotypal personality disorder, any anxiety disorder (the strongest Axis I predictor), and dysthymic disorder (Grilo et al., 2010; Skodol et al., 2011). From a cost-effective perspective, it would appear that patients with major depression and a comorbid personality disorder must be treated for both conditions to forestall recurrent and persistent depressive illness even though the treatment of the personality disorder may well require a longer, more intensive treatment.

For patients with a variety of common DSM4 Axis 1 and 2 diagnoses, studies of outcome and cost-effectiveness for several cohorts, the first of 861 outpatients (De Maat et al., 2007) and the second of 5,063 outpatients (De Maat et al., 2009), treated with either LTPP or psychoanalysis, show that both treatments yield large effect sizes in symptom reduction, personality change, and improvement in moderate pathology at termination and at follow-up, with larger effect sizes for psychoanalysis. Both LTPP and psychoanalysis also lead to reduced health care use and sick leave (De Maat et al., 2009, 2007). A meta-analysis of pre-post studies of psychoanalysis for complex mental disorders also showed a large effect size of 1.46 at follow-up for all outcome measures including symptoms, personality, and psychosocial functioning (De Maat et al., 2013). Psychoanalysis, with its greater frequency, is more costly but more cost-effective than LTPP from a health-related quality perspective (Berghout et al., 2010a, 2010b), and both treatments yield significantly reduced work absenteeism and lowered hospitalization at seven-year follow-up (Beutel et al., 2004). Psychodynamic psychotherapies have also been found to be effective for anxiety disorders, eating disorders, substance abuse, somatic symptoms, and marital discord (Levy et al., 2014).

Illegal insurance protocols and the lawsuit

In light of the above data with regard to the cost-effectiveness and need for extended and often intensive psychodynamic psychotherapy, Bendat (2014) has given us an analysis of inadequate insurance coverage in the context of MHPAEA and the ACA. Both MHPAEA and the ACA require parity for both "quantitative" (number of services) and "non-quantitative" (describing protocols) limitations on the scope or duration of mental health and substance use treatment eligible for coverage. These treatment limitations may not be applied in a more restrictive manner to mental health benefits than to medical/surgical benefits.

However, the mandate for parity is still being observed essentially in the breach since insurers have not really abandoned their decades-long rationing of mental health care using sub-standard, overly restrictive medical necessity guidelines that are not developed by recognized, nonprofit clinical specialty associations. In addition, they adjudicate benefits for other medical conditions based on more generally recognized standards.

National professional organizations' support is urgently needed for efforts to enforce genuine compliance with the requirements of the parity and affordable care act laws with respect to mental health care.

To protect patients, clinicians and advocates need to become familiar with the parity law and specific ways it is evaded by inappropriate treatment limitations and proprietary insurance company "medical necessity" guidelines that are not consistent with professional standards. There must be an insistence on the recognition of both professional expertise and the robust research base validating necessary treatment.

Below are excerpts from a federal court's liability findings in a recent class action suit against United Behavioral Health (UBH), which failed to apply medical necessity guidelines that were consistent with generally accepted standards of care:

The lawsuit – Wit vs. UBH

Excerpts from FINDINGS OF FACT AND CONCLUSIONS OF LAW in Wit vs. UBH (n.d.), UNITED STATES DISTRICT COURT NORTHERN DISTRICT OF CALIFORNIA, Judge Joseph Spero

UBH's conflicts of interest

Testimony that the Guidelines were developed solely to reflect generally accepted standards of care was not credible. Internal UBH communications … make it crystal clear that the *primary* focus of the Guideline development process ... was the implementation of a "utilization management" model

that keeps benefit expenses down by placing a heavy emphasis on crisis stabilization and an insufficient emphasis on the effective treatment of co-occurring and chronic conditions. (para. 33)

UBH's guidelines were viewed as an important tool for meeting utilization management targets, "mitigating" the impact of the 2008 Parity Act, and keeping "benex" *(benefit expenses)* down ... as the "Mitigation Strategy" for Parity's "removal of day and visit limits." (para. 182)

Financial self-interest was a critical consideration in deciding ... coverage decisions. (para. 184) UBH's Finance Department had veto power with respect to the Guidelines and used it to prohibit even a change in the Guidelines that all of its clinicians had recommended ... UBH has a conflict of interest that has had a significant impact on decision-making as to the development of the Guidelines. (para. 202)

(Author's Comment: Note the judge's explicit finding that cost-savings for UBH was prioritized over clinical need, flouting the intent of parity.)

Whether the UBH guidelines adhere to generally accepted standards of care

Many mental health and substance use disorders are long-term and chronic ... While current symptoms are typically related to a patient's chronic condition ... effective treatment of individuals with mental health or substance use disorders is not limited to the alleviation of the current symptoms ... effective treatment requires treatment of the chronic underlying condition as well. (para. 71)

Many individuals with a behavioral health diagnosis have multiple, co-occurring disorders ... Co-occurring disorders can interact in a "reciprocal way" that makes each of them "worse" ... Because co-occurring disorders can aggravate each other, treating any of them effectively requires a comprehensive, coordinated approach to all conditions. (para. 72)

The CMS Manual explains, "[f]or many psychiatric patients, particularly those with long-term, chronic conditions, control of symptoms and maintenance of a functional level to avoid further deterioration or hospitalization is an acceptable expectation of improvement." (para. 75)

It is a generally accepted standard of care that the appropriate duration of treatment for behavioral health disorders is based on the individual needs of the patient; there is *no specific limit on the duration of such treatment.* (section f, para. 76)

The Court finds an excessive emphasis on addressing acute symptoms and stabilizing crises while ignoring the effective treatment of members' underlying conditions. (para. 82)

Common Criteria applicable to continued service and discharge also make clear that coverage will end when the member's symptoms are no longer acute.

(para. 100) ... the Guidelines drove members to lower levels of care even when treatment of the member's overall and/or co-occurring conditions would have been more effective at the higher level of care. (para. 111)

It is well established that effective treatment of mental health and substance use disorders includes treatment aimed at preventing relapse or deterioration of the patient's condition and maintaining the patient's level of functioning. UBH Guidelines deviate from that standard by restricting the concept of "improvement" to "reduction or control of the acute symptoms that necessitated treatment in a level of care." (para. 117)

Improvement, under the UBH Guidelines, is about crisis stabilization rather than maintenance of function. (para. 119)

In sum, the Court concludes that the improvement criteria provision in the UBH Guidelines...is inconsistent with generally accepted standards of care. (para. 123)

(Author's Comment: Above we see the impact of a judge's reaction to proprietary insurance company medical necessity criteria that deviate from generally accepted standards of care as established by nonprofit clinical specialty associations and expert consensus. Plaintiffs were represented by Meiram Bendat, a psychoanalytically trained therapist. Plaintiffs' experts included Eric Plakun, Medical Director of Austen Riggs Center.)

Wrongful benefit denials

The Court finds, by a preponderance of the evidence, that UBH's Guidelines were unreasonable and an abuse of discretion because they were more restrictive than generally accepted standards of care. (para. 212)

For these reasons, the Court finds that UBH is liable with respect to the Denial of Benefits Claim. (para. 216)

Further developments

In an important development subsequent to the Wit vs. UBH decision, on September 25, 2020, Governor Gavin Newson of California signed into law SB855 (2019–2020), a bill that Meiram Bendat, attorney for the plaintiffs in the Wit case, helped draft and in support of which he testified at the California legislature. SB855 ushers in an era of accountability for commercial health insurers in California and sets the stage for national reform.

First, the law expands parity protections to all conditions described in the DSM, rather than to just nine previously identified mental health disorders. Second, by establishing a state-wide definition of "medical necessity" for coverage of mental health and substance disorder treatment, the law requires insurers to make benefit determinations that are consistent with "generally accepted standards of care," and codifies the generally accepted standards of care articulated in the landmark Wit decision. Notably, with respect to mental health and substance use disorders, the law requires insurers to apply exclusively medical necessity criteria developed by nonprofit clinical specialty associations (such as AACP and ASAM), to receive trainings from nonprofit clinical specialty associations in the application of such criteria, and to achieve inter-rater reliability scores of at least 90% when applying these criteria. The law expressly forbids insurers from limiting benefits or coverage for mental health and substance use disorders to short-term or acute treatment.

Additionally, the law requires insurers to cover out-of-network treatment so that patients are not subject to anything beyond in-network cost-sharing if medically necessary mental health or substance use services are not available in-network within geographical and timeliness standards set by law or regulation. The practical effect is that insurers will be incentivized to expand their network capacity by recruiting suitable providers based on competitive market (rather than artificially devalued) reimbursement rates.

Finally, the law prohibits discretionary clauses in insurance contracts that give rise to a deferential standard of judicial review. This provision will require courts to review legal claims against health insurers de novo and will serve as another deterrent against insurer misconduct.

The findings in the Wit vs. UBH lawsuit have thus prepared the ground for California's new, more detailed, and comprehensive legal standard for the equitable coverage of mental health services that have been unlawfully curtailed. It also indicates the potential of the Wit decision to pave the way for an increasingly broad national trend, beyond California, in mandates for the support of clinically proven and research supported care. In addition to its support for coverage of a broad range of mental health services, the Wit decision also furnishes additional legal ground for providers, advocates, and for patients for appropriate support for clinically necessary extended and intensive psychodynamic psychotherapy and psychoanalysis. These patients are clearly entitled to be included and protected by these findings; thus, providers must be aware of the research documenting its importance and the laws protecting the cohort of patients who need it and to be prepared to demand from insurers and, if necessary in court, the observance of the mandate for its provision at parity with other health care.

Acknowledgments

The presentation of psychotherapy research and related data in this chapter is expanded and updated from an analogous discussion in an earlier paper (Lazar, 2018).

References

Bateman, A. W. (2012). Treating borderline personality disorder in clinical practice. *American Journal of Psychiatry*, *169*(6), 560–563. https://doi.org/10.1176/appi.ajp.12030341

Bateman, A. W., & Fonagy, P. (1999). Effectiveness of partial hospitalization in the treatment of borderline personality disorder: A randomized controlled trial. *American Journal of Psychiatry*, *156*(10), 1563–1569. https://doi.org/10. 1176/ajp.156.10.1563

Bateman, A. W., & Fonagy, P. (2003). Health service utilization costs for borderline personality disorder patients treated with psychoanalytically oriented partial hospitalization versus general psychiatric care. *American Journal of Psychiatry*, *160*(1), 169–171. https://doi.org/10.1176/appi.ajp.160.1.169

Bateman, A., & Fonagy, P. (2008). 8-year follow-up of patients treated for borderline personality disorder: Mentalization-based treatment versus treatment as usual. *American Journal of Psychiatry*, *165*(5), 631–638. https://doi.org/10.1176/appi.ajp.2007.07040636

Bateman, A., & Fonagy, P. (2009). Randomized controlled trial of outpatient mentalization-based treatment versus structured clinical management for borderline personality disorder. *American Journal of Psychiatry*, *166*(12), 1355–1364. https://doi. org/10.1176/appi.ajp.2009.09040539

Bendat, M. (2014). In name only? Mental health parity or illusory reform. *Psychodynamic Psychiatry*, *42*(3), 353–375. https:// doi.org/10.1521/pdps.2014.42.3.353

Berghout, C. C., Zevalkink, J., & Hakkaart-van Roijen, L. (2010a). A cost-utility analysis of psychoanalysis versus psycho-analytic psychotherapy. *International Journal of Technology Assessment in Health Care*, *26*(1), 3–10. https://doi.org/10. 1017/s0266462309990791

Berghout, C. C., Zevalkink, J., & Hakkaart-Van Roijen, L. (2010b). The effects of long-term psychoanalytic treatment on healthcare utilization and work impairment and their associated costs. *Journal of Psychiatric Practice*, *16*(4), 209–216. https://doi.org/10.1097/01.pra.0000386907.99536.75

Beutel, M. E., Rasting, M., Stuhr, U., Ruger, B., & Leuzinger-Bohleber, M. (2004). Assessing the impact of psychoanalyses and long-term psychoanalytic therapies on health care utilization and costs. *Psychotherapy Research*, *14*(2), 146–160. https://doi.org/10.1093/ptr/kph014

Blatt, S. J. (1992). The differential effect of psychotherapy and psychoanalysis with anaclitic and introjective patients: The Menninger Psychotherapy-Research Project revisited. *Journal of the American Psychoanalytic Association*, *40*(3), 691–724. https://doi.org/10.1177/000306519204000303

Blatt, S. J., Quinlan, D. M., Pilkonis, P. A., & Shea, M. T. (1995). Impact of perfectionism and need for approval on the brief treatment of depression: The national institute of mental health treatment of depression collaborative research program revisited. *Journal of Consulting and Clinical Psychology*, *63*(1), 125–132. https://doi.org/10.1037/0022-006X.63.1.125

Buchheim, A., Viviani, R., Kessler, H., Kachele, H., Cierpka, M., Roth, G., George, C., Kernberg, O. F., Bruns, G., & Taubner, S. (2012). Changes in prefrontal-limbic function in major depression after 15 months of long-term psychotherapy. *PLoS One*, *7*(3), e33745. https://doi.org/10.1371/journal.pone.0033745

Casey, P. R., & Tyrer, P. J. (1986). Personality, functioning and symptomatology. *Journal of Psychiatric Research*, *20*(4), 363–374. https://doi.org/10.1016/0022-3956(86)90039-7

Cellini, S. R., & Kee, J. E. (2010). Cost-effectiveness and cost-benefit analysis. In Wholey, J. S., Hatry, H. P., & Newcomer, K. E. (Eds.), *Handbook of program evaluation* (3rd ed., pp. 493–530). Jossey-Bass.

Clarkin, J., Levy, K., Lenzenweger, M., & Kernberg, O. (2007). Evaluating three treatments for borderline personality disorder: A multiwave study. *American Journal of Psychiatry*, *164*(6), 922–928. https://doi.org/10.1176/ajp.2007.164.6.922

Clarkin, J. F., Foelsch, P. A., Levy, K. N., Hull, J. W., Delaney, J. C., & Kernberg, O. F. (2001). The development of a psychodynamic treatment for patients with borderline personality disorder: A preliminary study of behavioral change. *Journal of Personality Disorders*, *15*(6), 487–495. https://doi.org/10.1521/pedi.15.6.487.19190

Cristea, I., Gentil, C., Cotet, C., Palomba, D., Barbui, C., & Cuijpers, P. (2017). Efficacy of psychotherapies for borderline personality disorder: A systematic review and meta-analysis. *JAMA Psychiatry*, *74*(4), 319–328. https://doi.org/10.1001/jamapsychiatry.2016.4287

Crown, W. H., Finkelstein, S., Berndt, E. R., Ling, D., Poret, A. W., Rush, A. J., & Russell, J. M. (2002). The impact of treatment-resistant depression on health care utilization and costs. *The Journal of Clinical Psychiatry*, *63*(11), 963–971. https://doi.org/10.4088/JCP.v63n1102

Cuijpers, P., Cristea, I. A., Karyotaki, E., Reijnders, M., & Huibers, M. J. H. (2016, October). How effective are cognitive behavior therapies for major depression and anxiety disorders? A meta-analytic update of the evidence. *World Psychiatry*, *15*(3), 245–258. https://doi.org/10.1002/wps.20346

Cuijpers, P., Smit, F., Bohlmeijer, E., Hollon, S., & Andersson, G. (2010). Efficacy of cognitive–behavioural therapy and other psychological treatments for adult depression: Meta-analytic study of publication bias. *British Journal of Psychiatry*, *196*(3), 173–178. https://doi.org/10.1192/bjp.bp.109.066001

De Maat, S., Philipszoon, F., Schoevers, R., Dekker, J., & De Jonghe, F. (2007). Costs and benefits of long-term psychoanalytic therapy: Changes in health care use and work impairment. *Harvard Review of Psychiatry*, *15*(6), 289–300. https://doi.org/10.1080/10673220701811654

De Maat, S., De Jonghe, F., Schoevers, R., & Dekker, J. (2009). The effectiveness of long-term psychoanalytic therapy: A systematic review of empirical studies. *Harvard Review of Psychiatry*, *17*(1), 1–23. https://doi.org/10.1080/ 10673220902742476

De Maat, S., De Jonghe, F., de Kraker, R., Leichsenring, F., Abbass, A., Luyten, P., Barber, J. P., Van, R., & Dekker, J. (2013, May-June). The current state of the empirical evidence for psychoanalysis: A meta-analytic approach. *Harvard Review of Psychiatry*, *21*(3), 107–137. https://doi.org/10.1097/HRP.0b013e318294f5fd

Deykin, E. Y., Keane, T. M., Kaloupek, D., Fincke, G., Rothendler, J., Siegfried, M., & Creamer, K. (2001). Posttraumatic stress disorder and the use of health services. *Psychosomatic Medicine*, *63*(5), 835–841. https://doi. org/10.1097/00006842–200109000-00018

Dossmann, R., Kutter, P., Heinzel, R., & Wurmser, L. (1997). The long-term benefits of intensive psychotherapy: A view from Germany. *Psychoanalytic Inquiry*, *17*(suppl 1, ed. Lazar SG), 74–86. https://doi.org/10.1080/ 07351699709534159

Driessen, E., Van, H., Don, F., Peen, J., Kool, S., Westra, D., Hendriksen, M., Schoevers, R. A., Cuijpers, P., Twisk, J. W. R., & Dekker, J. J. M. (2014). The efficacy of cognitive-behavioral therapy and psychodynamic therapy in the outpatient treatment of major depression: A randomized clinical trial. *FOCUS*, *12*(3), 324–335. https://doi. org/10.1176/appi.focus.12.3.324

Duehrssen, A. (1962). Catamnestic results with 1004 patients following analytic psychotherapy. *Zeitschrift fur Psychosomatische Medizin*, *8*, 94–113. https://pubmed.ncbi.nlm.nih.gov/13888205/

Fava, G. A., Ruini, C., & Belaise, C. (2007). The concept of recovery in major depression. *Psychological Medicine*, *37*(3), 307–318.

Fonagy, P. (Ed). (2002). *An open door review of outcome studies in psychoanalysis* (2nd ed.). International Psychoanalytical Association.

Fonagy, P., Rost, F., Carlyle, J., McPherson, S., Thomas, R., Pasco Fearon, R. M., Goldberg, D., & Taylor, D. (2015). Pragmatic randomized controlled trial of long-term psychoanalytic psychotherapy for treatment-resistant depression: The Tavistock Adult Depression Study (TADS). *World Psychiatry*, *14*(3), 312–321. https://doi.org/10.1002/ wps.20267

Frank, R. G., & McGuire, T. G. (2000). Economics and mental health. In Culyer, A. J. & Newhouse, J. P. (Eds.), *Handbook of health economics* (Vol. 1, pp. 893–954). Elsevier.

Gabbard, G. O. (2000). Psychotherapy of personality disorders. *The Journal of Psychotherapy Practice and Research*, *9*(1), 1–6. https://www.ncbi.nlm.nih.gov/pmc/articles/PMC3330582

Grande, T., Dilg, R., Jakobsen, T., Keller, W., Krawietz, B., Langer, M., Oberbracht, C., Stehle, S., Stennes, M., & Rudolf, G. (2006). Differential effects of two forms of psychoanalytic therapy: Results of the Heidelberg-Berlin study. *Psychotherapy Research*, *16*(4), 470–485. https://doi.org/10.1080/10503300600608082

Grilo, C. M., Stout, R. L., Markowitz, J. C., Sanislow, C. A., Ansell, E. B., Skodol, A. E., Bender, D. S., Pinto, A., Shea, M. T., Yen, S., Gunderson, J. G., Morey, L. C., Hopwood, C. J., & McGlashan, T. H. (2010). Personality disorders predict relapse after remission from an episode of major depressive disorder: A 6-year prospective study. *Journal of Clinical Psychiatry*, *71* (12), 1629–1635. https://doi.org/10.4088/JCP.08m04200gre

Hadjipavlou, G., & Ogrodniczuk, J. S. (2010). Promising psychotherapies for personality disorders. *Canadian Journal of Psychiatry*, *55*(4): 202–210. https://doi.org/10.1177/070674371005500403

Hall, J., Caleo, S., Stevenson, J., & Meares, R. (2001). An economic analysis of psychotherapy for borderline personality disorder patients. *Journal of Mental Health Policy and Economics*, *4*(1), 3–8. https://psycnet.apa.org/record/2002-06288-003

Heinzel, R., Breyer, F., & Klein, T. (1996). Ambulante Psychoanalyse in Deutschland: Eine katamnestische evaluation studie (No. 281), Diskussionsbeitrage: Seriel. Baden-Wurtemmberg (Germany): Fakultat fur Wirtschaftswissenschaften und Statistik, Universitat Konstanz. RePEc:zbw:kondpl:281. https://www.econstor.eu/bitstream/10419/68878/1/686791754.pdf

Høglend, P. (1993). Personality disorders and long-term outcome after brief dynamic psychotherapy. *Journal of Personality Disorders*, *7*(2), 168–181. https://doi.org/10.1521/pedi.1993.7.2.168

Holt-Lunstad, J., Smith, T. B., & Layton, J. B. (2010). Social relationships and mortality risk: A meta-analytic review. *PLoS Medicine*, *7*(7), e1000316. https://doi.org/10.1371/journal.pmed.1000316

Howard, K. I., Kopta, S. M., Krause, M. S., & Orlinsky, D. E. (1986). The dose–effect relationship in psychotherapy. *American Psychologist*, *41*(2), 159–164. https://doi.org/10.1037/0003-066X.41.2.159

Huber, D., Zimmermann, J., Henrich, G., & Klug, G. (2012). Comparison of cognitive-behaviour therapy with psychoanalytic and psychodynamic therapy for depressed patients: A three-year follow-up study. *Zeitschrift Fur Psychosomatische Medizin Und Psychotherapie*, *58*(3), 299–316. https://doi.org/10.13109/zptm.2012.58.3.299

Katon, W., & Sullivan, M. D. (1990). Depression and chronic medical illness. *Journal of Clinical Psychiatry, 1990*, 15–22. Jun;51Suppl:3–11; discussion 12–4.4. https://pubmed.ncbi.nlm.nih.gov/2189874/

Keller, W., Westhoff, G., Dilg, R., Rohner, R., & Studt, H. H. (1998). Efficacy and cost effectiveness aspects of outpatient (Jungian) psychoanalysis and psychotherapy—A catamnestic study. In Leuzinger-Bohleber, M. & Target, M. (Eds.), *Outcomes of psychoanalytic treatment: Perspectives for therapists and researchers* (pp. 186–200). Whurr Publishers.

Kessler, R. C., Berglund, P., Demler, O., Jin, R., Koretz, D., Merikangas, K. R., Rush, A. J., Walters, E. E., & Wang, P. S. (2003). The epidemiology of major depressive disorder: Results from the National Comorbidity Survey Replication (NCS-R). *JAMA, 289*(23), 3095–3105. https://doi.org/10.1001/jama.289.23.3095

Kopta, S. M., Howard, K. I., Lowry, J. L., & Beutler, L. E. (1994). Patterns of symptomatic recovery in psychotherapy. *Journal of Consulting and Clinical Psychology, 62*(5), 1009–1016. https://doi.org/10.1037/0022-006X.62.5.1009

Landerman, L. R., Burns, B. J., Swartz, M. S., Wagner, H. R., & George, L. K. (1994, December). The relationship between insurance coverage and psychiatric disorder in predicting use of mental health services. *American Journal of Psychiatry, 151*(12), 1785–1790. https://psycnet.apa.org/record/1995-18792-001

Lazar, S. G. (ed). (2010). *Psychotherapy is worth it: A comprehensive review of its cost-effectiveness*. American Psychiatric Association Publishing.

Lazar, S. G. (2018). The place for psychodynamic therapy and obstacles to its provision. *Psychiatric Clinics of North America, 41*(2), 193–205. https://doi.org/10.1016/j.psc.2018.01.004

Lazar, S. G., & Yeomans, F. E. (eds). (2014). Psychotherapy, the Affordable Care Act, and mental health parity: Obstacles to implementation. *Psychodynamic Psychiatry, 42*(3). https://guilfordjournals.com/toc/pdps/42/3

Leichsenring, F., Abbass, A., Luyten, P., Hilsenroth, M., & Rabung, S. (2013). The emerging evidence for long-term psychodynamic therapy. *Psychodynamic Psychiatry, 41*(3), 361–364. https://doi.org/10.1521/pdps.2013.41.3.361

Leichsenring, F., Leweke, F., Klein, S., & Steinert, C. (2015). The empirical status of psychodynamic psychotherapy - an update: Bambi's alive and kicking. *Psychother Psychosom, 84*(3), 129–148. https://doi.org/10.1159/000376584 Epub Mar 28

Leichsenring, F., Luyten, P. J., Hilsenroth, M. J., Abbass, A., Barber, J. P., Keefe, J. R., Leweke, F., Rabung, S., & Steinert, C. (2015). Psychodynamic therapy meets evidence-based medicine: A systematic review using updated criteria. *The Lancet Psychiatry, 2*(7), 648–660. https://doi.org/10.1016/S2215-0366(15)00155-8

Leichsenring, F., & Rabung, S. (2008). Effectiveness of long-term psychodynamic psychotherapy: A meta-analysis. *Journal of the American Medical Association, 300*(13), 1551–1565. https://doi.org/10.1001/jama.300.13.1551

Leichsenring, F., & Rabung, S. (2011). Long-term psychodynamic psychotherapy in complex mental disorders: Update of a meta-analysis. *British Journal of Psychiatry, 199*(1), 15–22. https://doi.org/10.1192/bjp.bp.110.082776

Leichsenring, F., & Steinert, C. (2017). Is cognitive behavioral therapy the gold standard for psychotherapy?: The need for plurality in treatment and research. *JAMA, 318*(14), 1323–1324. https://doi.org/10.1001/jama.2017.13737

Lenzenweger, M. F. (2008). Epidemiology of personality disorders. *Psychiatric Clinics of North America, 31*(3), 395–403. https://doi.org/10.1016/j.psc.2008.03.003

Leuzinger-Bohleber, M., Hautzinger, M., Fiedler, G., Keller, W., Bahrke, U., Kallenbach, L., Kaufhold, J., Ernst, M., Negele, A., Schoett, M., Küchenhoff, H., Günther, F., Rüger, B., & Beutel, M. (2019, Jan). Outcome of psychoanalytic and cognitive-behavioural long-term therapy with chronically depressed patients: A controlled trial with preferential and randomized allocation, *The Canadian Journal of Psychiatry*, *64*(1), 47–58. Epub 2018 Nov 1 https://doi.org/10.1080/ 07351699709534159

Levy, K. N., Ehrenthal, J. C., Yeomans, F. E., & Caligor, E. (2014). Efficacy of psychotherapy: Psychodynamic psychotherapy as an example. *Psychodynamic Psychiatry*, *42*(3), 377–422. https://doi.org/10.1521/pdps.2014.42.3.377

Levy, K. N., Meehan, K. B., Kelly, K. M., Reynoso, J. S., Weber, M., Clarkin, J. F., & Kernberg, O. F. (2006). Change in attachment patterns and reflective function in a randomized control trial of transference-focused psychotherapy for borderline personality disorder. *Journal of Consulting and Clinical Psychology*, *74*(6), 1027–1040. https://doi.org/10.1037/0022-006X.74.6.1027

Levy, K. N., Meehan, K. B., & Yeomans, F. E. (2010). Transference-focused psychotherapy reduces treatment drop-out and suicide attempters compared with community psychotherapist treatment in borderline personality disorder. *Evidence Based Mental Health*, *13*(4), 119. https://doi.org/10.1136/ebmh1097

Linehan, M. M., Armstrong, H. E., Suarez, A., Allmon, D., & Heard, H. L. (1991). Cognitive-behavioral treatment of chronically parasuicidal borderline patients. *Archives of General Psychiatry*, *48*(12), 1060–1064. https://doi.org/10. 1001/archpsyc.1991. 01810360024003

Linehan, M. M., & Heard, H. I. (1999). Borderline personality disorder. In Miller, N. E. & Magruder, K. M. (Eds.), *Cost effectiveness of psychotherapy* (pp. 291–305). Oxford University Press.

Luber, M. P., Hollenberg, J. P., Williams-Russo, P., DiDomenico, T. N., Meyers, B. S., Alexopoulos, G. S., & Charlson, M. E. (2000). Diagnosis, treatment, comorbidity, and resource utilization of depressed patients in a general medical practice. *The International Journal of Psychiatry in Medicine*, *30*(1), 1–14. https://doi.org/10.2190/ YTRY-E86M-G1VC-LC79

Maier, W., Lichtermann, D., Klingler, T., Heun, R., & Hallmayer, J. (1992). Prevalences of personality disorders (DSM-III-R) in the community. *Journal of Personality Disorders*, *6*(3), 187–196. https://doi.org/10.1521/pedi.1992.6.3.187

Manning, W. G., Jr, Wells, K. B., Duan, N., Newhouse, J. P., & Ware, J. E., Jr. (1986). How cost sharing affects the use of ambulatory mental health services. *JAMA*, *256*(14), 1930–1934. https://doi.org/10.1001/jama.1986. 03380140100030

Markowitz, J. C., Skodol, A. E., Petkova, E., Cheng, J., Sanislow, C. A., Grilo, C. M., Gunderson, J. G., & McGlashan, T. H. (2007). Longitudinal effects of personality disorders on psychosocial functioning of patients with major depressive disorder. *Journal of Clinical Psychiatry*, *68*(2), 186–193. https://doi.org/10.4088/JCP. v68n0202

McHugh, R. K., Whitton, S. W., Peckham, A. D., Welge, J. A., & Otto, M. W. (2013). Patient preference for psychological vs. pharmacologic treatment of psychiatric disorders: A meta-analytic review. *The Journal of Clinical Psychiatry*, *74*(6), 595–602. https://doi.org/10.4088/JCP.12r07757

McMain, S. F., Guimond, T., Streiner, D. L., Cardish, R. J., & Links, P. S. (2012). Dialectical behavior therapy compared with general psychiatric management for borderline personality disorder: Clinical outcomes and functioning over a 2-year follow-up. *American Journal of Psychiatry*, *169*(6), 650–661. https://doi.org/10.1176/appi.ajp. 2012.11091416

Melek, S., & Norris, D. (2008). *Chronic conditions and comorbid psychological disorders*. Milliman.

Mullin, A., Hilsenroth, M., Gold, J., & Farber, B. (2016, May). Changes in object relations over the course of psychodynamic psychotherapy. *Clinical Psychology & Psychotherapy*, *24*(2), 501–511. https://doi.org/10.1002/cpp. 2021

National Institute for Health and Care Excellence. (2009). *Borderline personality disorder: Treatment and management*. NICE Clinical Guideline.

Pilkonis, P. A., Neighbors, B. D., & Corbitt, E. M. (1999). Personality disorders. In Miller, N. E. & Magruder, K. M. (Eds.), *Cost-effectiveness of psychotherapy* (pp. 279–290). Oxford University Press.

Ravesteijn, B., Schachar, E. B., Beekman, A. T. F., Janssen, R. T. J. M., & Jeurissen, P. P. T. (2017). Association of cost sharing with mental health care use, involuntary commitment, and acute care. *JAMA Psychiatry*, *74*(9), 932–939. https://doi.org/10.1001/jamapsychiatry.2017.1847

Reich, J., Yates, W., & Nduaguba, M. (1989). Prevalence of DSM-III personality disorders in the community. *Social Psychiatry and Psychiatric Epidemiology*, *24*(1), 12–16. https://doi.org/10.1007/BF01788194

Rosso, G., Aragno, E., Cuomo, A., Fagiolini, A., Di Salvoa, G., & Maina, G. (2019). Five-year follow-up of first-episode depression treated with psychodynamic psychotherapy or antidepressants. *Psychiatry Research Journal Homepage*, *275*(May), 27–30. https://doi.org/10.1016/j.psychres.2019.02.073

Rudolf, G., Manz, R., & Ori, C. (1994). Ergebnisse psychoanalytischer Therapie {Outcome of psychoanalytic therapy}. *Zeitschrift für Psychosomische Medizin und Psychotherapie*, *40*(1), 25–40. https://neuro.unboundmedicine.com/medline/citation/8147138/{Results_of_psychoanalytic_therapy}

Sandell, R., Blomberg, J., Lazar, A., Carlsson, J., Broberg, J., & Schubert, J. (2000). Varieties of long-term outcome among patients in psychoanalysis and longterm psychotherapy: A review of findings in the Stockholm outcome of psychoanalysis and psychotherapy project (STOPPP). *The International Journal of Psychoanalysis*, *81*(5), 921–942. https://doi.org/10.1516/0020757001600291

Seligman, M. E. (1995). The effectiveness of psychotherapy. *The Consumer Reports Study*, *50*(12), 965–974. https://psycnet.apa.org/record/1996-13324-001

Shedler, J. (2010). The efficacy of psychodynamic psychotherapy. *American Psychologist*, *65*(2), 98–109. https://doi.org/ 10.1037/a0018378

Shedler, J. (2015). Where is the evidence for "evidence-based" therapy? *Journal of Psychological Therapies in Primary Care*, *4*(May), 47–59. https://jonathanshedler.com/wp-content/uploads/2015/07/Shedler-2015-Where-is-the-evidence-for-evidence-based-therapy-R.pdf

Shedler, J. (2018). Where is the evidence for "evidence-based" therapy? *Psychiatric Clinics of North America*, *41*(2), 319–329. https://doi.org/10.1016/j.psc.2018.02.001

Simon, G. E., Grothaus, L., Durham, M. L., VonKorff, M., & Pabiniak, C. (1996). Impact of visit copayments on outpatient mental health utilization by members of a health maintenance organization. *American Journal of Psychiatry*, *153*(3), 331–338. https://doi.org/10.1176/ajp.153.3.331

Skodol, A. E., Grilo, C. M., Pagano, M. E., Bender, D. S., Gunderson, J. G., Shea, M. T., Yen, S., Zanarini, M. C., & McGlashan, T. H. (2005). Effects of personality disorders on functioning and well-being in major depressive disorder. *Journal of Psychiatric Practice*, *11*(6), 363–368. https://doi.org/10.1097/00131746-200511000-00002

Skodol, A. E., Grilo, C. M., Keyes, K. M., Geier, T., Grant, B. F., & Hasin, D. S. (2011). Relationship of personality disorders to the course of major depressive disorder in a nationally representative sample. *American Journal of Psychiatry*, *168*(3), 257–264. https://doi.org/10.1176/appi.ajp.2010.10050695

Steinert, C., Munder, T., Rabung, S., Hoyer, J., & Leichsenring, F. (2017, October 1). Psychodynamic therapy: As efficacious as other empirically supported treatments? A meta-analysis testing equivalence of outcomes. *American Journal of Psychiatry*, *174*(10), 943–953. https://doi.org/10.1176/appi.ajp.2017.17010057

Van Den Bosch, L., Verheul, R., Schippers, G. M., & Van Den Brink, W. (2002). Dialectical behavior therapy of borderline patients with and without substance use problems: Implementation and long-term effects. *Addictive Behaviors*, *27*(6), 911–923. https://doi.org/10.1016/S0306-4603(02)00293-9

Wampold, B., Budge, S., Laska, K., Del Re, A., Baardseth, T., Flűckiger, C., Minami, T., Kivlighan, D. M., & Gunn, W. (2011). Evidence-based treatments for depression and anxiety versus treatment-as-usual: A meta-analysis of direct comparisons. *Clinical Psychology Review*, *31*(8), 1304–1312. https://doi.org/10.1016/j.cpr.2011.07.012

Wang, P. S., Berglund, P., Olfson, M., Pincus, H. A., Wells, K. B., & Kessler, R. C. (2005). Failure and delay in initial treatment contact after first onset of mental disorders in the National Comorbidity Survey Replication. *Archives of General Psychiatry*, *62*(6), 603–613. https://doi.org/10.1001/archpsyc.62.6.603

Wang, P. S., Lane, M., Olfson, M., Pincus, H. A., Wells, K. B., & Kessler, R. C. (2005). Twelve-month use of mental health services in the United States: Results from the National Comorbidity Survey Replication. *Archives of General Psychiatry*, *62*(6), 629–640. https://doi.org/10.1001/archpsyc.62.6.629

Westen, D., Novotny, C., & Thompson-Brenner, H. (2004). The empirical status of empirically supported psychotherapies: Assumptions, findings, and reporting in controlled clinical trials. *Psychological Bulletin*, *130*(4), 631–663. https://doi.org/10.1037/0033-2909.130.4.631

Wit vs. United Behavioral Health (n.d.). United States District Court Northern District of California, Findings of Fact and Conclusions of Law, Judge Joseph Spero.

World Health Organization. (2008). *The global burden of disease*. WHO.

Young, M. (2018). Treatment-resistant depression: The importance of identifying and treating co-occurring personality disorders. *Psychiatric Clinics of North America*, *41*(2), 249–261. https://doi.org/10.1016/j.psc.2018.01.003

Zimmerman, M., & Coryell, W. H. (1990). Diagnosing personality disorders in the community: A comparison of self-report and interview measures. *Archives of General Psychiatry*, *47*(6), 527–531. https://doi.org/10.1001/archpsyc.1990.01810180027005

4

In name only? Mental health parity or illusory reform

Meiram Bendat

The Paul Wellstone and Pete Domenici Mental Health Parity and Addiction Equity Act of 2008 and the Affordable Care Act (ACA) mandate significant insurance and patient protection reforms. Despite these safeguards, lax regulatory enforcement and lack of consumer and provider sophistication have failed to remedy ongoing insurer abuses resulting in deprivation of crucial mental health and substance abuse treatment. Even with persistent and informed advocacy, including strategies outlined herein, any potential parity gains are negated by unreasonably low reimbursement benchmarks already used by insurers in many ACA-exchange plans. The need for legislative remediation is therefore urgent.Inadequate access to mental health[1] care has been an enduring blight lurking in the shadows of public awareness. "This situation has been tolerated far too long," said President John F. Kennedy in 1963. "It has troubled our national conscience—but only as a problem unpleasant to mention, easy to postpone, and despairing of solution." Since passage of the Community Mental Health Act during President Kennedy's administration, advances in psychopharmacology have made deinstitutionalization a reality for many. Yet in the absence of robust psychosocial supports to replace locked facilities, the care of many chronically and severely ill patients has been improperly relegated to prisons, charities, and emergency rooms ill-equipped to handle their needs.

Compounding inadequate access to community mental health resources has been historic discrimination against mental health coverage by private insurers, managed behavioral healthcare organizations, and employers,[2] based largely on irrational and disproven fears of rapacious benefits consumption by a patient population culpable of psychic infirmity and pathological dysregulation preyed on, at best, by misguided practitioners with dubious clinical methods. Consequently, in the United States, where an estimated quarter of the population suffers from mental health conditions in any given year (Kessler, Chiu, Demler, & Walters, 2005) and where the lifetime incidence of mental illness is estimated at 50% (Kessler, Berglund, Demler, Jin, Merikangas, & Walters, 2005), insurers have balked at covering mental health conditions by either altogether excluding or greatly limiting treatment.[3] Ironically, despite tremendous need for treatment, mental healthcare spending accounted for only 7.3% of total health costs

DOI: 10.4324/9781003325512-6

in 2009, dropping from 8.7% in 1990.[4] Yet the mental health administrative share (including the costs and profits of private insurers) of all healthcare administrative expenditures ballooned from 10% in 1990 to 17.2% in 2009.[5]

Not until passage of the Paul Wellstone and Pete Domenici Mental Health Parity and Addiction Equity Act of 2008 ("Federal Parity Act")[6] were large group health plans that offered benefits for mental health and/or substance use disorders required, with limited exceptions,[7] to administer them on par with medical/surgical benefits. In 2011, the General Accounting Office reported on findings "that the implementation of [mental health] parity requirements led to reduced enrollee expenditure" (GAO-12–63, 2011, p. 20). A 2013 report commissioned by the US Department of Health and Human Services (HHS) reinforced that "[e]valuations of [Federal Employees Health Benefits Program] parity found no significant increase in total behavioral health spending. Nor did evaluations find an increased probability of any [mental health/substance use disorder] service utilization resulting from parity. In fact, the quantity of [mental health/substance use disorder] services patients received may have decreased slightly after parity was introduced" (Goplerud, 2013, p. 6).

It took full implementation of the Affordable Care Act ("ACA")[8] in 2014, however, to require insurers to include "essential health benefits," encompassing treatment for mental health, substance abuse, and behavioral disorders, in plans sold on the individual and small group markets.[9] Notably, while large group plans choosing to offer mental health benefits and individual/small-group plans required to include essential mental health benefits must be parity-compliant, by no means has parity been achieved. Due to the public's unfamiliarity with these intricate laws, stigma and fatigue inhibiting patients, and lax surveillance, it is unsurprising that meaningful mental health treatment remains out of reach for so many insureds.

While one need not scratch hard beneath the surface to find rampant mental health parity violations, reliance on governmental intervention appears misplaced. Regulatory oversight and public enforcement campaigns have been sporadic and anemic at best. Given the profound, current need for treatment and continued insurer impediments to meaningful care, this chapter will expound on the ACA and parity laws with an eye toward patient advocacy and empowerment of mental health professionals. Recommendations for reform will follow.

Mandates for reform: The ACA and federal parity act

According to the US Census Bureau's 2011 American Communities Survey, 47.5 million Americans were found to lack health insurance coverage altogether, and 25% of uninsured adults suffer from a mental health condition, substance use disorder, or both (Garfield, Lave, & Donahue, 2010). Responding to these chilling statistics, President Obama's signature piece of legislation, the ACA, forever altered the American health insurance landscape. Among other things, the ACA eliminated insurability barriers like pre-existing conditions and provided for ten categories of "essential health benefits" that insurers must cover in all non-grandfathered individual and small group plans:[10]

- Ambulatory patient services
- Emergency services
- Hospitalization
- Maternity and newborn care
- Mental health and substance use disorder services, including behavioral health treatment
- Prescription drugs
- Rehabilitative and habilitative services and devices
- Laboratory services
- Preventive and wellness services and chronic disease management
- Pediatric services, including oral and vision care

While the ACA requires that "health benefits established as essential not be subject to denial to individuals against their wishes on the basis of the individuals' age or expected length of life or of the individuals' present or predicted disability, degree of medical dependency, or quality of life,"[11] states regulating insurance marketplaces are nonetheless permitted to establish the scope of essential health benefits based on benchmark plans[12] from which "substantially equal" and "actuarially equivalent" deviations are permitted (see Table 4.1).[13]

Though all such plans include in- and outpatient care for mental health, substance abuse, and behavioral disorders, exactly which conditions are covered are inherently subject to deviation. Furthermore, in the absence of state-specific definitions of "habilitative services," insurers may define such coverage on their own and may substitute greater "rehabilitative" services with lesser "habilitative" services.[14] Thus, even with the ACA's mandate for inclusion of essential health benefits, plans may not necessarily be required to cover the same mental health conditions or offer a uniform continuum of services across all states.

In 2008, the Federal Parity Act amended the Employee Retirement Income Security Act of 1974 ("ERISA"), regulating private-employer–sponsored welfare benefit plans, and the Public Health Service Act ("PHSA"), which applies to individual and non-federal governmental health plans regulated by the

Table 4.1 Variability of "Essential" Mental Health Benefits across ACA-Exchange Plans

States are free to establish their own scope of:
Inpatient and outpatient services, defining covered conditions of habilitative and rehabilitative services

states. While the Federal Parity Act initially applied only to large group health plans that chose to offer mental health benefits, the ACA further wrapped the Federal Parity Act into all non-grandfathered individual and small group insurance plans required to include essential mental health benefits. Moreover, the Federal Parity Act is intended to work in tandem with state laws applicable to individual and group insurance that may mandate coverage for certain mental health conditions and confer greater protections than provided by the Federal Parity Act.[15] Thus, stakeholders must be attuned to the possibility of concurrent and separate application of the Federal Parity Act and state mental health parity laws (See Table 4.2).[16] While the Federal Parity Act contains numerous provisions, the most relevant for purposes of this discussion is its unequivocal prohibition of separate treatment limitations applicable only to benefits for mental health or substance use disorders.[17] The Federal Parity Act's implementing regulations define "treatment limitations" as either "quantitative,"

Table 4.2 Applicability of Parity Laws to Health Plans

Plan Type	*Federal Parity Act*	*State Parity Laws*
Private-Employer–Sponsored		
Large group (both grandfathered and non-grandfathered under ACA)		
Self-funded	Generally yes, if MH/SA benefits are offered	Not possibly
Fully insured	Generally yes, if MH/SA benefits are offered	
Small group (generally <50 employees but increased in 2016 to <100)		
Non-grandfathered under ACA		
Self-funded	Yes, with respect to essential mental health benefits	Not possibly
Fully insured	Yes, with respect to essential mental health benefits	
Grandfathered under ACA		
Fully insured	No	Possibly
Privately Obtained Individual Coverage		
Non-grandfathered under ACA	Yes, with respect to essential mental health benefits	Possibly
Grandfathered under ACA	No	Possibly

expressed numerically, or "non-quantitative," expressed as protocols limiting the scope or duration of benefits for treatment. Because non-quantitative treatment limitations ("NQTL") can theoretically take many forms, the implementing regulations identify an "illustrative list":[18]

- Medical management standards
- Formulary design for prescription drugs
- For plans with multiple network tiers (such as preferred providers and participating providers), network tier design
- Standards for provider admission to participate in a network, including reimbursement rates
- Methods for determining usual, customary, and reasonable charges
- Refusal to pay for higher cost therapies until it can be shown that a lower cost therapy is not effective (also known as fail-first policies or step therapy protocols)
- Exclusions based on failure to complete a course of treatment
- Restrictions based on geographic location, facility type, provider specialty, and other criteria that limit the scope or duration of benefits

Additionally, while not enumerated in the "illustrative list," the regulations cite the following as NQTL:[19]

- Limitations on inpatient services for situations where the participant is a threat to self or others
- Exclusions for court-ordered and involuntary holds
- Experimental treatment limitations
- Service coding limitations
- Exclusions for services provided by non-psychiatrists
- Network limitations

When applied exclusively to mental health benefits, the above NQTL are, without exception, proscribed. Recognizing that NQTL may also be employed in the medical/surgical context, however, the regulations further expound that, as written and in operation, NQTL may not be imposed on mental health or substance use disorder benefits unless any *processes*, *strategies*, *evidentiary standards*, or *other factors* used in applying them are *comparable* to and *no more stringent than* the processes, strategies, evidentiary standards, or other factors applied to medical/surgical benefits. The regulations operationalize the parity analysis within each of six classifications:[20]

- In-network, outpatient
- In-network, inpatient
- Out-of-network, outpatient
- Out-of-network, inpatient

- Emergency care
- Prescription drugs

The regulations further emphasize:

> The classifications are intended to be comprehensive and cover the complete range of medical/surgical benefits and mental health or substance use disorder benefits offered by health plans and issuers. Medical/surgical benefits and mental health or substance use disorder benefits cannot be categorized as being offered outside of these classifications and therefore not subject to the parity analysis.
>
> Cross-walking or pairing specific mental health or substance use disorder benefits with specific medical/surgical benefits is a static approach that the Departments do not believe is feasible, given the difficulty in determining "equivalency" between specific medical/surgical benefits and specific mental health and substance use disorder benefits and because of the differences in the types of benefits that may be offered by any particular plan.[21]

In rejecting "that specific mental health or substance use disorder benefits be crosswalked or paired with specific medical/surgical benefits (e.g., physical rehabilitation with substance use disorder rehabilitation) for purposes of parity analyses,"[22] the regulations leave little doubt that the processes, strategies, evidentiary standards, or other factors used in applying NQTL for mental health benefits must be the same for *all* medical/surgical benefits within each of the six benefits classifications. For example, concurrent medical necessity reviews applied to outpatient (in- or out-of-network) psychotherapy and only to select outpatient (in- or out-of-network) services (like physical rehabilitation) are impermissible if such concurrent medical necessity reviews are not otherwise applied to *all* outpatient (in- or out-of-network) medical/surgical benefits.

It should come as no surprise that when the Federal Parity Act's nearly identical interim final regulations were unearthed in 2010, the managed care industry waged war.[23]

Cloaking the identities of managed behavioral healthcare organizations opposed to the rules, the "Coalition for Parity, Inc." sued the secretaries of Health and Human Services, Labor, and Treasury, along with their respective departments. The plaintiffs unsuccessfully challenged the duration of the public comment period, which they had been amply accorded, in an effort to nullify the most substantial provision in the interim final regulations, namely the prohibition against disparate NQTL and their implementing processes, strategies, evidentiary standards, or other factors (See Table 4.3). Without legal sanction to circumvent parity, liability for discriminating against mental health treatment became much more tangible. Or so it appeared.

Table 4.3 Prohibitions on Treatment Limitations Imposed by Federal Parity

Act Treatment Limitation	*Rule*
Quantitative or Non-Quantitative Applied Only to MH/SA benefits within each of six classifications	Strictly prohibited
Non-Quantitative Applied to MH/SA and medical benefits within each of six classifications	Prohibited if processes, strategies, evidentiary standards, or other factors are not comparable or more stringent than those applied to medical benefits within each classification

Enforcement challenges

Despite official confirmation that "plans frequently employ NQTLs for behavioral health conditions that are more restrictive than those used for other medical/surgical conditions,"[24] to date, not a single parity enforcement action against a health plan, insurer, or managed behavioral healthcare organization has been publicly announced by either the HHS or the Department of Labor ("DOL").[25] Moreover, few states with mental health parity laws of their own, including those which have incorporated the Federal Parity Act into state law, have taken robust, public measures to enforce them (and particularly, their prohibition of disparate NQTL).[26] In the absence of regulatory scrutiny, one might imagine that private individuals adversely impacted by insurer discrimination would at least have the opportunity to bring their claims to light through the courts. While individuals with employer-sponsored mental health benefits can assert a private right to enforce parity and due process remedies conferred by the Federal Parity Act and ACA under ERISA, beneficiaries of ERISA-exempt plans such as non-federal governmental employees (i.e., first responders, legislators, judges) and privately insured individuals (now including members of Congress) cannot. This is because the Federal Parity Act and ACA apply to their health plans through the PHSA, which does not explicitly confer a private right of enforcement.[27] Thus, an estimated 30 million Americans covered by non-federal governmental plans currently subject to the Federal Parity Act cannot directly invoke its protections and must assert alternative, indirect, and potentially less effective legal theories to try to enforce their rights.[28] As previously uninsured individuals gain coverage through the ACA-exchanges, the number of ERISA-exempt beneficiaries lacking an explicit private right to enforce the Federal Parity Act and ACA will substantially increase.

While insurers obviously take solace from ERISA-exempt beneficiaries lacking an explicit private right of action to enforce their rights (See Table 4.4), they

Table 4.4 Explicit Private Rights of Action to Enforce the Federal Parity Act

Plan Type	*Private Right of Action*	*Available Remedy*
Private Employer Sponsored (ERISA)	Yes	Award of benefit, Injunction
Non-Federal Governmental (PHSA)	No	Unclear
Individual Coverage (PHSA)	No	Unclear

are also emboldened by ERISA beneficiaries not being able to sue for anything more than owed benefits, injunctive relief, and at best, attorney fees—assuming that individual litigants can even find counsel to represent them in individual benefit cases since, under ERISA, damages for denial of benefits are nonexistent. Thus, even if mental health patients can overcome the stigma and psychic toils of initiating litigation, insurers need not worry much about the potential impact of unlawful claims practices resulting in non-jury damage awards.

With little to fear, insurers have brazenly continued to apply proscribed, discriminatory policies toward mental health benefits. These discriminatory practices include adhering to substandard, unjustifiably restrictive (proprietary) medical necessity guidelines that are not recognized by practitioners and medical specialty groups while otherwise adhering to generally recognized medical guidelines for non-mental health conditions. They also include fail-first protocols that require patients to attempt and fail at lower (or no) levels of care before more robust treatments are considered. Rather than approving treatments consistent with assessed needs, insurers demand proof of treatment failures, imminent regression, or risk of requiring even higher levels of care. Perversely, under this schema, failed suicide attempts become the *sine qua non* for intensive or continued care at any level. It is hard to imagine how such an inhumane protocol could square with the ACA's "essential" re/habilitation benefit mandate or be comparably applied and tolerated in the medical context. Equally problematic is the application of involuntary commitment standards (danger to self/others, grave disability) to voluntary levels of care, and the corresponding, self-serving exclusion of involuntary (legally mandated or court-ordered) treatment from coverage.

Capping these abuses is the application of concealed algorithms to restrict higher needs patients from receiving ongoing care. These undisclosed algorithms flag patients whose service needs deviate from industry-determined "norms,"[29] often set by "in-house" utilization frequency trends from the pre-parity era when routine access to mental healthcare was excluded, quantitatively capped, or otherwise financially disincentivized by unequal copays or rates of reimbursement. Circumventing (for now) the Federal Parity Act's unequivocal prohibition on disparate quantitative treatment limits (such as predetermined visit maximums), undisclosed algorithms do not purport to be an absolute treatment cap.

Rather, a wolf in sheep's clothing, they ostensibly safeguard "quality control" and deter "fraud and abuse" by triggering insurer reviews intended to prospectively ration care under the guise of "medical necessity."

While these discriminatory protocols apply throughout the continuum of mental health services, they most consistently target psychotherapy and residential treatment, two modalities that are often long-term and intensive in the care of complex or chronic psychopathology.

Private enforcement: "Independent" review organizations (IROs)

Theoretically, the ACA has sought to bypass the need for litigation by providing claimants of all non-grandfathered health plans subject to ERISA or PHSA the right to expeditiously challenge insurer denials of mental health claims through independent external reviews. Moreover, regulations implementing the ACA have vested IROs with the responsibility of verifying plan compliance with the Federal Parity Act's prohibitions against disparate application of NQTL.[30] Thus, IROs have been charged with overturning adverse insurer determinations based on unlawful NQTL.

Regrettably, the DOL has simultaneously unrolled a federal external review process for self-funded health plans,[31] providing nearly half of all health benefits in this country, which is laden with conflicts of interest undermining the independence and efficacy of external reviews. Under current DOL rules implementing external reviews, self-funded health plans (primarily through their managed behavioral healthcare organizations) privately contract with IROs to adjudicate external appeals. Whereas, in theory, fully insured health plans are subject to oversight by state insurance departments that facilitate external reviews of denied claims through contracts with IROs, IROs contracted with self-funded health plans are self-policing and accountable to no one but their large volume clients, the managed behavioral healthcare organizations. Therefore, not only are IROs implicitly incentivized to not reverse medical necessity denials by the hiring managed behavioral healthcare organizations, they also routinely fail to discharge their fiduciary duties to insureds by overlooking parity and due process violations, even when explicitly alerted to such. The inference is clear—findings of non-compliance with parity laws and procedural safeguards would likely doom any contractual relationships between managed behavioral healthcare organizations and their cherry-picked external review agents.

All this is not to suggest that state-run external review programs are free of taint. Because many of the IROs contracted with managed behavioral healthcare organizations are also contracted with state insurance departments, their incentive to reverse insurer denials is equally diminished in the fully insured context. IROs are keenly aware that their decisions in fully insured cases result in direct liability to insurers (rather than employers) and that expensive or frequent reversals will almost certainly be met with retaliation in the form of contractual terminations by insurers (acting as managed behavioral healthcare organizations) in the self-funded context.

Furthermore, while state insurance departments have primary authority to enforce parity compliance in fully insured cases, no state, as a matter of course, routinely scrutinizes mental health claims denials based on parity considerations before assigning external appeals to many of the very same IROs contracted with the managed behavioral healthcare organizations. Some states even immunize IROs from liability except in cases of gross negligence, resulting in complete lack of accountability. And most states as well as all insurers contracted with IROs rely on managed behavioral healthcare organizations to transmit internal case files to external reviewers—often without any advance opportunity for claimants to ensure that all relevant plan, clinical, and insurer files have been forwarded for review. Regrettably, IROs rarely provide claimants with copies of documents received from managed behavioral healthcare organizations prior to adjudication of external appeals, if at all.

Additionally, the external review process for both fully insured and self-funded plans does not require transparency with regard to medical necessity criteria and guidelines used by IROs *before* external appeals are submitted. Thus, it is not infrequent for mental health claimants to challenge adverse medical necessity determinations (based on proprietary managed behavioral healthcare organization guidelines) only to be sandbagged by final rulings from IROs using the same or other proprietary guidelines (i.e., Milliman or InterQual) or unexpected rationales, potentially also in violation of mental health parity laws and the terms of claimants' health plans.

Because self-funded health plan sponsors with the ultimate responsibility to ensure IROs' compliance with the Federal Parity Act and ACA defer to their conflict-riddled managed behavioral healthcare organizations to safeguard the external appeals process, and because most state-administered external review programs neither adequately insulate patients from insurer-external review agent conflicts of interest nor routinely tackle parity violations, the external appeals process as currently constituted is an inadequate enforcement remedy for mental health claimants.

Enforcement strategies: Litigation

One strategy, however, carries substantial promise for deterrence of abuse and implementation of reform: impact litigation. In opposing uniform, discriminatory policies through associational challenges and class action suits, providers and beneficiaries can wield substantial leverage. To date, several associational and class action suits invoking mental health parity protections have been filed against insurers and managed behavioral healthcare organizations. These include cases challenging: preauthorization requirements for outpatient psychotherapy; disparate evidentiary burdens imposed by insurer-developed mental health guidelines; fail-first protocol applied to all levels of mental healthcare; and coverage exclusions.[32] These cases highlight the fact that while insurers routinely balk at authorizing higher levels of care such as psychiatric hospitalization and residential treatment, they simultaneously try to limit access to the least restrictive levels of care, including outpatient psychotherapy. Furthermore, these cases also unearth procedural abuses such as the failure to respond to appeals, the use of subordinates to review claims denied by their superiors, and the termination of benefits pending adjudication of final appeals.

Proposed solutions

It is axiomatic that systemic insurer abuses flourish in the absence of enforcement of antidiscrimination and patient protection laws. To make parity a reality, a multi-pronged response is required. First, Congress should extend an explicit private right of action to ERISA-exempt beneficiaries ostensibly protected by the Federal Parity Act and ACA through the PHSA. Now that members of Congress must purchase insurance through ACA exchanges, their own self-interest may actually prompt such relief. If Congress cannot be convinced to add an explicit private right of action to the PHSA applicable to these policies, individual states can certainly do so since the PHSA sections incorporating the Federal Parity Act and ACA also apply to them. Thus, states can simply pass statutes incorporating the PHSA provisions related to the Federal Parity Act and ACA while adding explicit private rights of action to enforce these statutes as well as any applicable state parity laws. Second, the DOL should amend the federal external review process for self-funded plans. By prohibiting self-funded plans and managed behavioral healthcare organizations from directly contracting with IROs, external review agents will have far less to fear in holding insurers and managed behavioral healthcare organizations accountable. In fact, the HHS has adopted such a strategy by specifically designating an IRO for appeals of Medicare and federal ACA exchange plans which is not available for hire by self-funded plans or managed behavioral health care organizations. Furthermore, by requiring all IROs to publicly post their medical necessity guidelines, redacted rulings, and relevant determination statistics, independent review organizations can be made much more accountable for the fairness of their decisions.

Meanwhile, the DOL, HHS, and employers sponsoring self-funded plans can be further sensitized to NQTL and their implementing processes, strategies, evidentiary standards, or factors improperly impacting mental health and substance abuse benefits. Currently, it appears that the DOL routinely rejects complaints of adverse benefit determinations based on medical necessity without comprehensively analyzing underlying NQTL and implementing protocols. To facilitate transparency and the parity analysis, then, the following information should also be required with all adverse benefit determinations as a matter of course:

- A description of any NQTL that a health *plan* (or insurance policy) has authorized for Mental Health/Substance Abuse (MH/SA) services within the relevant classification (in- or out-of-network, in- or outpatient) to the claim. This should also include the exact written reference to such within the plan (or insurance policy) documents (as distinguished from a managed behavioral healthcare organization's clinical guidelines implementing the NQTL);
- A description of any NQTL that the *insurer* or *managed behavioral healthcare organization* believes have been used in any given MH/SA service adverse benefit determination within the relevant classification based on the plan (or insurance policy);
- A description of any NQTL implementing processes, strategies, evidentiary standards, or factors that a *plan* (or insurance policy) has authorized for MH/SA services within the relevant classification to the claim. This should also include the exact written reference to such within the plan documents (as distinguished from a managed behavioral healthcare organization's clinical guidelines);
- A description of any non-quantitative treatment implementing processes, strategies, evidentiary standards, or factors that the *insurer* or *managed behavioral healthcare organization* believes have been used in any given MH/SA service adverse benefit determination within the relevant classification;
- A description of the NQTL and their implementing processes, strategies, evidentiary standards, or factors that a health *plan* (or insurance policy) has authorized for use with respect to *each and every* medical/surgical service within the same classification as the MH/SA claim. This should also include the exact written reference to such within the plan documents (as distinguished from a managed behavioral healthcare organization's clinical guidelines);
- A description of the NQTL and their implementing processes, strategies, evidentiary standards, or factors that the *insurer* or *managed behavioral healthcare organization* believes are used with respect to *each and every* medical/surgical service within the same classification as the MH/SA claim. Because insurers and claims administrators are required to provide all clinical guidelines and rationales in adverse benefit determinations, there is little reason why they cannot be required to post all medical necessity guidelines for medical/surgical procedures broken down by in- and outpatient bases on their websites.
- The frequencies with which the itemized NQTL and their implementing processes, strategies, evidentiary standards, or factors are used in both the MH/SA and medical/surgical contexts, by classification.

Effectively, by requiring that adverse benefit determinations explicitly reference the NQTL/protocols *authorized* by insurance policies and the NQTL/protocols *actually operationalized* by insurers, insurers would be far more likely to scrutinize their own conduct while policy holders could at least attempt to evaluate the consistency and comprehensiveness of insurer disclosures.

Another important remedy would be for legislators and regulators to prohibit discretionary clauses in health plans. Such clauses effectively require courts to defer to adverse determinations in the absence of insurers' "abuse of discretion," a highly deferential legal standard extremely difficult for patients to surmount. Rather than accord insurers any deference, courts should be required to review health claims denials afresh and in a truly even-handed manner—as they would scrutinize most legal claims. Moreover, rather than claimants being required to justify the medical necessity of healthcare prescribed in good faith, insurers should uniformly bear the burden of disproving medical necessity. Only then will insurers be systematically disincentivized from disregarding potential liability due to deliberate or negligent claims mishandling.

While the above proposals will certainly be met with stiff insurer resistance, there are numerous strategies for clinicians and their patients to employ to facilitate such change. First, establishing and maintaining contacts with federal and state officials is paramount. Important issues too often fail to gain traction due to collective fatigue or worse yet, passivity and submission. If members of Congress and state legislatures are not inundated with concerns that now equally affect them, then they cannot be held as readily accountable for inertia. Since many, if not most, clinicians belong to professional associations with potentially far greater resources, leveraging the power of associational standing is an underutilized and highly effective reform tool. While numerous professional associations have actively lobbied for mental health parity, to date only the New York State Psychiatric Association and the American Psychiatric Association have sued to enforce the Federal Parity Act. With more insistent calls for action from impacted members and their patients, however, professional mental health associations can and will do more.

Of course, lobbying for systemic reform is an aspirational (albeit critical) task. Insisting on immediate recourse for patients is an entirely different matter.

A word of caution

Ethical, contractual, and legal principles compel advocacy of patient access to mental health treatment. Clearly, the greater custody and control clinicians and facilities exercise over patients, the greater the imperative to avoid abandonment through effective advocacy.[33] This imperative increases commensurate with the degree of patients' mental impairments. Moreover, network contracts, often ignored by clinicians and facilities upon being signed, may also require providers to submit clinical appeals on behalf of patients. While clinicians are not expected to employ attorney skills in contesting denials, they should be readily familiar with the following due process rights, which are now standard across ERISA and non-grandfathered health plans and which must generally be "exhausted" (a term of art for "fully undertaken and completed") as a prerequisite to filing external appeals with IROs or to commencing legal actions.

When possible, appeals should be written to preserve the integrity of the clinical record, to articulate the precise issues being challenged, and to invite a meaningful exchange with insurers. With limited exceptions, the time frame for internally appealing denied claims is no less than 180 days from the date of a benefits denial, though some plans provide for subsequent levels of internal appeals that must be pursued within even shorter time frames, typically 60 days after an initial appeal denial. In urgent cases, insurers must respond to any claims and appeals within 72 hours and must treat any claims or appeals as "urgent" if designated as such by treating clinicians—at least in theory.

Since insurers, managed behavioral healthcare organizations, IROs, and regulators are not usually available to process urgent mental health appeals on evenings, weekends, and holidays, and while their unavailability obviously obstructs access to urgent care and defeats the purpose of expedited reviews, clinicians and patients must hold these entities accountable to their legal obligations. Thus, clinicians and patients should not delay submitting (urgent) appeals through tracked means, placing the onus on regulators and insurers to justify non-compliance with mandated processing time frames.

Moreover, while patients and their designated representatives are entitled to obtain copies of their claims files from insurers and managed behavioral health organizations prior to submitting their appeals, it is rarely the case that these records are made available, let alone on expedited bases. Because such records can be extremely helpful in proving parity violations and demonstrating procedural irregularities, insurers and managed behavioral healthcare organizations make it difficult to obtain this information by, at best, providing fax numbers for requests that are routinely ignored or delayed. Nonetheless, in non-urgent cases, patients or their authorized representatives (i.e., parents of minors, guardians, and conservators) should directly request their case files from insurers while, in urgent cases, providers are legally deemed "authorized representatives" and should likewise attempt to review insurer case management records prior to appealing.

Appealing

While no particular format is prescribed for appealing denied claims, appeals of mental health claims should ideally strike an appropriate balance between maintaining patient privacy and facilitating necessary disclosure. Because the Health Insurance Portability and Accountability Act of 1996 ("HIPAA") grants providers (and not insurers) the discretion to decide what constitutes a "minimally necessary disclosure," patients and providers submitting claims and appealing denials should not succumb to insurer coercion for gratuitous detail. By identifying the bases for a claim or appeal in advance, providers and patients can set limits on what will be revealed. For example, while insurers may deny care as "not medically necessary," all too frequently such denials occur in the context of prospective reviews that violate parity laws. Thus, while medical necessity may be relevant to an appeal, challenging adverse determinations may more suitably center on the disparate application of medical management techniques. In other words, challenging insurers' oracular forecasts of long-term needs in the outpatient mental health context (when such is not the case in the outpatient medical/surgical context) may suffice without further clinical disclosures.

That said, standards do matter and comprehensive appeals should often (though not always) refute adverse determinations of medical necessity based on clinical rationales that do not comport with case facts or prevailing national standards (i.e., published guidelines or research). Thus, it matters little which clinical rationales insurers offer if they are selectively tailored or not congruent with prevailing clinical standards. Moreover, insurers cannot rely on clinical definitions of "medical necessity" that conflict with contractual language in health plans. Therefore, in addition to procuring insurer case files for purposes of identifying proscribed denial rationales, procedural irregularities (i.e., appeals decisions made by subordinates of initial claims reviewers), or more thoroughly dissecting flawed conclusions, the most vigilant appellants should compare definitions of medical necessity in policy documents with clinical protocols employed by insurers. Hypothetically, then, insurer denials predicated exclusively on internally developed clinical guidelines that ignore health plan definitions of "medically necessary" as "services recognized by peer-reviewed literature" might be particularly susceptible to legal challenge. It is hoped that the succeeding articles in this installment will lay out a comprehensive base of research from which support for psychotherapy can be reliably cited in "medical necessity" appeals.

Apart from providing a brief clinical history, the reasons for current treatment, and diagnostic information, appeals should carefully weigh how to respond to insurers' insistence on "progress." While inefficacious mental health treatment, including psychotherapy, should not be offered (let alone reimbursed), the idea that "progress" rather than "prevention" should serve as the benchmark for treatment is a red herring. Obviously, in the case of severe mental illness, psychotherapy is frequently necessary to prevent further deterioration or to sustain any gains. Given that many chronic medical disorders only result in death and that insurers would be hard-pressed to ration their outpatient care in the interim, parity would mandate similar treatment. Thus, while expounding on progress may be warranted in some circumstances, appeals should at least emphasize the role of treatment in maintaining patient functioning that would erode in its reduction.

Of course, no appeal is complete without adequate confirmation of its receipt. Since insurers often fail to dispose of appeals within proper time frames, if at all, verification of their receipt is critical when other remedies must be sought (i.e., external appeals or lawsuits). Some courts punish belated, incomplete, or non-responses by insurers by not according any deference to their prior determinations, thereby increasing the likelihood of successful legal challenges.

Clinical considerations

While most outpatient medical claims are never reviewed beyond coding, it has become all too common a practice for insurers to demand ongoing reviews of even the most basic level of mental healthcare, out-patient psychotherapy. Often, these reviews are prospective (rather than retrospective) such that their very use offends the parity laws. They also consume enormous clinical resources on the part of providers and dramatically unsettle patients.

Thus, it is unsurprising that attending providers would reflexively balk at being critiqued by "peer reviewers" of materially different professional backgrounds (and often of far less experience or stature) who have never even encountered the same clinical situations or diagnostic groups of patients. Since most, if not all, providers are loathe to pleading their patients' cases to outside parties intent on rationing care and lecturing them on appropriate treatment standards, providers must be mindful of their understandable hostility before engaging in clinical reviews affecting their patients. Likewise, providers must be careful to resist defending against their hostility by allowing peer reviewers to use a "collegial" approach masquerading as a false alliance by means of which more than "minimally necessary" disclosures are elicited and then used to substantiate the denial of care.

To further contain their indignation and manage incursions into the therapeutic milieu, providers should plan a strategy for managing insurer reviews before they occur. By addressing the implications for privacy and the burden of insurance reviews with patients at the onset of treatment, providers can attempt to establish protective parameters in advance. Thus, how much time providers can be reasonably expected to devote to claims without charging their patients and what to charge for administrative work can be negotiated in advance. In the out-of-network context, where no contractual relationship exists between providers and insurers, it may also be reasonable for providers to bill insurers for their professional time allotted to "peer reviews." While insurers may refuse to reimburse these charges, their accounting certainly may prove valuable in litigation, when insurers might be ordered to compensate providers for their trouble, especially if brought on by unlawful claims review procedures.

Last, it is worth mentioning that providers must remain attuned to the particular patient fantasy of providers as "hero-rescuers" when insurance is at stake. While reasonable expectations must be set for clinical roles, expectations of omnipotence, benevolence, or futility of insurance negotiations are worthy of clinical exploration as they may all color patient dynamics and contribute to the psychotherapeutic task at hand.

Conclusion

Even with the promise of mental health parity and "essential health benefits," access to care is meaningless in the absence of reasonable reimbursement benchmarks. While the ACA has mandated a reduction in healthcare costs, including administrative fees, the ACA does not set uniform reimbursement benchmarks for any size plan, whether fully insured or self-funded. Instead, insurers are required to simply establish actuarial values based on total premium amounts that must be used to reimburse clinical services. With little more than self-interest in mind, many insurers have set the reimbursement bar so low that some leading facilities and providers have refused their compensation terms. Perhaps nowhere is this problem more acutely demonstrated than in the nation's most populous state, California, where the absence of state law establishing reasonable reimbursement benchmarks has encouraged insurers to apply Medicaid reimbursement rates to ACA-exchange plans. In turn, ACA-exchange provider networks in California are a fraction of large-group provider networks, which often establish far more favorable reimbursement benchmarks (based on either Medicare or the Fair Database). Access to leading facilities and healthcare providers is therefore severely restricted (Terhune, 2013), even when insureds opt for out-of-network benefits made equally illusory by the same Medicaid caps. Ironically, then, while we may finally have the tools to end insidious insurer discrimination in the mental health context, any parity advances are negated by strangulation of reasonable reimbursement for all "essential health benefits" in many, if not most, ACA-exchange plans. Without Congress and the states acting swiftly to establish minimum reimbursement benchmarks, private insurance will be nothing more than an extension of Medicaid—with meaningful care effectively out of reach for premium-paying patients lured into the ACA exchanges by the promise of access, affordability, and quality.

Dedicated to my dear friend and mentor, Elyn Saks.
*See Appendix for a list of acronyms used throughout the chapter.

Notes

1 For convenience, "mental health" shall encompass "substance abuse" in this chapter.
2 For convenience, these entities shall be collectively referred to as "insurers" in this chapter. Technically, insurers underwrite and generally administer health plans. Managed behavioral healthcare organizations are generally owned by insurers, and while they may not underwrite plans, they are responsible for most, if not all, aspects of plan administration, including development and implementation of clinical protocols. Employers, as group sponsors of health plans, either purchase coverage from insurers or contract with managed care organizations to administer health plan benefits.
3 Until 2014, about one-third of insureds in the individual market had no coverage for substance use disorder services and nearly 20% had no coverage for mental

health services, including outpatient therapy visits and inpatient crisis intervention and stabilization. (See ASPE Issue Brief, 2011.)

4 Specifically, in 2009, the mental health and substance abuse shares of all health expenditures were 6.3% and 1.0%, respectively. In 1990, they were 6.9% and 1.8%, respectively (Substance Abuse and Mental Health Services Administration, 2013, p. 255).

5 Substance Abuse and Mental Health Services Administration, 2013, p. 261.

6 Pub. L. No. 110-343, Div. C, Tit. V, Sub. B, §§ 511-512, 122 Stat. 3765, 3881-3893 (Oct. 3, 2008), passed as part of the Emergency Economic Stabilization Act of 2008, expands the parity requirements established by the Mental Health Parity Act of 1996 (Pub. L. No. 104-204, Tit. VII, §§ 701–702, 100 Stat. 2874, 2944-2950 (Sept. 26, 1996), the first federal mental health parity law, which required parity in annual and aggregate lifetime dollar limits.

7 Large group plans demonstrating that the Federal Parity Act's requirements have increased health care costs by 2% in the first year that the Federal Parity Act applies to the plan, or by at least 1% in subsequent years, may seek exemption for the following year. Self-insured non-federal government employee plans can opt out of compliance with the federal parity law but few have done so. Church-based plans, TriCare, Medicare, and traditional Medicaid are subject to different regulatory schema forming the basis for separate discussion.

8 Pub. L. No. 111-148, 124 Stat. 119 (2010), amended by the Health Care and Education Reconciliation Act of 2010, Pub. L. No. 111-152, 124 Stat. 1029 (2010), (codified in scattered sections of 29 U.S.C. & 42 U.S.C.). See Appendix for a list of acronyms used throughout the chapter.

9 Employer-sponsored large-group plans and "grandfathered" individual and small group plans are not currently required to include "essential health benefits." Grandfathered plans are those created before March 23, 2010. See 45 CFR § 147.140.

10 42 U.S.C. § 18022(b)(1).

11 42 U.S.C. § 18022(b)(4)(D)

12 Benchmark plans are based on a plan from: (1) Any of the largest three plans in the state's small group insurance market (by enrollment); (2) Any of the largest three state employee health benefit plans (by enrollment); (3) Any of the largest three national federal employee health plans (by enrollment); (4) The largest commercial non-Medicaid Health Maintenance Organization (HMO) operating in the state.

13 42 U.S.C. § 18022(b)(1) and 45 C.F.R. § 156.115.

14 *Id.*

15 Final Rules under the Paul Wellstone and Pete Domenici Mental Health Parity and Addiction Equity Act of 2008, 78 Fed. Reg. 68240, 68252 (Nov. 13, 2013).

16 Since it is beyond the scope of this chapter to address state mental health parity laws, data maintained at www.ncsl.org/research/health/mental-health-benefits-state-mandates.aspx by the National Conference of State Legislatures may prove useful.

17 The Federal Parity Act permits large group plans to exclude all or any mental health conditions from coverage and does not consider this to be a "treatment limitation." Any mental health or substance use disorder conditions that are covered by large group plans, however, must be covered on par with medical/surgical conditions. The Federal Parity Act does not allow plans to exclude specific non-experimental/investigational treatments for covered conditions. Furthermore, fully insured large group plans are still subject to state mental health parity laws, which may require coverage for certain conditions that must then be administered according to the Federal Parity Act and any applicable state laws.

18 Final Rules under the Paul Wellstone and Pete Domenici Mental Health Parity and Addiction Equity Act of 2008, 78 Fed. Reg. 68240, 68272 (Nov. 13, 2013).
19 *Id.* at 68246.
20 The regulations permit splitting the outpatient classification into two subclassifications: (1) office visits and (2) all other outpatient items and services. See *id.* at 68242.
21 *Id.* at 68243.
22 *Id.* at 68243.
23 See *Coalition for Parity v. Sebelius,* 709 F.Supp.2d 10 (LEXIS 2010).
24 See Gopelrud, 2013, p. x ["Analyses of large employer benefits in 2010 found numerous examples of NQTLs that were stricter for MH/SUD than for medical/surgical services. Some of the most common NQTLs include MH/SUD precertification requirements that were more stringent than medical/surgical requirements (28% of tested plans), medical necessity criteria that were applied to MH/SUD benefits but not to medical/surgical benefits (8% of tested plans), the use of routine retrospective reviews for MH/SUD services, and not for medical/surgical services, and reimbursement rates that were based on lower percentages of UCR rates for MH/SUD services than those provided for medical/surgical services."] Also see p. xiii, "Although we were able to identify areas where the application of NQTLs appeared to be inconsistent with the IFR, it is likely that our reliance on these limited sources of information drawn primarily from large employers' health plans resulted in a significant under-identification of problematic NQTLs."
25 The DOL has, however, expressed support for allowing private plaintiffs to sue a managed behavioral healthcare organization for various parity violations in an amicus brief submitted to the United States Court of Appeals for the Second Circuit. See *New York State Psychiatric Association, Inc. et al. v. UnitedHealthGroup, Inc. et al.,* April 22, 2014.
26 Most notably, in 2014, the New York State Attorney General publically announced several high-profile settlements with insurers Emblem Health, Cigna Health and Life Insurance Company, and MVP Health Care (operating contractually with Value Options) for parity violations, including disparate treatment caps for nutritional counseling, disproportionately high (40% more) denials of coverage in behavioral health cases than in medical cases, and exclusions of residential treatment for behavioral health conditions when subacute medical care was otherwise covered.
27 See August 17, 2012 Technical Guidance for Non-Federal Governmental Plans by the United States Department of Health & Human Services: "The ERISA private right of action under section 502(a) is not available to participants or beneficiaries of non-federal governmental plans...HHS will not enforce the requirement that non-federal governmental plans provide notice of the ERISA private right of action."
28 See estimates cited in Final Rules under the Paul Wellstone and Pete Domenici Mental Health Parity and Addiction Equity Act of 2008, 78 Fed. Reg. 68240, 68257 (Nov. 13, 2013).
29 See, for example, *C.M. v. Fletcher Allen Healthcare,* 2013 U.S. Dist. LEXIS 120469, (Cigna Health Insurance Company informed the patient, "[M]ost Cigna customers complete routine outpatient treatment in 8 sessions. Should claims exceed 25 sessions for this customer [C.M.], a case review based on medical necessity and the benefit plan design will be necessary. In addition, at that point, claim payment for this customer will be pulled from the automatic process and require prior authorization for additional sessions.")

30 See 76 Fed. Reg. 37208, 37216 (June 4, 2011) ("Additional examples of situations in which a claim is considered to involve medical judgment include adverse benefit determinations based on:....Whether a plan is complying with the nonquantitative treatment limitation provisions of the Mental Health Parity and Addiction Equity Act and its implementing regulations, which generally require, among other things, parity in the application of medical management techniques.")
31 See United States Department of Labor August 23, 2010 Technical Release 2010–01, Interim Procedures for Federal External Review Relating to Internal Claims and Appeals and External Review Under the Patient Protection and Affordable Care Act.
32 See New York State Psychiatric Association, Inc. et al. v. UnitedHealth Group et al., March 11, 2013 (complaint filed). Also See K.M. et al. v. Regence BlueShield et al., July 11, 2013 (complaint filed). Also See A. F. ex rel. Legaard v. Providence Health Plan (decided on Aug. 8, 2014).
33 *See Wickline v. California*, 192 Cal. App. 3d 1630 (1986).

References

ASPE Issue Brief. (2011). *Essential health benefits: Individual market coverage*. U.S. Department of Health & Human Services. Retrieved from http://aspe.hhs.gov/ health/ reports/2011/IndividualMarket/ib.shtml.

GAO-12-63. (2011). *Mental health and substance use: Employers' insurance coverage maintained or enhanced since parity act, but effect of coverage on enrollees varied.* Retrieved from http://www.gao.gov/assets/590/586551.html.

Garfield, R. L., Lave, J. R., & Donahue, J. M. (2010). Health reform and the scope of benefits for mental health and substance use disorder services. *Psychiatric Services, 61,* 1081–1086.

Goplerud, E. (2013). *Consistency of large employer and group health plan benefits with requirements of the Paul Wellstone and Pete Domenici Mental Health Parity and Addiction Equity Act of 2008.* Chicago: NORC and U.S. Department of Health and Human Services.

Kessler, R. C., Berglund, P., Demler, O., Jin, R., Merikangas, K. R., & Walters, E. E. (2005). Lifetime prevalence and age-of-onset distributions of *DSM-IV* disorders in the National Comorbidity Survey Replication. *Archives of General Psychiatry, 62,* 593–602.

Kessler, R. C., Chiu, W. T., Demler, O., & Walters, E. E. (2005). Prevalence, severity, and comorbidity of twelve-month *DSM-IV* disorders in the National Comorbidity Survey Replication (NCS-R). *Archives of General Psychiatry, 62*(6), 617–627.

Substance Abuse and Mental Health Services Administration. (2013). *Behavioral health, United States, 2012.* HHS Publication No. (SMA) 13–4797. Rockville, MD: Substance Abuse and Mental Health Services Administration.

Terhune, C. (2013, September 14). Insurers limiting doctors, hospitals in health insurance market. *Los Angeles Times.* Retrieved from http://articles.latimes.com/2013/sep/14/business/la-fi-insure-doctor-networks-20130915.

APPENDIX

Acronyms

ABD	Adverse Benefit Determination
ACA	Affordable Care Act
DOL	United States Department of Labor
ERISA	Employee Retirement Income Security Act of 1974
FEHBP	Federal Employees Health Benefits Program
HHS	United States Department of Health and Human Services
HIPAA	Health Insurance Portability and Accountability Act of 1996
IFR	Interim Final Regulation
IRO	Independent Review Organization
MH/SA (SUD)	Mental Health/Substance Abuse
MBHO	Managed Behavioral Healthcare Organization
MHPAEA	Paul Wellstone and Pete Domenici Mental Health Parity and Addiction Equity Act of 2008
NQTL	Non-Quantitative Treatment Limitation
PHSA	Public Health Service Act
UCR	Usual, Customary, and Reasonable

This chapter has been cited by:

1 Norman A. Clemens, Eric M. Plakun, Susan G. Lazar, Lisa Mellman. 2014. Obstacles to Early Career Psychiatrists Practicing Psychotherapy. *Psychodynamic Psychiatry* 42:3, 479–495.

2 Susan G. Lazar. 2014. The Cost-Effectiveness of Psychotherapy for the Major Psychiatric Diagnoses. *Psychodynamic Psychiatry* 42:3, 423–457.

3 Susan G. Lazar. 2014. The Mental Health Needs of Military Service Members and Veterans. *Psychodynamic Psychiatry* 42:3, 459–478.

4 Richard C. Friedman. 2014. Introduction to the Special Issue on Psychotherapy, the Affordable Care Act, and Mental Health Parity: Obstacles to Implementation. *Psychodynamic Psychiatry* 42:3, 339–342.

The exclusion of psychoanalysis in academic and organized U.S. psychology

On voodooism, witch-hunts, and the legion of followers

Oksana Yakushko

Introduction

Most psychoanalytic scholars and historians agree that psychoanalysis and related approaches have held a precarious place in American psychology since the introduction of Freud's ideas to this country (Aron & Starr, 2013; Cordón, 2012; Danto, 2005; Hale, 1995; Scharff, 2001). Yet despite continued attacks on psychoanalysis (and specifically Freud) by some historians and scholars (Cordón, 2012), the broader American culture and non-psychology disciplines have shown marked interest in its ideas and methods (Cordón, 2012; Scharff, 2001; Zaretsky, 2004). Psychoanalysis also continues to be recognized as among the first and most influential forces in psychology (Cordón, 2012; Zaretsky, 2005) and has been recognized as a dynamic and vibrant theoretical school, which has shaped multiple disciplines (Aron & Starr, 2013; Hale, 1995).

In spite of these contributions, marginalization and exclusion of psychoanalysis within organized academic U.S. psychology has been pervasive, as is apparent to most American-based psychoanalytic clinicians and scholars within the discipline of psychology. This rejection of psychoanalysis has been described as spiteful because of its focus on the devaluation of psychoanalysis and psychoanalysts, even earning its own distinctive term, "Freud-bashing" (Cordón, 2012). This professional ostracism has led to noticeable consequences, including a lack of psychoanalytic ideas in psychology academic training, practice guidelines, grants, and scholarship, despite the evidence of their significant value. In this contribution, I seek to examine this exclusion, like other forms of social sidelining, within the historical context of values embraced by American psychology since its inception. In concert with Freud's (1916/1977) own assertion: "I wish to stimulate thought and to upset prejudices" (p. 302), this contribution seeks to scrutinize prejudicial attitudes toward psychoanalysis in organized academic and professional psychology in the U.S., as well as to assess the impact of this exclusion on the discipline of psychology as a whole. Because this contribution is directed at a psychoanalytic community itself, I also wish to contribute toward greater contextual understanding of this exclusion so as to develop strategies that may aid in fighting this marginalization.

DOI: 10.4324/9781003325512-7

The history of responses to psychoanalysis in the U.S.

The century-long history of attitudes toward psychoanalysis and related approaches in the U.S., specifically within academia and organized psychology (i.e., the American Psychological Association), offers insights into some of the reasons for the long-standing marginalization and vilification of psychodynamic perspectives. William James, viewed as one of the founders of American psychology as a discipline, may have been the first to introduce Freud's work to U.S. scholars and the public by highlighting the possible importance of its key constructs, such as the unconscious (Cordón, 2012). James (1920), who attended the lectures by Freud and his colleagues at Clark University, noted in his letters that "They [psychoanalytic scholars] can't fail to throw light on human nature" (p. 213). However, he was dismayed at Freud's criticism of religion: "Freud had condemned the American religious therapy (which has such extensive results) as very 'dangerous' because so 'unscientific.' Bah!" (p. 213).

G. Stanley Hall, who had invited Freud and his colleagues to Clark in 1909, also appeared to be interested in the examination of unconscious aspects of human behavior (Cordón, 2012; Hall, 1923). In his *Life and Confessions as a Psychologist*, Hall (1923) states that, in his view, explorations of unconscious "mechanisms" may have "immense fruitfulness" and are "likely to prove significant in the world of psychology" (p. 411). However, Hall decried that the psychoanalytic focus on "sex," in addition to this approach's "rapid growth," made it a "cult" (p. 412). By the 1920s, Hall's books, such as *Jesus, the Christ, In the Light of Psychology* (1917), express a clear rejection of psychoanalytic therapy. He states that the "Freudian theory of therapy… is mistaken" (p. 12). Individuals, rather than being "cured by their very modesty" as offered by religious counseling, would have their "morality" destroyed by psychoanalysis (p. 13).

John B. Watson, also a founding pillar of American psychology, likewise used his academic, professional, and public position as a scientist to disparage Freud and psychoanalysis. In his commitment to an exclusively animal-based, experimental vision of psychology, Watson's (1914) Behaviorist Manifesto was an open call toward the goal of rooting out psychoanalytic interests in "introspection" and "consciousness" from American psychological sciences. According to Watson (1914), American psychology must become a "purely objective experimental branch of natural science," holding firmly to "its goal of prediction and control of behavior" (p. 1). This form of psychology, Watson stated, "recognizes no dividing line between man [human] and brute [animal]" and hence, "introspection forms no essential part of its methods" (p. 1).

Watson (1919, 1928), however, acceded to several of Freud's points, including the idea that early childhood is an influential developmental time, although, unlike Freud, Watson insisted that childhood was a time to "socially engineer" happy and efficient people to resist feeble-minded behaviors (e.g., lack of emotional and behavioral self-control) through laboratory experiments.

Unsurprisingly, Watson's public and private correspondence showed open disregard for psychoanalysis (Bakan, 1998; Buckley, 1989; Rilling, 2000), branding it as "voodooism" (Watson, 1924, p. 18). Watson and Rayner (1920) energetically mocked psychoanalysis; someday in the future, they snidely cautioned, [little] "Albert's fear" would result in an analysis of the little boy attempting "to play with the pubic hair of the mother" (p. 317) rather than an appreciation of his laboratory-conditioned fears. Watson and Rayner (1920) also openly discussed their experimentations on erogenous, including genital, areas of orphans and children in their scientific investigations, claiming that infants' craving for certain types of human touch resulted in their vulnerability to feeble-minded dependency and adult incapacity to control sexual urges. Like Hall (1923), Watson (1912) called psychoanalysis a "cult" (p. 916), and in his book, *Behaviorism*, Watson (1930) offered a "prediction" that "in twenty years an analyst using Freudian concepts and Freudian terminology will be placed in the same category as phrenologist" (p. 243).

Interestingly, like James and Hall, Watson (1930) routinely acknowledged that psychoanalytic scholars produced plenty of scientific work; the objected only that this work was mistaken:

> Indeed the awe-inspiring number of volumes and papers and journals produced by Freudians and post-Freudians in the last 20 years would fill a good-sized room. And yet the behaviorist, as he reads through this great mass of literature, cannot but feel in it a lack of any central scientific viewpoint. Not until his own genetic studies, started less than 10 years ago, began to bear fruit, did it become apparent to the behaviorist that he could simplify the problems of emotion and apply objective experimental methods to their solution. (p. 108)

Continuing on in this seminal volume, *Behaviorism*, Watson (1930) declared that psychoanalytic theories and scientific concepts in fact are not only useful, but are responsible for *major problems* in the field of psychology:

> Much of the confusion we have today dates back to Freud. His adherents cannot see this. Most of them through having to undergo analysis at his hands (either first, second, or third hand) have formed a strong positive 'father' organization. They have been unwilling to have their 'father' spoken of in criticism. This unwillingness to accept criticism and to find progress through it has brought the crumbling at the top of what started out to be the most significant movement in modern times. I venture to predict that 20 years from now an analyst using Freudian concepts and Freudian terminology will be placed upon the same plane as a phrenologist. And yet analysis based upon behavioristic principles is here to stay and is a necessary profession in society to be placed upon a par with internal medicine and surgery. By analysis I mean studying the cross section of

> personality in some such way as I have outlined it. This will be the equivalent of diagnosis. Combined with this will go unconditioning and then conditioning. These will constitute the curative side. Analysis as such has no virtue, no curative value. New habits, verbal, manual and visceral, of such and such kinds, will be the prescriptions the psychopathologist will write. (p. 243)

B. F. Skinner added to the rising chorus of attacks on Freud and psychoanalysis. Skinner, like James, Hall, and Watson, tended to acknowledge some value in Freud's concepts as a spring board for supposedly more "scholarly" ideas and experiments (Overskeid, 2007; Skinner, 1956). Nonetheless, Skinner similarly predicted that psychoanalysis, as a non-experimental discipline, would decline and die. In his essay on the future of psychology, Skinner (1961) stated, "It is possible that theories of behavior derived from the clinic or from field studies, rather than from the laboratory, are on the wane. A strict Freudian psychology, for example, is no longer stoutly defended" (p. 242).

During the subsequent history of American psychology, reactions to psychoanalysis continued to be negative and vitriolic. Albert Ellis proclaimed that Freud "was full of horseshit" (Neukrug, 2015, p. 120), and described his training and experiences with psychoanalysis as leaving him disillusioned and discontented. Psychoanalysis, according to Ellis's best-selling *Guide to Rational Living* (Ellis & Harper, 1961), is confused and confusing, wasteful of psychotherapy's time and focus. According to "modern authorities," Ellis claims, "intensive psychotherapy" such as psychoanalytic psychotherapy erroneously emphasizes the need for "therapeutic conditions" in order for "personality change to occur" in treatment (Ellis & Harper, 1961, p. 5). Ellis (1965) proclaimed that while "Freudian psychoanalytic methods are next to useless and are often harmful in treatment of homosexuals," his own rational emotive behavioral method, a form of conversion therapy, offers superior results in "curing" same-sex behaviors and their "causes" (p. 265).

A. T. Beck, trained as a psychiatrist, similarly claimed to have been initially committed to psychoanalytic clinical care until he saw the futility and ineffectiveness of such an approach (Beck, 1970, 1976; Hollon, 2010). Seligman (2002), a colleague and ardent admirer of Beck's work, summarized Beck's transition from psychoanalysis to cognitivism in terms of "his disenchantment with the premise of emotional hydraulics [proposed by psychoanalysis]" (p. 69). Seligman noted that Beck "had completed his Freudian training... and found that there was no problem getting depressed people to re-air past wrongs and to dwell on them at length," which apparently "occasionally" could be problematic, even leading "to suicide attempts, some fatal" (p. 69).

In an escalated attack on psychoanalysis, Wolpe (1981), a contemporary behaviorist, proclaimed in an article in the *American Psychologist*, a flagship APA journal, not only that psychoanalysis has been scientifically proven to be ineffective but also that psychoanalysis is "an immoral practice and a social blot on the psychological profession" (p. 163). "We are all tainted," Wolpe (1981, p. 163) declared, demanding that psychoanalytic treatments be banned and behaviorism be instituted as the only state-of-the-art approach in therapy rooms and therapy training programs.

Such critiques and dismissals of Freud and psychoanalysis have not waned. Many recent assaults have taken inspiration from the writings of Seligman (2002, 2006, 2011), the founder of positive psychology. Seligman's writings invariably involve attacks of Freud and "his legion of followers" (Seligman, 2002, p. 66). According to Seligman (2002), "Freud's philosophy, as bizarre as it sounds when laid out so starkly [the idea that past individual and social conflicts influence people's lives], finds its way into daily psychological and psychiatric practice, wherein patient scour their past for the negative impulses and events that have formed their identities" (p. xii). Seligman (2006) decries the continuation of psychoanalytic approaches to clinical care:

> For all its hold over the American (particularly in Manhattan) imagination, I have to say that this view [psychoanalytic treatment] is preposterous… Although many thousands of patients have had hundreds of thousands of sessions, psychoanalytic therapy has not been demonstrated to work for depression. (p. 11)

Seligman (2006) offers the following summary of a psychoanalytic formulation: "You want to have sex with your mother. You want to kill your father. Your harbor fantasies that your newborn baby might die – because you want him to die. You want to spend your days in endless misery. Your most loathsome, inner secrets are what is most basic to you" (p. 11). These statements not only reflect a concerted effort to discredit psychoanalysis and its applications, but have been used systematically to mislead both lay consumers and mental health professionals themselves about psychoanalysis.

These negative and disrespectful representations of psychoanalysts and psychoanalysts are also visible in contemporary textbooks on psychology for undergraduate and graduate students. For example, Schultz and Schultz (2015), in their recent version of *A History of Modern Psychology*, introduced Freud as a person who "loved detective stories and cheese," and further described his interests in the unconscious, dreams, and intrapsychic processes as related to his problematic upbringing and personality flaws (p. 297). Another notable method of dismissing psychoanalysis within American mainstream psychology can be found in the intentional stripping of influential figures or significant approaches in psychotherapy of their psychoanalytic foundations. Direct influences of psychoanalytic theories on key psychology figures such as Erickson, Piaget, Vygotsky, Luria, and Frankl who were openly affiliated with psychoanalysis are typically omitted or minimized in psychology textbooks (Cordón, 2012).

The socio-historical origins of attitudes toward psychoanalysis in the US academy

Since Freud and his colleagues' initial lectures at Clark University in 1909, cultural fascination with psychoanalysis and related approaches became significant in the U.S. (Burnham, 2012; Hale, 1995; Samuel, L. R., 2013; Strenger, 2015; Zaretsky, 2004). American journalism, literature, movie production, advertising, parenting, philosophy, and the arts are among many cultural areas influenced by psychoanalysis (Burnham, 2012; Scharff, 2001; Zaretsky, 2004). American medical schools and the psychiatric profession were closely aligned with psychoanalysis in its early days, which made it a visible and legitimate part of the mental health fabric of the country during the past century, especially in terms of the practice of psychotherapy (Hale, 1995; Samuel, 2013). Danto (2009) highlighted the centrality of early psychoanalytic work to the development of such mental health fields and movements as social work, child guidance, and other forms of public social care in Europe and the U.S. Among the most popular psychoanalytic voices in American society were scholars who addressed broader social issues. Psychiatrists such as Karen Horney (1936, 1937) and Erich Fromm (1941, 1955) questioned the ways in which individuals' conformity, narcissism, and adherence to patriarchal capitalist and racist values contributed to violent and disconnected societies that further produced personal suffering. Sullivan (1953) introduced the theory of interpersonal psychoanalysis, specifically emphasizing how culture created and reinforced mental disorders. Sullivan was known for the establishment of gay-affirmative psychiatric wards and for openly questioning homonegative cultural practices such barring gay men from the service in the U.S. military (Blechner, 2005; Wake, 2007). Frantz Fanon (1959/2008), an African psychoanalytic psychiatrist, applied psychoanalytic theories to questioning racist colonialism and its socio-psychological impact, initiating anti-colonial movements and theories worldwide.

In contrast, one of the most significant influences on American psychology as a new discipline stemmed from its alignment with the eugenics movement, which was defined as the science of racial betterment (Davenport, 1910; Goddard, 1911, 1912, 1917; Gould, 1996; Hall, 1903, 1920; McDougall, 1921; Tucker, 1996; Yerkes, 1923). Eugenics fully embraced a social Darwinist perspective that the survival of the fittest through natural and sexual selection accurately represented both individual and collective human development, and was to be studied through experimental and supposedly neutral statistical approaches (Davenport, 1911; Norton, 1978; Pearson, 1911; Yerkes, 1920). Intelligence and its correlates with moral, social, and physical levels of functioning (i.e., Anglo-Saxon ethnicity, wealth, good health, productivity, optimism, and heterosexual monogamy) were viewed as central to the determination of racial hereditary fitness (Popenoe & Johnson, 1935). Thus, American psychologists took on the task of examining, classifying, and improving American society through mental testing and behaviorist management of supposedly negative emotions or actions, for which they received access to government and private grants, public visibility, and academic prominence (Brigham, 1923; Popenoe & Johnson, 1935; Watson, 1919; Yerkes, 1920, 1923). The majority of early influential psychologists, APA presidents, editors of journals, and heads of top psychology departments openly published eugenics-based scholarship and served as leaders of multiple eugenic organizations (*Eugenical News*, 1916–1922; Tucker, 1996). For example, when the American Eugenics Research Association was formed, Hall, Yerkes, Thorndike, and Watson were listed among many other notable psychologists as its founding and leading members (*Eugenical News*, 1916–1922). Promises of eugenically based Utopias, created through the efforts of scientific psychology, were among the most common talking points in the effort to popularize psychology as a discipline to the American public, the academy, and political leaders (Hall, 1920; McDougall, 1921; Watson, 1919; Yerkes, 1921). Research conducted by eugenicists became well-funded (e.g., Army Mental tests) and provided these scholars with access to political and cultural power (Tucker, 1996). Supposedly racially parasitic characteristics actively studied by psychologists included the lack of intelligence and morality among non-Anglo-Saxons and economically marginalized individuals, as well as other social dangers such as those associated with "feeble-mindedness" such as non-normative sexuality, non-optimistic mental states, and lack of self-control or productivity (Brigham, 1923; Goddard, 1912, 1917; Popenoe & Johnson, 1935; Tucker, 1996; Yerkes, 1920).

These concerns, viewed by American psychologists as specific targets for experimental research, testing, and action, were fundamentally different in their foundational assumptions and methods from the perspectives on human psychology articulated by psychoanalysis (Aron & Starr, 2013; Greenwood, 2015; Hale, 1995). Because psychoanalysts rejected the notions that humans and animals are essentially alike, that socio-cultural context and complex consciousness or subjectivity played no part in individual functioning, and that human psychology could be understood through experimentation on animals in research laboratories, their work was excluded from academic psychology (Cordón, 2012). Bakan (1998) in his historical review of psychology in the U.S. stated that from the establishment of American psychology as an academic field and throughout last century, "Freudian psychology found virtually no institutional support in America. It was either neglected or rejected in the academy" (p. 222).

In contrast to American psychologists' appeals to the public in regard to the power of psychology to protect them from the dangers of feeble-mindedness (Goddard, 1912; Watson, 1928; Yerkes, 1920, 1923), psychoanalysts did not offer to "engineer" human beings who were self-controlled, optimistic, and productive. In fact, academic psychologists and the public alike were warned that psychoanalysis could be *dangerous* to eugenic goals: in the opening issue of the *Journal of Applied Psychology*, Hall's (1917) editorial explicitly warned against the "revisionary conceptions of Freud… that it is… normal for man at times to plunge back and down the evolutionary ladder" (p. 12). Note the contrast Watson (1914, 1919, 1930) routinely placed on science produced by psychoanalysis (e.g., introspective, subjective, non-biological) versus behaviorist American psychology (e.g., genetic, animal-based, experimental). Indeed, it was not therapy but testing and behavioral manipulation, especially of military recruits, animals, and young children, that were well funded and well received by governmental, academic, and newly formed granting agencies in the U.S. from the early 1900s until long after the World War II (Gould, 1996; Smith, 1985; Tucker, 1996; Watson, 1919). According to Balkan (1998), even "in the decades following World War II, huge amounts of money from the government were funneled into psychological research, but almost none of it went to the support of psychoanalytic research" (p. 222).

It is also notable that Freud and psychoanalysis were openly branded as "Jewish sciences," and anti-Semitic governments, including Nazi Germany, actively persecuted psychoanalysts during the early 20th century (Aron & Starr, 2013; Frosh, 2004, 2015; Gay, 1989). Markedly, anti-Semitism was just as common in the U.S. as in Europe during the turn of the 20th century (Aron & Starr, 2013; Cordón, 2012; Dinnerstein, 1995; Gerber, 1988). Steiner (1909), a Jewish immigrant to the U.S. who converted to Christianity and became a professor of Christian Theology, offered a summary of early 20th-century American attitudes toward immigrant Jews in the U.S. in his xenophobic book, *The Immigrant Tide: Its Ebb and Flow*. He argued that Jewish people rejected the true religion of Christianity by turning toward "Mammon" (i.e., financial gain), which in turn resulted in their comfort with "sexual immorality" (p. 286) and criminality by being "too shrewd to be caught" (p. 287). Thus, Freud, who was referred to as a "godless Jew," (Gay, 1989, p. 1), like Karl Marx, was suspected of inciting social movements that treacherously undermined morality and the functioning of Western cultures, individuals, and communities (Hall, 1881, 1920; Phillips, 2014; Steiner, 1909).

The American eugenics movement frequently produced anti-Semitic scholarship and promoted anti-Semitic social and political practices, including deriding any contributions by Jewish scientists or thinkers (Cordón, 2012; Tucker, 1996). In his book *Aspects of German Culture*, G. Stanley Hall (1881) warned that although Jews contributed to the world specifically via being a stepping stone for Christianity, they were mercenary and marked by their commercialism. H. H. Goddard (1917), who ran a well-known eugenics laboratory in Vineland, NJ, further produced empirical data to show that over 80% of Jews seeking immigrant entry to the U.S. were feeble-minded and should be barred admission. The Army Mental tests, developed by top psychologists as well as APA presidents, all of them eugenicists (e.g., Yerkes, Watson, Thorndike, and Terman), were used to prove lack of intelligence among the Jews along with all other individuals from non-Anglo-Saxon ethnic groups. According to Brigham (1923), a Princeton psychologist and collaborator on the Army tests, their study produced "figures" which "tend to disprove the popular belief that the Jew is highly intelligent" (p. 190), advocating for the immigration ban to include Jewish immigrants. These racist assumptions about Jewish culture and Jewish individuals were frequently directed at Freud, psychoanalysis, and psychoanalysts, many of whom were European Jews (Aron & Starr, 2013; Cordón, 2012; Frosh, 2004, 2015; Gay, 1989). The echoes of anti-Semitism, including stereotypes that all of psychoanalysis focuses exclusively on sex and violence, or that psychoanalysts are avaricious, remain visible in its contemporary critique within American psychology (Shedler, 2010).

Moreover, many of the immigrant European analysts entering the U.S. were not only Jewish but also espoused socialist and communist leanings (Altman, 1995; Aron & Starr, 2013; Danto, 2005) and thus were often excluded from top academic posts through processes which historians have termed intellectual witch-hunts (Schrecker, 1986). In contrast to European psychoanalytic writings that integrated socialist values and psychoanalytic practice (Danto, 2005), the American context of anti-communist and anti-Marxist academia, communism, and Marxism often also considered "Jewish," marginalized many psychoanalysts and did not permit the development of a socially progressive psychoanalysis (Aron & Starr, 2013). Erik Erickson (1995), for one, a staunchly Freudian psychoanalyst and a socialist, refused to sign a McCarthy era "loyalty oath," resulting in his removal from a position at the University of California-Berkeley. Indeed, critiques of Freud and psychoanalysis routinely appear connected to criticisms of Karl Marx and other theorists, including in the writings of Hall (1881), Watson (1919), Skinner (1953), and Seligman (2002).

The history of psychoanalysis in the American Psychological Association

The theoretical hegemony in training and practice guidelines noted above undoubtedly reflects the role of organizational dynamics in determining the course of professional psychology, and specifically the role of the American Psychological Association in the exclusion of psychoanalysis. As noted earlier, many APA leaders held openly anti-psychoanalytic commitments while placing their professional credibility in the service of the eugenics movement (Guthrie, 2004; Tucker, 1996). Their emphasis on exclusively laboratory-based animal behavioral or testing-focused models of human experience came in opposition to views, such as that of psychoanalysis, which typically relied on case-focused, subjective, and socio-historical contextual models (Aron & Starr, 2013; Cushman, 1996). In the U.S., the practice of psychotherapy was mostly associated with psychiatry (often synonymous with psychoanalysis), although over time it came to be widely accepted among psychologists, who began to practice psychotherapy in greater numbers during the 1950s (Freedheim & Wachtel, 1992).

Efforts to create a Division of Psychoanalysis within APA were met with significant resistance, even though a substantial number of APA members throughout the organization expressed interest in and adherence to psychoanalytic perspectives (Lane & Meisels, 2013). Psychoanalysis officially received a sanctioned standing as an APA division (Division 39) only in 1979, despite the long-standing presence of psychoanalysis in the American mental health landscape and repeated requests of psychoanalytic psychologists for such representation (Lane & Meisels, 2013; Lawrence, 1994). From its inception to the present time, this division has remained among the largest within the APA in terms of membership while notably lacking in any significant organizational influence or visible respect and promotion to the public (Lane & Meisels, 2013; Lawrence, 1994).

Divisions within psychology with a focus on clinical practice continue to show psychoanalytic and psychodynamic interests, often as their primary theoretical tradition within an integrative or eclectic framework (Norcross et al., 2005). Recently available studies show that nearly 30% of the membership of the psychotherapy division (Division 29) described themselves as primarily psychodynamic/ psychoanalytic in their orientation (in addition, another 30% describe themselves as "integrative," which appears to include mainly psychodynamic theories) (Norcross et al., 2002). Even within Division 12 (Clinical Psychology), a division that is openly committed to the promotion of primarily "evidence-based" CBT treatments, almost 18% identified themselves as exclusively psychodynamic/psychoanalytic (Norcross & Karpiak, 2012). In a cross-national study with a sample of over 4,000 psychotherapists, the two largest groups, comprising over 2,700 individuals, were primarily analytic/ psychodynamic (over 1,000 psychotherapists) and broadly integrative, including an analytic-psychodynamic interest as a primary focus (over 1,700 psychotherapists). These data show that analytic-psychodynamic therapist identification is widespread both in the U.S. and worldwide (Heinonen & Orlinsky, 2013). Nevertheless, visible or supportive representation of psychoanalytic theoretical and scholarly interests appears to be minimal within the APA.

One way to examine the level of a group's prominence, influence, and professional attitudes can be deduced from the organization's most visible professional publications, which include *The American Psychologist* and *The APA Monitor* as the official journals of the American Psychological Association. Since the inception of *The American Psychologist* in 1946, less than 1% (0.07%) of all of its contributions mention psychoanalysis or related concepts (e.g., psychodynamic, psychoanalytic, Freudian). Among this limited number of contributions, approximately three-fifths are comments (brief responses to major contributions), one-fifth are obituaries or awards, and one-fifth are articles with an actual focus on psychoanalysis to some degree. However, this latter number includes articles that are negative or even hostile toward psychoanalysis. For example, Wolpe's (1981) anti-psychoanalytic screed is counted among these 0.7% of contributions.

The representation of psychoanalysis and related approaches in *The APA Monitor* is even more problematic. In its nearly 20-year-long history, less than 1% of its short or long contributions have acknowledged psychoanalysis or related approaches. The majority of these publications included announcements by APA's Division of Psychoanalysis. Removing these Division announcements resulted in 0.01% representation, most of which included only brief or indirect mentions of psychoanalysis or related concepts. Moreover, as in *The American Psychologist*, even this meager number of contributions encompassed several openly adversarial articles. For example, a full page was dedicated to an article about Freud's nephew, Bernays, who utilized psychoanalytic principles to develop manipulative consumer techniques (Held, 2009). Although the article acknowledges that Freud, in fact, was neither close to his nephew nor supported such applications of psychoanalysis, nevertheless this contribution appeared to represent both Freud and psychoanalysis negatively. Only a single article discussing psychoanalysis appeared recently in the *Monitor* (Novotney, 2017).

The exclusion of psychoanalytically identified approaches, studies, ideas, and individuals as well as misrepresentation or selective historical accounts is visible throughout the APA's organizational structure. Organizational leadership within the APA appears to have been openly skewed toward non-psychoanalytic divisions and ideas (Evans et al., 1992). APA's current public information efforts, whether lobbying or offering continuing education, emphasize to an almost exclusive extent only cognitive, behavioral, and biological orientations to psychology. In a search of announcements and messages to the public, APA-sponsored studies, lobbying on behalf of psychologists by the APA, and descriptions of its educational training focus reveal a nearly complete absence of reference to psychoanalysis or related work.

Recent notable examples of psychoanalysis' exclusion

As we have seen, various attempts to exclude psychoanalysis have been openly and subtly attempted within American academia throughout the last century and today. But perhaps most prominent today among these forms of exclusion are claims that psychoanalysis and all forms of psychoanalytic care are not empirically validated or scientifically grounded. Contemporary methods of marginalizing psychoanalysis in organized American psychology on the basis of scientific *bona fides* include restricting psychoanalysis's accreditation development, excluding its input from practice guidelines, and its non-representation in grant-based studies, among many other forms of exclusion.

As noted earlier, after the 1950s, psychology education in the U.S. moved toward embracing psychoanalytic and psychodynamic perspectives because of their fundamental contributions to practice of psychotherapy (Freedheim & Wachtel, 1992). Meanwhile, the formal inclusion of psychoanalysis in the APA and psychologists' efforts to gain designation as psychoanalysts resulted in greater participation of psychoanalytic psychologists in U.S. undergraduate and graduate training between 1950s and 1980s (Bakan, 2013; Hale, 1995). However, the inception and further development of accreditation guidelines for training in applied psychology, which once again emphasize experimental and biological views of psychology, appears to have returned academic American psychology to dominance by behaviorism-based theoretical orientations. Recent analysis of accredited programs in psychology (Levy & Anderson, 2013) shows that over the last several decades since the institutionalization of accreditation "standards," the field experienced a dramatic decline of especially psychoanalytic traditions in all accredited programs, with a parallel dramatic increase in cognitive-behavioral and behavioral orientation across the entire accreditation spectrum. This new form of exclusion of psychoanalysis is striking, and is documented in both research-based (Ph.D.) and professional schools of psychology (PsyD), (Levy & Anderson, 2013). Representation of psychoanalysis in contemporary undergraduate psychology education has once again become marginal or non-existent (Yakushko & Hook, 2017). Likewise, "here are hardly any graduate programs in clinical psychology that are psychoanalytically oriented, and there are very few professorships in psychology that are in the hands of psychoanalysts" (Strenger, 2010, p. 8).

The process of creating supposedly theoretically neutral, research-driven, and clinically helpful guidelines on the treatments of various disorders, for use by all clinicians and in all clinical care organizations (e.g., insurance companies, federal mental health systems), is distorted by a similar bias. For example, the *Clinical Practice Guidelines for the Treatment of PTSD* (APA, 2017b), which are contained in a 139-page document, do not mention or even include terms such as "psychodynamic," "psychoanalytic," or "psychoanalysis." Of the four recommended treatments in these Guidelines, three are cognitive or cognitive-behavioral and one is behavioral. Separate appendices to this document include a single approach, brief eclectic therapy, which is recommended for the treatment of PTSD "conditionally" and is described as a "manualized treatment that combines cognitive behavior therapy techniques and psychodynamic strategies including psychoeducation, relaxation, imaginal exposure, writing, learning from the trauma, meaning and integration and an ending ritual" (APA, 2017a, p. 125). The approach has not been published in psychodynamic or psychoanalytic scholarly literature and bears no relationship to standard brief psychoanalytic treatments, which value the "affect and the expression of patients' emotions," "an emphasis on past experiences," "patients' interpersonal experiences," and "the therapeutic relationship" (Blagys & Hilsenroth, 2000, p. 167). Moreover, whereas published meta-analyses of short- and long-term psychodynamic approaches include summaries of statistically and clinically significant results in its utility in treatment of PTSD (Abbass et al., 2014; Leichsenring & Klein, 2014; Levi et al., 2016), these were not included in the APA Guidelines.

The exclusion of psychoanalysis and psychodynamic treatments on the basis of their supposed lack of evidence appears to reflect not only the denial of evidence of their effectiveness but also a misrepresentation of the clinical utility of currently hailed "evidence-based" approaches (Holmes, 2002; Holmes et al., 2006; Shedler, 2015; Wachtel, 2010; Westen et al., 2004). Researchers increasingly highlight that such standards and guidelines reflect theoretical hegemony rather than actual scientific data (Leichsenring & Steinert, 2017; Shedler, 2015; Wampold & Imel, 2015) while openly ignoring evidence that psychoanalytic and related approaches have indisputably strong empirical support (Abbas et al., 2014; de Maat et al., 2009; Fonagy, 2015; Leichsenring et al., 2013, 2015; Leichsenring & Rabung, 2008; Levy et al., 2014; Shedler, 2010; Zimmermann et al., 2015). Not unexpectedly, this exclusion of psychoanalysis is also reflected in the attitudes of granting organizations and federal agencies, which are influenced by their connections to both academic and organized American psychology, such as the Veterans Administration system and the National Institute of Mental Health. In short, continued disregard for psychoanalytic and psychodynamic treatments, including their absence in the training of psychologists and in the creation of recommendations for practitioners, seems to reflect long-standing organizational and professional bias rather than actual evidence of what works with diverse clients in diverse communities presenting with complex psychological concerns.

The evidence presented in this manuscript reflects only a fraction of the systematic and institutionalized anti-psychoanalytic practices within American academic and organized professional psychology. The circular justifications for the marginalization of psychoanalysis in American psychology are noteworthy: psychoanalysis is presented de-facto as nonscientific or wrongly scientific, and this disregard for psychoanalysis in psychology within the academy is then directly related to its absence in training, scholarship, or funding, which in turn is used as a rationale for its further professional rejection. Psychoanalysis continues to be represented as malevolent and harmful, as psychology trainees, practicing psychotherapists, policy makers, and the public are systematically misinformed regarding its values, practices, and assumptions.

Alternative historical perspectives on psychoanalysis

One of the dominant claims made to both psychologists and the general public is that psychoanalysis is not relevant to the practice of psychology (Seligman, 2002, 2006, 2011; Watson, 1930; Wolpe, 1981). In contrast, as noted above, a significant number of psychologists within the APA and around the globe draw on psychoanalytic and related orientations, especially in their clinical work (Heinonen & Orlinsky, 2013; Norcross et al., 2002). Moreover, data by (Bike et al. 2009; Norcross et al. 1988) show that regardless of their own theoretical orientation, psychologists who seek their own psychotherapeutic care for personal or professional reasons (approximately 85% of all psychologists) appear drastically to prefer psychodynamic or psychoanalytic forms of treatments to all others for their own therapeutic care.

Similarly, the history of the role of psychoanalysis in the lives of noted figures in psychology who are famous for maligning it appears to have been forgotten or systematically hidden. One of the most concealed histories is that of John B. Watson's children, on whom he experimented to develop his still-standing behavioral treatments (Buckley, 1989). For example, Jimmy, Watson's youngest son, a subject of intense experimentation by John B. Watson, described in interviews that by age 30 he had made a decision to end his life based on his feelings of profound inner emptiness and unexplained somatic concerns. In his video interview with Walker (1990), James Watson shared what finally facilitated his recovery: "Six years of analysis four times a week were very helpful to me. They helped me to begin to understand the impact of what emotional depravation [due to Watson's treatments] did to my life" (n.p.). Jimmy concluded that "I never would have made it if I hadn't gone into [analysis]" (n.p.). Similarly, the granddaughter of John B. Watson, child of Watson's eldest daughter Polly, condemned behaviorism and discussed her recovery through psychoanalytic care in her autobiography entitled *Breaking the Silence* (Hartley & Commire, 1991).

Even more surprising are occasional accounts of interest or even participation in analysis by the leaders of psychology who publicly denounced and maligned it. Overskeid (2007) provided evidence of Skinner's discussions of either being open to or seeking psychoanalytic treatment following the death of his brother. Rosner (2014) used archival evidence based on A. T. Beck's correspondence to show that Beck, after being rejected several times from acceptance into psychoanalytic associations and making a move to develop his new theory of cognitivism, persisted in using psychoanalysis as a defining theoretical framework for his theory of CBT. Rosner highlighted that, "There is something scandalous to a contemporary clinical ear in suggesting that Beck needed Freud... so much rhetoric has been invested in keeping the wall between him and Freud firm" (p. 16).

Regardless the extensive history of psychoanalysis' influence on U.S. mental health and its cultural fabric, and discounting significant empirical evidence noted above of its effectiveness, psychoanalysis is often blamed for being a profession dedicated to the care of neurotic wealthy White people. Sexism, racism, homophobia, and other social problems are easily and continually attached to psychoanalysis. Undoubtedly, psychoanalysis and psychoanalytic treatments, just as the rest of psychology and, in fact, American society, are complicit in the perpetuation of social injustices (i.e., see psychoanalysts' own questioning of their practices in Jacoby, 1975; Layton et al., 2006; Tummala-Narra, 2013). However, what is being dismissed in the appraisals common in mainstream American psychology is that psychoanalysis also has been a theoretical platform from which the most powerful critiques of oppression were developed, including feminism (Horney, 1936, 1967), anti-racism and anti-colonialism (Fanon, 1959/2008; Hook, 2012; Said, 2003), critiques of social class inequalities and ideologies (Danto, 2005; Zizek, 2004), questioning of gender normativity (Butler, 1995, 2011; Chodorow, 1978), and challenges to the proliferation of neo-liberal capitalist values (Layton, 2006; Parker, 2016; Sloan, 1996). In fact, outside of mainstream psychology, psychoanalysis is thriving precisely because of its focus on deconstructing implicitly embedded structures of oppression and power (Hollander, 1997; Pick, 2016).

In contrast, continued attacks on psychoanalysis in contemporary Western psychology reflect lingering epistemological privileging of animal-based, experimental, de-contextualized, and evolutionary explanations of human behavior. This reduction of motivation to "character and heredity," which is at base profoundly anti-psychological, and to which psychoanalysis represents perhaps its most significant challenge, easily lends itself to be used by those who aim to justify their superiority along racial and religious lines. For example, Eysenck (1985), known for his eugenic commitments, who emphasized the heritability of personality traits, openly attacked psychoanalysis for its theories of the social and relational origins of personality. Eysenck was praised by Rushton (2001) for not only promoting "the biological bases of personality" (p. 32), including intelligence, aggression, and optimism, but also for supposedly replacing "psychodynamic dogma" with "an empirically tested and scientifically based psychotherapy – now called 'cognitive-behavioral therapy'"(p. 35).[1] Moreover, Freud continues to be critiqued by contemporary apologists for eugenics and social Darwinism who draw on predominately evolutionary and genetic explanations of human behavior (Pinker, 1997). Whitney, a behavioral geneticist and American psychologist who wrote the Forward to one of the most infamous contemporary White supremacy books – David Duke's (1999) *My Awakening* – singled out "Freudian psychoanalytic theory" as a key "dogmatic belief system" (p. 2). Duke (1999), who referred to multiple scientific studies produced by psychologists to justify his racist positions, specifically decried the "Freudian assault," which in his view necessitated psychology's struggle with "the Jewish onslaught" and the supposed psychoanalytic "attack on our [American Christian] cultural values" (pp. 4–6). Meanwhile, positive psychologists who rely on evolutionary, experimental, and animal explanatory models not only critique psychoanalysis and Freud while minimizing the role of history or social context but also insist that only "character and heredity" account for "what people do" (Seligman, 2011, p. 104).

In contrast to these Western psychological and cultural anti-psychoanalytic perspectives, significant number of clinicians and scholars in Central and South America, the Middle East, Africa, and Asia embrace psychoanalysis (Hollander, 1997; Hook, 2012; Pick, 2016; Said, 2003; Smith, 2014). South and Central America remain among the global nuclei for psychoanalytic perspectives, viewing them as central to both the practice and science of psychology as well as to social and political cultural critique (Hollander, 1997). In China, where official emphasis upon control of subjective individual emotional life (common to behavioral and CBT treatments) remains, the growth of interest in psychoanalysis has been "surging" as a method not only for addressing "personal suffering" but also "as a way to understand and metabolize historical traumas" (Gerlach et al., 2013, p. xiii). As noted earlier, the analytic-psychodynamic theoretical orientation remains consistently the most endorsed approach for psychotherapists worldwide (Heinonen & Orlinsky, 2013).

Conclusions

I believe it is vital to recognize that psychoanalysis has been perceived as a threat to American academic psychology since its inception because of its radical challenge to American psychology's open adherence to social Darwinism, eugenics, industrial capitalism, and Protestant religious morality. Anti-Semitism and racism, which was central to social Darwinism, eugenics, and American Christian religiosity, also served as an explicit and implicit rationale for vehemently rejecting psychoanalytic theories by American psychology academics. The continued reduction of psychoanalysis to an exclusive focus on supposedly perverse forms of sexual desire and aggression reflects neither the entirety of original Freudian theory nor contemporary psychoanalytic traditions (Aron & Starr, 2013; Hale, 1995; Phillips, 2014). Despite long-standing and voluminous scholarship by psychoanalysts since Freud, psychoanalytic empirical evidence and clinical utility are dismissed, minimized, or openly disparaged. These prolonged biases point to long-standing worldviews embedded within American psychology itself in relation to human experience, i.e., the minimization of social context, the denial of social oppression, and the reluctance to discuss the dynamics of human sexuality beyond the hetero-normative and procreative. In Freud's (1920) words, "Society thus brands what is unpleasant as untrue, denying the conclusions of psychoanalysis with logical and pertinent arguments. These arguments originate from affective sources, however, and society holds to these prejudices against all attempts at refutation" (p. 43).

Note

1 Southern Poverty Law Center (2012) identified Rushton as "probably the most important race scientist at work today" whose scholarship supports White extremism.

References

Abbass, A. A., Kisely, S. R., Town, J. M., Leichsenring, F., Driessen, E., De Maat, S.,... Crowe, E. (2014). Short-term psychodynamic psychotherapies for common mental disorders. *Cochrane Database of Systematic Reviews*, (7). https://doi.org/10.1002/14651858.CD004687.pub4

Altman, N. (1995). *The analyst in the inner city: Race, class, and culture through a psychoanalytic lens*. The Analytic Press.

APA. (2017a). *Appendices: Clinical practice guidelines for PTSD*. American Psychological Association. Retrieved November 2, 2017, from http://www.apa.org/ptsd-guideline/appendices.pdf

APA. (2017b). *Clinical practice guidelines for the treatment of PTSD*. American Psychological Association. Retrieved November 2, 2017, from http://www.apa.org/ptsd-guideline/ptsd.pdf

Aron, L., & Starr, K. (2013). *A psychotherapy for the people: Toward a progressive psychoanalysis*. Routledge.

Bakan, D. (1998). American culture and psychology. In Rieber, R. W., & Salzinger, K. (Eds.). *Psychology: Theoretical– historical perspectives* (pp. 217–225.) Academic Press.
Bakan, D. (2013). Politics and American psychology. In Rieber, R. W. & Salzinger, K. (Eds.), *Psychology: Theoretical– historical perspectives* (pp. 125–144). Academic Press.
Beck, A. T. (1970). Cognitive therapy: Nature and relation to behavior therapy. *Behavior Therapy*, *1*(2), 184–200. https://doi.org/10.1016/s0005-7894(70)80030-2
Beck, A. T. (1976). *Cognitive therapy and the emotional disorders*. International Universities Press.
Bike, D. H., Norcross, J. C., & Schatz, D. M. (2009). Processes and outcomes of psychotherapists' personal therapy: Replication and extension 20 years later. *Psychotherapy: Theory, Research, Practice, Training*, *46*(1), 19.
Blagys, M. D., & Hilsenroth, M. J. (2000). Distinctive features of short-term psychodynamic-interpersonal psychotherapy: A review of the comparative psychotherapy process literature. *Clinical Psychology: Science and Practice*, *7*(2), 167–188. https://doi.org/10.1093/clipsy.7.2.167
Blechner, M. J. (2005). The gay Harry Stack Sullivan: Interactions between his life, clinical work, and theory. *Contemporary Psychoanalysis*, *41*(1), 1–19. https://doi.org/10.1080/00107530.2005.10745845
Brigham, C. C. (1923). *A study of American intelligence*. Oxford University Press.
Buckley, K. W. (1989). *Mechanical man: John Broadus Watson and the beginnings of behaviorism*. Guilford Press.
Burnham, J. (Ed.). (2012). *After Freud left: A century of psychoanalysis in America*. University of Chicago Press.
Butler, J. (1995). Melancholy gender-refused identification. *Psychoanalytic Dialogues*, *5*(2), 165–180. https://doi.org/10.1080/10481889509539059
Butler, J. (2011). *Gender trouble: Feminism and the subversion of identity*. Routledge.
Chodorow, N. (1978). *The reproduction of mothering*. University of California.
Cordón, L. A. (2012). *Freud's world: An encyclopedia of his life and times*. Greenwood.
Cushman, P. (1996). *Constructing the self, constructing America: A cultural history of psychotherapy*. Addison-Wesley/Addison Wesley Longman.
Danto, E. A. (2005). *Freud's free clinics: Psychoanalysis & social justice, 1918–1938*. Columbia University Press.
Danto, E. A. (2009). "A new sort of 'Salvation Army'": Historical perspectives on the confluence of psychoanalysis and social work. *Clinical Social Work Journal*, *37*(1), 67–76.
Davenport, C. B. (1910). *Eugenics. The science of human improvement by better breeding*. Henry Holt.
Davenport, C. B. (1911). *Heredity in relation to eugenics*. H. Holt.
de Maat, S., De Jonghe, F., Schoevers, R., & Dekker, J. (2009). The effectiveness of long-term psychoanalytic therapy: A systematic review of empirical studies. *Harvard Review of Psychiatry*, *17*(1), 1–23. https://doi.org/10.1080/ 10673220902742476
Dinnerstein, L. (1995). *Anti-semitism in America*. Oxford University Press.
Duke, D. E. (1999). *My awakening: A path to racial understanding*. Free Speech Press.
Ellis, A. (1965). *Homosexuality: Its causes and cure*. L. Stuart.
Ellis, A., & Harper, R. A. (1961). *A guide to rational living*. Prentice Hall.
Erickson, E. H. (1995). *Statement to the committee on privilege and tenure of the University of California concerning the California loyalty oath*. E.H. Erikson, A way of looking at things: Selected papers from, 618–620.

Eugenical News. (1916–1922). *Monthly publication of the Eugenics record office*. Retrieved February 22, 2018, from https://babel.hathitrust.org/cgi/pt?id=coo.31924063788834

Evans, R. B., Sexton, V. S. E., & Cadwallader, T. C. (1992). *The American Psychological Association: A historical perspective*. APA.

Eysenck, H. J. (1985). *Decline and fall of the Freudian empire*. Viking.

Fanon, F. (1959/2008). *Black skin, white masks*. Grove Press.

Fonagy, P. (2015). The effectiveness of psychodynamic psychotherapies: An update. *World Psychiatry*, *14*(2), 137–150. https:// doi.org/10.1002/wps.20235

Freedheim, D. K., & Wachtel, P. L. (1992). *History of psychotherapy: A century of change*. American Psychological Association.

Freud, S. (1916/1977). *Introductory lectures on psychoanalysis*. W.W. Norton.

Freud, S. (1920). *A general introduction to psychoanalysis*. Horace Liveright.

Fromm, E. (1941). *Escape from freedom*. Farrar & Rinehart.

Fromm, E. (1955). *The sane society*. Rinehart & Co.

Frosh, S. (2004). Freud, psychoanalysis and anti-semitism. *The Psychoanalytic Review*, *91*(3), 309–330. https://doi.org/ 10.1521/prev.91.3.309.38302

Frosh, S. (2015). *Hate and the 'Jewish science': Anti-Semitism, Nazism and psychoanalysis*. Springer.

Gay, P. (1989). *A godless Jew: Freud, atheism, and the making of psychoanalysis*. Yale University Press.

Gerber, D. A. (1988). Anti-semitism in American history. *Science and Society*, *52*(3), 365–367. https://philpapers.org/ rec/GERAIA-2

Gerlach, A., Hooke, M. T., & Varvin, S. (Eds.). (2013). *Psychoanalysis in Asia: China, India, Japan, South Korea, Taiwan*. Karnac Books.

Goddard, H. H. (1911). The elimination of feeble-mindedness. *The Annals of the American Academy of Political and Social Science*, *37*(2), 261–272. https://doi.org/10.1177/000271621103700222

Goddard, H. H. (1912). *The Kallikak family: A study in the heredity of feeble-mindedness*. Macmillan.

Goddard, H. H. (1917). Mental tests and the immigrant. *Journal of Deliquincy*, *2*(2), 243–277. https://www.gwern.net/ docs/iq/1917-goddard.pdf

Gould, S. J. (1996). *The mismeasure of man*. WW. Norton.

Greenwood, J. D. (2015). *A conceptual history of psychology: Exploring the tangled web*. Cambridge University Press.

Guthrie, R. V. (2004). *Even the rat was white: A historical view of psychology*. Pearson Education.

Hale, N. G. (1995). *The rise and crisis of psychoanalysis in the United States: Freud and the Americans, 1917–1985*. Oxford University Press.

Hall, G. S. (1881). *Aspects of German culture*. J.R. Osgood.

Hall, G. S. (1903). The white man's burden versus indigenous development of the lower races. *The Journal of Education*, *58*(4), 83. https://doi.org/10.1177/002205740305800415

Hall, G. S. (1917). *Jesus, the Christ, in the light of psychology*. Doubleday, Page & Company.

Hall, G. S. (1920). *Recreations of a psychologist*. D. Appleton.

Hall, G. S. (1923). *Life and confessions of a psychologist*. D. Appleton.

Hartley, M., & Commire, A. (1991). *Breaking the silence*. Signet Book.

Heinonen, E., & Orlinsky, D. E. (2013). Psychotherapists' personal identities, theoretical orientations, and professional relationships: Elective affinity and role adjustment as modes of congruence. *Psychotherapy Research*, *23*(6), 718–731. https://doi.org/10.1080/10503307.2013.814926

Held, L. (2009). Psychoanalysis shapes consumer culture: Or how Sigmund Freud, his nephew and a box of cigars forever changed American marketing. *The APA Monitor*, *40*(11), 32. https://www.apa.org/monitor/2009/12/consumer

Hollander, N. C. (1997). *Love in a time of hate: Liberation psychology in Latin America*. Rutgers University Press.

Hollon, S. D. (2010). Aaron T. Beck: The cognitive revolution in theory and therapy. In Castonguay, L., Muran, J. C., Angus, L., Hayes, J. A., Ladany, N., & Anderson, T. (Eds.), *Bringing psychotherapy research to life* (pp. 63–74). APA.

Holmes, D., Murray, S. J., Perron, A., & Rail, G. (2006). Deconstructing the evidence-based discourse in health sciences: Truth, power and fascism. *International Journal of Evidence-Based Healthcare*, *4*(3), 180–186. https://doi.org/10.1097/01258363-200609000-00003

Holmes, J. (2002). All you need is cognitive behaviour therapy? *British Medical Journal*, *324*(7332), 288–294. https://doi.org/ 10.1136/bmj.324.7352.1522

Hook, D. (2012). *A critical psychology of the postcolonial: The mind of apartheid*. Routledge.

Horney, K. (1936). Culture and neurosis. *American Sociological Review*, *1*(2), 221–230. https://doi.org/10.2307/2084481

Horney, K. (1937). *The neurotic personality of our time*. W.W. Norton & Company.

Horney, K. (1967). *Feminine psychology*. Springer.

Jacoby, R. (1975). *Social amnesia: A critique of conformist psychology from Adler to Laing*. Beacon Press.

James, W. (1920). *The letters of William James* (Vol. 1). Little, Brown.

Lane, R. C., & Meisels, M. (Eds.). (2013). *A history of the division of psychoanalysis of the American Psychological Association*. Routledge.

Lawrence, E. S. (1994). Section I: Psychologist-Psychoanalyst Practitioners: A history, 1982–1992. A history of the Division of Psychoanalysis of the American Psychological Association, 167–175.

Layton, L. (2006). Racial identities, racial enactments, and normative unconscious processes. *Psychoanalytic Quarterly*, *75*(1), 237–269. https://doi.org/10.1002/j.2167-4086.2006.tb00039.x

Layton, L., Hollander, N. C., & Gutwill, S. (Eds.). (2006). *Psychoanalysis, class and politics: Encounters in the clinical setting*. Routledge.

Leichsenring, F., Abbass, A., Luyten, P., Hilsenroth, M., & Rabung, S. (2013). The emerging evidence for long-term psychodynamic therapy. *Psychodynamic Psychiatry*, *41*(3), 361–384. https://doi.org/10.1521/pdps.2013.41.3.361

Leichsenring, F., & Klein, S. (2014). Evidence for psychodynamic psychotherapy in specific mental disorders: A systematic review. *Psychoanalytic Psychotherapy*, *28*(1), 4–32. https://doi.org/10.1080/02668734.2013.865428

Leichsenring, F., Luyten, P., Hilsenroth, M. J., Abbass, A., Barber, J. P., Keefe, J. R.,... Steinert, C. (2015). Psychodynamic therapy meets evidence-based medicine: A systematic review using updated criteria. *The Lancet Psychiatry*, *2*(7), 648–660. https://doi.org/10.1016/s2215-

Leichsenring, F., & Rabung, S. (2008). Effectiveness of long-term psychodynamic psychotherapy: A meta-analysis. *Journal of American Medical Association*, *300*(13), 1551–1565. https://doi.org/10.1001/jama.300.13.1551

Leichsenring, F., & Steinert, C. (2017). Is cognitive behavioral therapy the gold standard for psychotherapy?: The need for plurality in treatment and research. *Journal of the American Medical Association*, *318*(14), 1323–1324. https://doi.org/10.1001/jama.2017.13737

Levi, O., Bar-Haim, Y., Kreiss, Y., & Fruchter, E. (2016). Cognitive–behavioural therapy and psychodynamic psychotherapy in the treatment of combat-related post-traumatic stress disorder: A comparative effectiveness study. *Clinical Psychology & Psychotherapy*, *23*(4), 298–307. https://doi.org/10.1002/cpp.1969

Levy, K. N., & Anderson, T. (2013). Is clinical psychology doctoral training becoming less intellectually diverse? And if so, what can be done? *Clinical Psychology: Science and Practice*, *20*(2), 211–220. https://doi.org/10.1111/cpsp.12035

Levy, K. N., Ehrenthal, J. C., Yeomans, F. E., & Caligor, E. (2014). The efficacy of psychotherapy: Focus on psychodynamic psychotherapy as an example. *Psychodynamic Psychiatry*, *42*(3), 377–421. https://doi.org/10.1521/pdps.2014.42.3.377

McDougall, W. (1921). *National welfare and national decay*. Methuen & Co. ltd.

Neukrug, E. (2015). *The world of the counselor: An introduction to the counseling profession*. Brooks/Cole Publishing Company.

Norcross, J. C., Hedges, M., & Castle, P. H. (2002). Psychologists conducting psychotherapy in 2001: A study of the Division 29 membership. *Psychotherapy: Theory, Research, Practice, Training*, *39*(1), 97–102. https://doi.org/10. 1037//0033–3204.39.1.97

Norcross, J. C., & Karpiak, C. P. (2012). Clinical psychologists in the 2010s: 50 years of the APA division of clinical psychology. *Clinical Psychology: Science and Practice*, *19*(1), 1–12. https://doi.org/10.1111/j.1468-2850.2012.01269.x

Norcross, J. C., Karpiak, C. P., & Lister, K. M. (2005). What's an integrationist? A study of self-identified integrative and (occasionally) eclectic psychologists. *Journal of Clinical Psychology*, *61*(12), 1587–1594. https://doi.org/10.1002/jclp.20203

Norcross, J. C., Strausser, D. J., & Faltus, F. J. (1988). The therapist's therapist. *American Journal of Psychotherapy*, *46*(1), 32–41. https://doi.org/10.1037/a0015140

Norton, B. J. (1978). Karl Pearson and statistics: The social origins of scientific innovation. *Social Studies of Science*, *8*(1), 3–34. https://doi.org/10.1177/030631277800800101

Novotney, A. (2017). Not your father's psychoanalysis. *The Monitor in Psychology*, *48*(11), 40–44. https://acapnj.org/ not-great-grandfathers-psychoanalysis/

Overskeid, G. (2007). Looking for Skinner and finding Freud. *American Psychologist*, *62*(6), 590–595. https://doi.org/ 10.1037/0003–066x.62.6.590

Parker, I. (2016). *Critical discursive psychology*. Springer.

Pearson, K. (1911). *The scope and importance to the state of the science of national eugenics*. Dulau and Company.

Phillips, A. (2014). *Becoming Freud: The making of a psychoanalyst*. Yale University Press.

Pick, D. (Ed.). (2016). *Psychoanalysis in the age of totalitarianism*. Routledge.

Pinker, S. (1997). *How the mind works*. Norton.

Popenoe, P., & Johnson, R. H. (1935). *Applied eugenics*. The MacMillan Company.

Rilling, M. (2000). John Watson's paradoxical struggle to explain Freud. *American Psychologist*, *55*(3), 301–312. https:// doi.org/10.1037/0003–066X.55.3.301

Rosner, R. I. (2014). The "splendid isolation" of Aaron T. Beck. *Isis*, *105*(4), 734–758. https://doi.org/10.1086/679421

Rushton, J. P. (2001). A scientometric appreciation of H.J. Eysenck's contributions to psychology. *Personality and Individual Differences*, *31*(1), 17–39. https://doi.org/10.1016/S0191-8869(00)00235-X

Said, E. W. (2003). *Freud and the non-European*. Verso.
Samuel, L. R. (2013). *Shrink: A cultural history of psychoanalysis in America*. University of Nebraska Press.
Scharff, D. E. (2001). *The psychoanalytic century: Freud's legacy for the future*. Other.
Schrecker, E. W. (1986). *No Ivory tower: McCarthyism and the universities*. Oxford University Press.
Schultz, D. P., & Schultz, S. E. (2015). *A history of modern psychology*. Cengage.
Seligman, M. E. (2002). *Learned optimism: How to change your mind and your life*. Vintage.
Seligman, M. E. (2006). *Authentic happiness: Using the new positive psychology to realize your potential for lasting fulfillment*. Simon and Schuster.
Seligman, M. E. (2011). *Flourish: A visionary new understanding of happiness and well-being*. Simon and Schuster.
Shedler, J. (2010). The efficacy of psychodynamic psychotherapy. *The American Psychologist*, *65*(2), 98–109. https://doi.org/10.1037/a0018378
Shedler, J. (2015). Where is the evidence for "evidence-based" therapy? *The Journal of Psychological Therapies in Primary Care*, *4*(1), 47–59. https://jonathanshedler.com/wp-content/uploads/2015/07/Shedler-2015-Where-is-the-evidence-for-evidence-based-therapy-R.pdf
Skinner, B. F. (1953). *Science and human behavior*. Simon and Schuster.
Skinner, B. F. (1956). A case history in scientific method. *American Psychologist*, *11*(5), 221–233. https://doi.org/10.1037/h0047662
Skinner, B. F. (1961). The flight from the laboratory. In Dennis, W. (Ed.), *Current trends in psychological theory* (pp. 50–69). University of Pittsburgh Press.
Sloan, T. (1996). *Damaged life. The crisis of the modern psyche*. Routledge.
Smith, C. (2014). Training of psychoanalytic psychotherapy in contemporary South Africa: Theoretical dilemmas, clinical debates and diverse contexts. *Psycho-analytic Psychotherapy in South Africa*, *22*(1), 26–70.
Smith, J. D. (1985). *Minds made feeble: The myth and legacy of the Kallikaks*. Aspen.
Southern Poverty Law Center. (2012). *Jean-Philippe Rushton*. Retrieved August 30, 2018, from https://www.splcenter. org/fighting-hate/extremist-files/individual/jean-philippe-rushton
Steiner, E. A. (1909). *The immigrant tide: Its ebb and flow*. F.H. Revell.
Strenger, C. (2010). Review of Psychoanalysis at the margins [Review of the book Psychoanalysis at the margins, by P. E. Stepansky]. *Psychoanalytic Psychology*, *27*(3), 376–388. https://doi.org/10.1037/a0020536
Strenger, C. (2015). *Freud's Legacy in the Global Era*. Routledge.
Sullivan, H. S. (1953). *Interpersonal theory of personality*. Norton.
Tucker, W. H. (1996). *The science and politics of racial research*. University of Illinois Press.
Tummala-Narra, P. (2013). Psychoanalytic application in a diverse society. *Psychoanalytic Psychology*, *30*(3), 471–487. https:// doi.org/10.1037/a0031375
Wachtel, P. L. (2010). Beyond "ESTs": Problematic assumptions in the pursuit of evidence-based practice. *Psychoanalytic Psychology*, *27*(3), 251–272. https://doi.org/10.1037/a0020532
Wake, N. (2007). The military, psychiatry, and "unfit" soldiers, 1939–1942. *Journal of the History of Medicine and Allied Sciences*, *62*(4), 461–494. https://doi.org/10.1093/jhmas/jrm002
Walker, E. (1990). *Interview with James Watson*. [Video recording]. American Psychological Association Archives.

Wampold, B. E., & Imel, Z. E. (2015). *The great psychotherapy debate: The evidence for what makes psychotherapy work.* Routledge.

Watson, J. B. (1912). Content of a course in psychology for medical students. *Journal of the American Medical Association, 58*(13), 916–918. https://doi.org/10.1001/jama.1912.04260030314005

Watson, J. B. (1914). *Behavior: An introduction to comparative psychology.* H. Holt.

Watson, J. B. (1919). *Psychology: From the standpoint of a behaviorist.* Lippincott.

Watson, J. B. (1924). *Behaviorism.* Norton.

Watson, J. B. (1928). *Psychological care of infant and child.* W W Norton & Co.

Watson, J. B. (1930). *Behaviorism* (Rev. ed.). W W Norton & Co.

Watson, J. B., & Rayner, R. (1920). Conditioned emotional reactions. *Journal of Experimental Psychology, 3*(1), 1–14. http://dx. doi.org/10.1037/h0069608

Westen, D., Novotny, C. M., & Thompson-Brenner, H. (2004). The empirical status of empirically supported psychotherapies: Assumptions, findings, and reporting in controlled clinical trials. *Psychological Bulletin, 130*(4), 631–663. https://doi.org/10.1037/0033–2909.130.4.631

Wolpe, J. (1981). Behavior therapy versus psychoanalysis: Therapeutic and social implications. *American Psychologist, 36*(2), 159–164. https://doi.org/10.1037//0003-066x.36.2.159

Yakushko, O., & Hook, D. (2017). Whatever happened to the human experience in undergraduate psychology? Comment on the special issue on undergraduate education in psychology (2016). *American Psychologist, 72*(2), 173–175. https://doi.org/10.1037/amp0000055

Yerkes, R. M. (1920). *The New World of Science: its development during the war.* The Century Company.

Yerkes, R. M. (Ed.). (1921). *Psychological examining in the United States Army.* Washington Government Printing Office: Memoirs of the National Academic of Sciences.

Yerkes, R. M. (1923). Eugenic bearing of measurements of intelligence. *The Eugenics Review, 14*(4), 225–229.

Zaretsky, E. (2004). *Secrets of the soul: A social and cultural history of psychoanalysis.* Knopf.

Zaretsky, E. (2005). *Secrets of the soul: A social and cultural history of psychoanalysis.* Vintage Books.

Zimmermann, J., Löffler-Stastka, H., Huber, D., Klug, G., Alhabbo, S., Bock, A., & Benecke, C. (2015). Is it all about the higher dose? Why psychoanalytic therapy is an effective treatment for major depression. *Clinical Psychology and Psychotherapy, 22*(6), 469–487. https://doi.org/10.1002/cpp.1917

Zizek, S. (2004). What can psychoanalysis tell us about cyberspace? *Psychoanalytic Review, 91*(6), 801–830. https://doi. org/10.1521/prev.91.6.801.55957

6

The psycho-politics of evidence-based practice and the assault on our mental health and mental health care

Allan Scholom

My purpose in addressing the concept of evidence-based practice (EBP) is to contribute to the developing perspective that psychoanalysis offers a methodology and a morality that can and should be directed toward understanding how individual dynamics and social forces interact. The history of psychoanalysis has been saturated with a splitting off of the personal from the societal. This began with Freud, who in his early years believed it was necessary for the survival of the psychoanalytic movement. Yet there have been significant movements within the psychoanalytic world throughout its history, as in the Frankfurt School, the Free Clinics and, between the World Wars, "Red Vienna," to integrate societal developments. These struggles were all in the pursuit of social and economic justice and embracing socialist values.

In fact, we might consider that psychoanalysis (along with social work) arose as a counterforce to preserve human subjectivity as a consequence of the alienation and fragmentation resulting from the industrial revolution (Scholom, 2017). From this perspective, psychoanalysis has ultimately and intrinsically been historically and politically embedded (as is everything else), albeit without sufficiently recognizing that this must be so. While invariably analyzing the role of personal history with our patients, we have not paid the same kind of attention to our own, the history of psychoanalysis, such that we might act more vigorously on our own behalf (Young-Bruehl & Schwartz, 2012).

Moreover, without an analysis of the historical, political and economic forces driving societal development, we are left without the necessary theoretical and clinical tools to address more fully the myriad issues facing us. The capitalism of the late 19th century driven by the industrial revolution is far different from that of the current stage of monopoly capitalism or neoliberalism. The Self of Freud's late 19th century Vienna is different from the Self of the mid-20th or that of the early 21st century owing to changing historical forces (Cushman, 2019). Nevertheless, capitalism as such has defining characteristics within which all human development since at least the time of the industrial revolution is formed.

While there are seeds throughout Freud's work inclusive of social forces, in his later years, he came to consider that psychoanalysis might have more

DOI: 10.4324/9781003325512-8

to contribute toward addressing social problems and how they impact individual psychic life than as a method of treatment. Recently, we have begun again to connect the individual to the societal. In order to understand the rise and fall of various movements within the field, we must analyze their historical contexts.

With our field threatened by professional and economic forces and humanity itself imperiled due to the pandemic and climate change, no doubt the time is upon us to engage more actively and consistently with the world. Among the consequences of our failure to do so has been a marginalization of psychoanalysis both professionally, in our theory and practice, as well as in our relevance to the world our patients inhabit (Tolleson, 2009).

An overarching question concerns why people do not act in their self-interest. My goal here is to provide a framework organized around the concept of evidence-based practice (EBP) that can help patients, the public and practitioners understand how societal forces and individual dynamics interact, toward a better understanding of both. We can then talk about how psychic reality is influenced by forces outside the family. In a sense, social forces act as a kind of third parent in both current and historical terms, with myriad transference possibilities. The pandemic by which we are now being victimized and traumatized surely has universal consequences, but it also has individual psychic impact based on each person's history and dynamics.

To illustrate the nexus between the personal and the social, we may view the current pandemic as the revenge of Mother Nature in acute terms (versus climate change as a chronic manifestation) against the systemic forces inherent in capitalism wherein the earth is an object of exploitation. Reactions to the pandemic range from denial – "the problem is overstated and a plot to undermine Donald Trump" – to horror and bewilderment at the failure of the federal government to address the crisis (in that the US has 4.5% of the world's population and 30% of its Covid cases). How people come to these positions and what we do to address them is surely a proper subject for psychoanalysis.

I'm using psychoanalysis in a broad sense meant to include all psychotherapies based upon depth, insight and relationship. More focally, my purpose is to address how approaches to human experience and societal organization that place subjectivity and emerging development as foundational have been under assault for the last five decades. Hence, I'll be speaking in the spirit of consciousness raising and activism in the psychoanalytic world, as well as for our citizenry more broadly.

EBP: All that glitters?

The term evidence-based practice has the ring of science, rationality and common sense. After all, who could be against using evidence and thereby science as a basis for judgment, action or practice? EBP dominates the landscape in the health care world as essentially valid and valuable. In mental health, it has become synonymous with cognitive behavioral therapy (CBT), which has become code for the short-term treatment approaches that most easily fit the flawed empirical requirements that constitute so-called scientific evidence today.

Those who do not practice what is referred to as EBP are left vulnerable to treatment denials, audits and lawsuits (Walls & Scholom, 1998, Shean, 2015). Depth oriented, longer term therapy as embodied by psychoanalysis has been especially damaged, as have educational and training programs offering psychoanalytic approaches. Experientially, there is stigma, shame, defensiveness and marginalization haunting those in the psychoanalytic, humanistic/existential and family systems clinical worlds.

The reality of EBP is, however, quite another matter. In a recent analysis of the empirical literature, Shedler (2015) has found that "evidenced based therapies are ineffective for most people most of the time" (p. 320). In a related review, Johnsen and Friborg (2015) have found that CBT is half as effective as it used to be in treating depression. This is even more striking in light of Shedler's conclusion that "evidenced based therapies are weak… their benefits trivial… and even the trivial benefits do not last" (p. 48).

Thus, even if we concede that empiricism, in the form of null hypothesis testing and randomized control trial designs undergirding CBT approaches, is the highest forms of evidence, a highly debatable claim which is statistically and methodologically questionable (Cohen, 1994, Meehl, 1978, Shean, 2015), the grounds for widespread acceptance of CBT were never there to begin with.

Furthermore, in January of 2018, the U.S. Substance Abuse and Mental Health Services Administration (SAMHSA) shut down their National Registry of Evidence-Based Programs and Practices (NREPP) website. Health and Human Services Assistant Secretary Elinore McCance-Katz issued a statement expressing her concern about incomplete and flawed research supporting the EBPs on the list. Moreover, 87 of 112 (78%) newly reviewed evidence-based programs involved some sort of conflict of interest, i.e., financial gain, research undertaken by program developers themselves, and so on (Gorman, 2017). Even more problematically, members of the APA practice guideline panel were strong-armed to make recommendations that ignore patients and therapists, as well as the far stronger evidence for relationship-based therapy vs. specific interventions, as in CBT (Courtois & Brown, 2019).

By contrast, there has been a great deal of empirical support for psychodynamic treatment (Shedler, 2010) as well as a long history of psychotherapy research prior to the EBP era demonstrating its general effectiveness. In fact, psychotherapy, including psychoanalytically oriented approaches, has historically been one of the most research-supported treatments in the health care world. In this sense, the EBP movement is an attempt to rewrite, if not eliminate, the research-rich history of the general effectiveness of psychotherapy. So we are left with a critical question – how and why has the EBP movement come to dominate the health care landscape?

EBP and the free market economy

To understand the dominance of EBP, we must turn our attention to history and begin with the broader social and economic forces that set the stage. Until the 1980s health care was essentially a "Ma and Pa" operation, with services provided by private practitioners, stand-alone hospitals and medical centers, some with a religious affiliation. In the 1980s, health care, the largest industry in the country, accounting for over 17% of GDP, essentially became the target of a corporate takeover because of its potential for great profit (Scholom, 1998, 2013). Health insurers, pharmaceutical companies and large hospital chains came to dominate the health care world as it galloped toward oligopoly.

The overarching result has been that the US has the most expensive system in the world, costing about twice as much in GDP and per capita health care as systems in nations with single-payer or non-market-based systems (as in all other first world and many third-world countries). The current system is ranked worst in the world among developed countries (Executive Summary, 2014b). Americans suffer poorer health, and this downward spiral has continued since the 1970s (Institute of Medicine, Woolf & Aron, 2013) in almost all categories, compared with the citizens of every other industrialized nation. The US is ranked 70th out of 132 nations worldwide in health and wellness (Executive Summary, 2014b). Life expectancy and the birth rate in the US have been declining over the last several years. In short, Americans get fewer services, including outpatient visits, hospital days and surgeries, for far greater cost and with far worse results.

In essence, it is the costs of the for-profit/market-based system that are responsible. These include administrative costs (about 30% to the health insurance industry versus less than 5% for traditional Medicare), excessive profit to corporations, such as insurance companies, not providing direct health care services (Scholom, 1997, 2013), pharmaceutical costs (due largely to drugs costing more than twice what other countries pay) and profit unrelated to health care service delivery (for stockholders, advertising and marketing, debt repayment from mergers and acquisitions and executive compensation). The bottom line is that in health care, the market works neither effectively nor humanely. In fact, the market IS the problem.

Set against this backdrop, EBP, when equivalent to short-term, manualized treatment, serves an important function as a vehicle to curtail services and thereby increase the profit of the health insurance and drug industries while also cutting government costs. One of the prime objectives of the ACA is to eliminate the fee-for-service system and replace it with "products" using a capitation model, now referred to as "accountable care organizations" (a new version of HMOs). Capitation is often referred to as "value over volume." In reality, capitation shifts financial risk onto practitioners, such that the incentive is to provide less service under the guise of "accountability." Essentially, this is code for austerity, or people getting less. Under the rubric of "medical necessity," a term created by the health insurance industry to control cost and increase profit, services that are not deemed to be "evidence-based" can more easily be denied.

Thus, EBP (as in short-term, often manualized therapy) provides a "scientific" rationale or cover for providing less service while garnering greater profit. Since Americans do not receive more services (in fact generally fewer, but do pay more for those they get) compared to people in other countries, the current fee-for-service system is not the problem. The so-called free market is the problem in health care – too many entities/middlemen making too much money while contributing little or nothing to service delivery.

While 75% of Americans believe the U.S. health care system requires fundamental change (Commonwealth Fund, 2014), the public debate in the mainstream media centers on the role of big government and not on the limits of the market. Media discussion of tax increases to pay for health care for all ignores the fact that overall costs to almost all Americans would decrease substantially. Furthermore, the current system is misrepresented as offering more choice, despite the fact that "provider networks'" and employers' control over plans offered do in fact provide less choice than single-payer systems like traditional Medicare, which allow people to consult with professionals and go to whatever hospitals they choose.

So how is it that we continue to act against our own best interests by allowing a system to remain in place that is harmful to us? The situation is not unlike the one we confront as practitioners when a patient arrives at our office knowing something is wrong with her/his life but having little to no awareness of what the real problems may be. We are charged with helping our patients look more deeply into their struggles to facilitate understanding and acting on their own behalf.

Political mythology through a psychoanalytic lens: Big government and the free market

Herein lies the potential for the psychoanalytic approach to aid us in understanding the connection of the individual to the social world. Layton (2006) has called attention to the unconscious pull in the US to dissociate individuals from their social milieu. In seeking to comprehend this unconscious pull in the health care context, it is essential to consider the mythologies and belief systems that are at issue here. Let us start by taking up those concerning big government and the free market and elucidating the individual and group fantasies and illusions that permit such myths to go unchallenged:

Regarding big government, the actual size of the government, and spending by the government, has not changed appreciably over recent history. This has been the case whether Republicans or Democrats were in power. What varies are the directions one party takes in contrast to the other regarding how resources are used and which laws are passed. For instance, when Republicans (generally seen as against big government) push to control women's choice or marital freedom, or determine what children are taught and tested on in school, or decide who can vote, they use big government for their own ends despite their alleged objections to "big" in other circumstances.

The free market, too, is dependent on the rules made by the government as to how it should conduct itself. For example, when the rules allowing banks to consolidate banking and commercial activities were changed under a Democrat (generally seen as more protective of individuals and the environment against the excesses of the market), the stage was set for the economic crisis of 2008. Similarly, when the various free-trade agreements starting in the 1990s were written favoring corporations without sufficient labor or environmental protections, jobs were lost, and the environment degraded.

I cite these examples to illustrate that there is no such thing as "big government" or the "free market." Rather, these are myths that serve to confuse and mystify us such that we cannot see our own self-interest. Big government and the free market become potent oversimplifications, illusions or mythologies used by both parties to manipulate public opinion and perceptions for political ends. This is largely to preserve their own influence, the status of which is vastly dependent upon serving the interests of those corporate entities which provide the financial resources necessary to gain power.

From a psychoanalytic perspective, we can endeavor to explicate the underlying fantasies these myths speak to. Regarding big government, fantasies regarding the dangers of dependency and vulnerability are foremost. The tension played out on the political stage concerns the clash between one narrative that presents the government as a parent on which we can depend and another narrative that reaffirms our autonomy and denies that sense of need. We might remind ourselves how we typically view patients who are afraid of and yet are desperately in need of close relationships (for understandable historical reasons) such that being influenced by others can become threatening or coercive. Many may seek the illusion of independence or self-reliance as a potential solution. This may find some expression in an idealization of the free market as an embodiment of individualism and safety, free of external threat. Of course, the opposite may also be true, in that some people may seek to be overly dependent so as to avoid the perils of separation/individuation.

To be sure, I am oversimplifying, as the fantasies around independence and dependence underlying the myths of "big government" and the "free market" can take myriad forms in the same person and certainly in a collective sense as well. My point is not to map, in some one-to-one fashion, how a given person or group may travel from fantasy to myth and back, but rather to illustrate that fantasies exist that make us vulnerable to political mystification. Furthermore, we in the psychoanalytic world are uniquely positioned to help resolve processes of demystification on an individual and collective level (Scholom, 2015).

The neoliberal exploitation of unconscious myths

The unconscious wish to deny dependency and to avoid the sense of being controlled offers fertile soil for the rise of neoliberalism taking place over the last 40 years. Neoliberalism entails free market economic fundamentalism, or basically little to no control over corporate power. This is in contrast to traditional Keynesian liberalism where the government contained corporate excess and provided a social safety net. In essence, neoliberalism represents a corresponding ideological assault on consciousness and subjectivity (Layton, 2010). A critical aspect of the mystification process involves the creation of a new language that leads us to think, feel and act in commodified and objectified terms. This mystification has given rise to the creation of a "neoliberal consciousness."

Importantly, the grip of neoliberal consciousness holds tight our beliefs not only regarding who we are, but who we *should* be. For instance, "multi-tasking" has become a worthwhile end, as if doing more than one thing at a time somehow makes us better, more capable people (assuming, from the point of view of mental processing, we could do this, which of course we cannot). More broadly, we tend to think of ourselves as good or virtuous, depending upon how much we can "accomplish" in a given day (Peltz, 2005). Over and above the stress and pressure this engenders, it places responsibility on us to do more, while at the same time estranging us from present experience, fostering a splitting off of our inner selves. This vision of who we should be has stark implications for our views of mental illness and thus how it should be treated.

The belief in the "productivity gospel" is reinforced and multiplied by the assumptions of the broader systems in which it is embedded. For instance, the rise of neoliberal free market fundamentalism with its key value of productivity corresponds to the rapid expansion of religious fundamentalism throughout the world. A key connection here is the belief in innate human sinfulness, an ultimate form of blame-the-victim self-hatred. As we are born in sin, it is our individual responsibility to overcome this state, regardless of how the deck is stacked against us by the system in which our lives are embedded. It follows, then, that we have come to approach life in productivity terms, as embodiments of this free market fundamentalist ideology, or what has been called "*homo entreprenaurus*."

In essence, our subjectivity has become a commodity. Unwittingly, we are increasingly objectified and objectifying entities embedded in this formative social reality, without our realizing what is happening. Of course, if we don't do this very well, it is our own fault. As we know all too well from our work with patients, this is a kind of defensive lie that covers or disavows a more painful truth (Freud, 1927). In this case, the painful truth is that government has ceased to function as the caretaker of last resort. Instead, it is increasingly merging with and serving the interests of large corporate entities – the corporate takeover of government.

The loss of the government as the caretaker of last resort is exemplified in the shredding of our social safety net over the last 30 years (i.e., cuts to Medicare and Medicaid, Social Security, the loss of private retirement programs, gauging in student loans, etc.). In light of this loss of an institutional caretaker, a collective trauma has been visited upon our citizenry, leaving us increasingly to our own devices. Thus more, we are more thoroughly dependent upon the myth of our own individualism even while we are increasingly pressured, often without knowing it, to sacrifice for the so-called common good. This sacrifice is valorized, as we are told that people *ought* to be more responsible or accountable or sacrifice for the greater good. In essence, we are a country organized around the fear of being controlled, of which our individualism is but a symptom.

Broader political movements make use of relational techniques that psychoanalysts understand clearly. Gaslighting (Welch, 2008) means being told that the bad things that are happening to you are not really happening, are not so bad or are actually good for you. This mystification is a pathogenic process that renders us more vulnerable to being controlled as our grip on reality is assaulted. To illustrate, the mainstream media tell us that the economy is healthy! But for whom? The true measure of unemployment is actually the workforce participation rate, a number about double the unemployment rate. Moreover, economic inequality has been inexorably increasing over the 40 years. Thus, our struggles become internalized as our own individual problems, as if unrelated to the neoliberal socio-economic order – the defensive lie that conceals the deeper truth that it is the larger system that is failing most of us (Layton, 2010).

Perhaps nowhere is gaslighting more evident than in the election of Donald Trump, in which fantasies of the American Dream and American Exceptionalism were used to delude voters into denying their current realities. "Make America Great Again" was a successful campaign slogan, meant to arouse a fantasy to cover over the fact that in essential economic respects, America's "greatness" has been relentlessly and significantly disappearing since the 1970s. Declining real wages and accelerating downward mobility are buried under the weight of the seductive delusion of this fantasy America, while in fact, the US is now the most economically unequal of all Western nations and has significantly less social mobility than Canada or Europe. What is most striking, though, is that Americans are both unaware of the extent of the inequality here and do not believe that it is as bad as it actually is (Fitz, 2015). Clearly, the public is in widespread cultural denial about the vanishing American Dream. As comedian George Carlin joked, "The reason they call it the American Dream is that you have to be asleep to believe it."

As the facts that need to be denied accumulate, the grip of the illusion of the American Dream must be that much further tightened. While we have been taught that the American Dream was responsible for waves of immigration to the US, the facts are otherwise, as 30–40% of immigrants from Europe before the First World War ultimately returned home and many more were unhappy that they had come (Zahra, 2015). Surely, we must also consider that the US was built upon a legacy of genocide of 9–10 million indigenous peoples and 25–30 million Blacks, not including those who lived in slavery (Zinn, 1980). Add to this the fact that the US is the most war-mongering country the world has ever known and that most polls taken in other countries reveal that the US is seen as the country posing the greatest threat to world peace. We are outraged at Russian interference in our elections at the same time as we fail to acknowledge that the US interferes in far more extensive ways both militarily, as in Vietnam and Iraq, and covertly in the internal affairs of countless nations around the world. Meanwhile, Trump's Tax Bill is but one domestic egregious example, which has done little else but increase economic inequality, benefiting the wealthy at the expense of most everyone else. This dissociated, disavowed and denied history further necessitates the intensification of American Exceptionalism.

EBP and the neoliberal illusion

If we are tempted to subscribe to the illusion that the discipline and practice of psychology have little to do with these broader political movements, we might best think again. Understanding their interconnection, however, necessitates an appreciation as to how these practices are determined, and that necessity, in turn, brings us to the history of EBP, both to illustrate how it came to dominate our field and how we ourselves, like most everyone else, have been unwittingly implicated.

EBP originated in the field of medicine, concurrently with the rise of neoliberalism, and the same systemic forces discussed above were at play. In medicine, EBP is defined as the **integration of the best available research with clinical expertise in the context of patient characteristics, culture and preferences**. Psychology followed medicine's lead; its earlier iteration, called empirically validated treatment (EVT), later evolved into its own version of the definition of EBP that the Institute of Medicine endorsed in 2001, adapted from Sackett and colleagues (2000): "Evidence-based practice is the integration of best research evidence with clinical expertise and patient values" (p. 1). The American Psychological Association formally adopted this broader definition of EBP in 2006, which includes therapist expertise and patient characteristics in addition to empirically validated/supported treatments (EVT/EST).

While the wish for treatment recommendations to reflect evidence of their effectiveness seems reasonable, however, there are difficulties built into the very concept that may not be apparent to the uninformed observer. For one, there is the question of what constitutes evidence itself, which was effectively narrowed to include only randomized control trials, or, in starker terms, studies involving standardized protocols, a symptom focus and short-term duration, parameters which are too narrow to allow for the inclusion of research into more in-depth treatments. Furthermore, the APA has offered no oversight in determining whether a treatment can be called evidence based by insurance companies or the government, thereby allowing the evidence for psychoanalytic treatment to be ignored by insurers. Worse yet, APA is now developing practice guidelines based on this narrow definition of evidence that will further limit public access to psychodynamic and depth oriented or longer-term treatment. To complete the CBT takeover of non-drug mental health care, APA is actively promulgating the near monopoly of CBT as "evidence-based treatment" in graduate training, internship placements and undergraduate education.

It is here that we can see the role of our professional organizations in colluding with broader systems, whether government or corporate. This is not surprising in view of the fact that professional organizations are authorized by the government to provide surveillance and control functions over their membership, presumably to "protect the public." There are economic guild interests at issue as well, such that those members who are more aligned with broader political and economic forces will be better served. Thus, those who practice from an EBP framework, such as CBT, will benefit, as these treatments are short term and cost less in the short run. This serves the financial interests of the government and health insurance industry. Historically, the narrower definition of EBP as EVT/EST represented the beginning of the collusion with the cost-cutting and service-limiting ideology and actuality of managed care.

Certainly, we in the psychoanalytic world do educate, suggest and otherwise directly try to influence our patients (some have called CBT a subset of analytic methodology). However, it is critical to understand that CBT fits the neoliberal paradigm economically, costing less and shifting the financial burden on to patients and practitioners. Moreover, it is consistent with neoliberal ideology that values the triumph, however illusory, of individual control over relationship and interdependence. Put another way, the illusion and fantasy of control over our psyches embodied by CBT triumph over the acceptance of vulnerability and interdependency via self-understanding embodied by psychoanalysis.

CBT is in essence a top-down approach to human experience that is undemocratic, if not oppressive, in relation to the rest of the mind. Even those of a CBT orientation who do enter into the relational world, rather than embracing manualized treatment, have generally been taught that the goal of therapy involves the erasure or marginalization of problematic thoughts. It is a model of domination and control, in contrast to psychoanalysis, a methodology that works from the bottom up... by analogy, much as we would want for our citizenry. In this sense, CBT is an extension of the neoliberal top/trickle down approach to human experience in the service of the economic, political and cultural aims of the current system. It is ahistorical and non-contextual and serves to split off the personal from the political: the source of distress and illness is narrowly attributed to the patient alone, and not to the efforts to metabolize the effects of the greater surround in which the patient is embedded.

Much of the drama around the establishment of the APA's adoption of the EBP mantra took place under the radar within the guild organization itself. As noted above, in the mid-1990s, under the auspices of the American Psychological Association's Division of Clinical Psychology's Task Force on Promotion and Dissemination of Empirically Validated Psychological Procedures (Division 12, 1993 as cited by Brooke, 2006), which paralleled the Association's Board of Professional Affairs (BPA) Template for Developing Guidelines: Interventions for Mental Disorders and Psychosocial Aspects of Physical Disorders (APA, 1995), the formalization of EBP began to take shape. Empirically validated/supported treatments became synonymous with good treatments. The only treatments that work, we were told, were those that are "evidenced-based." The government and health insurance companies compiled lengthy lists of EVTs and used them to limit therapy to shorter term approaches.

Within the context of APA politics, there had been a shift in the organization toward a more clinical/professional as opposed to academic/scientific orientation due to the growth of membership in the practitioner community in the 1980s. Rather than broadening an appreciation for in-depth treatment models that support patients' long-term growth and quality of life, however, this clinician-academic division sparked the formation of a separate organization, the Association for Psychological Science, in 1988. It also precipitated a backlash within APA, which spurred the academic community toward the promulgation of empirical research, over which it had power, as the exclusive criteria for professional practice. Worth highlighting is that the BPA and Division 12 consisted largely of academic psychologists during this period. The President of Division 12 was also chair of the BPA and had published an approved manual for the treatment of Panic Disorder. Hence, he and others stood to gain both professionally and financially from these efforts, just as psychiatric consultants to drug companies do.

There was a successful movement within APA by practitioners of psychoanalytic, humanistic and family therapy traditions arguing for the re-inclusion of therapist expertise and patient characteristics in the definition of EBP, but this victory has been undermined by APA's general stance toward the creation of treatment recommendations and guidelines. Part of the stimulus for this response was an attack waged by psychologists in the academic community, as they pushed to make it unethical for practitioners not to use so-called EVTs in their work. When the role of therapist expertise is taken in to account, however, many treatments that were not considered "evidence-based" turn out to have an additional wealth of evidence to support them. APA reluctantly included these additional criteria, but has consistently shirked responsibility to inform the public when the full EBP criteria are not being met, deliberately misleading the uninformed by passing off manualized and other forms of CBT as if they fulfilled all the requirements. In short, the development of EBP has been rife with personal and political power and influence and is far from representing a pure product of scientific progress.

EBP and the landscape of mental health

The so-called "revolution" in EBP dovetails with other developments in the last 40 years related to top-down, market-based social engineering in health care that similarly embody the neoliberal assault in social and economic reality terms on our subjectivity. A major thrust of the Affordable Care Act involves a shift from fee-for-service to a so-called "value"-based approach toward reimbursement for health care services. This is grounded on the flawed neoliberal market ideology that blames fee-for-service as the major cause of the failures of our expensive and ineffective health care system instead of acknowledging that the market itself is the problem – too many entities making too much money while delivering limited or no useful health care services.

This approach, often called "pay for performance," relies upon the Physician Quality Reporting System (PQRS), essentially a system of classifying conditions that determines which treatments will be paid for and how much they should cost. This means that a given diagnosis will get a pre-defined reimbursement and no more, regardless of the complexity and specific nature of the case. Thus, payment is capitated and legitimate individual needs for service are limited or denied. In fact, there are reimbursement penalties for those practitioners who do not follow these guidelines.

PQRS is based on standards derived from studies now largely discredited (Gourguechon, 2007), yet are still considered to be evidenced-based. Rather than questioning the validity of this system or, more importantly, the cost cutting agenda it serves, APA is now offering training for psychologists to teach them to comply with it. Consequently, while EBP masquerades under the banner of accountability, it is actually a disguise for austerity. We are getting far less than what we need despite our having paid in advance in the form of taxes and premiums for it. Lastly, there is no evidence that "pay for performance" schemes improve quality of care or save money (Snyder and Anderson, 2005). What we surely do know is that these schemes do increase the potential for profit through cost cutting.

Nowhere are the effects more evident than in mental health over the last 40 years. During this time, spending on mental health services has remained at about 1% of the gross domestic product from 1986 to 2009 while total health care costs have increased from 10% to 17% (Rampell, 2013). Put another way, while mental health spending remained about the same during this period, all health care expenditures went up by 70%! More focally, both the total numbers of psychotherapy sessions and the reimbursements for treatment sessions have continued to decline over the last decades (Gnaulati, 2019). Our professional organizations have offered little to no opposition to or even education about this deteriorating situation. Neither practitioners nor the public have been made sufficiently aware of the extent of the destructive reality of this situation.

This current situation illustrates how science, or more accurately scientism, can be used for political and economic purposes (Hoffman, 2009). It is in the realm of science where we can see a critical fantasy constellation whose promulgation enables the neoliberal assault to take hold. I will call this the "science as savior" fantasy – the fantasy that science and technology will provide the answers to our problems in living. Of course, science has had a profound effect on the quality of our lives, particularly materially. However, when it comes to human interactions, our relationships to one another and to ourselves, science has its limits. Yet still, in light of our collective trauma over the last 40 years, exemplified by the loss of the government as caretaker of last resort, we look to science, in a form of religious fundamentalism, for compensation if not salvation. As Nebula Award winning science fiction author Richard Chwedyk views it, "what we want from science is magic" (2015, personal communication).

We can think of scientism as a way of characterizing science as a belief system. As we now know, EBP is based upon virtually non-existent or corrupted science. At the same time, it was used as a rationale for carrying out the cost cutting/austerity aims of the government and the profit requirements of the health insurance, hospital and drug industries. Thus, the "science as salvation" fantasy moves us toward participation in our own exploitation, via our embrace of the defensive, surface level, less painful truth. The deeper truth, that we are being done in by the neoliberal system itself, remains split off.

To complete the picture of how the corporate/government control over mental/health care takes place, we need to look at National Provider Identifier numbers (NPI) and the move toward Electronic Medical Records (EMR). The NPI evolved out of the Health Insurance Portability and Accountability Act (HIPPA) of 1996 and was implemented in 2006. Note that HIPPA is not so much about protecting individual privacy but rather to inform people as to how their privacy could be breached. Contrary to pressure by our professional organizations, we are not required to have an NPI unless we file insurance forms electronically, are Medicare providers or are on insurance panels. In essence, NPIs allow insurance companies and the government to have access to our practice patterns and likely clinical orientation. The reality of coercion, treatment denials, therapist audits and violations of privacy by these entities are profound. The benefits for our patients and for us are yet to be found.

Similarly regarding EMRs, the notion that such information would improve quality of care and help control costs is not born out by any substantive evidence (Himmelstein and Woolhandler, 2005). On the other hand, there is much data attesting to the enormous cost – in the tens of billions of dollars – of creating electronic records. Yet there are hundreds of EMR systems in hospitals, government and insurance companies that do not and likely cannot ever communicate effectively with one another. Moreover, the ever-present reality of breaches of security via leaks and hacking, which have occurred with increasing frequency and scope over the last years, are undeniably a pernicious threat to the right to privacy. Nevertheless, health insurance companies are actively using this information to scrutinize claims and practice patterns and to deny care. Surely, this contributes to professional burnout, as M.Ds spend two hours on paperwork for every hour of patient contact (Young and Fairchild, 2016). A similar plight plagues all professionals dealing with the impossible demands of health insurers.

These electronic methods of enforcement and surveillance work together to reinforce the work of EBP as a neoliberal imperative. Gourguechon (2007) concludes that Pay for Performance relies on standards derived from EBP, which cannot be fully implemented without EMR, and I would add without NPI. The bottom line is an effort toward top-down social engineering that serves the profitability of the health insurance industry and allows for hidden austerity measures on the part of the government under the guise of accountability and technological efficiency. As a result, we are all getting less and paying more, which in the final analysis results in income redistribution from most of us to the very few.

Psychoanalysis: The compulsion to sleep and waking from the dream

Now we come to the most difficult and painful questions. Why don't we already know this and what are we going to do now that we do? We in the psychoanalytic world have much to contribute to the analysis of broader systemic issues and the ways they interact with individual psychodynamics. The trauma and resulting fantasies, illusions and defensive configurations yielded by neoliberalism's incursions into all our lives call out for further elucidation and discourse amongst us, with our patients and in the broader world.

Of course we do talk a great deal about the outside world with our patients. However, without sufficient understanding, our frame of reference is limited, as is our therapeutic discourse. Whether with our struggles with health insurance, burdens related to job stresses or familial pressures, the system we live in is inevitably implicated. Without an adequate comprehension of social reality, it is harder to parse out psychic reality. We run the risk indirectly of blaming the victim for matters beyond the individual's control, thereby reproducing the very trauma s/he came to us to address. We may, in fact, suffer the same illusions as our patients, by not sufficiently recognizing the external organizing realities of our shared trauma. Surely the current pandemic shows how profoundly a shared collective trauma has differing impacts on individuals based upon their own histories and transferences. Yet we can turn this shared experience toward therapeutic ends. It is critical that we be able to offer a perspective or point of view to our patients. Patients find hearing my views and analyses about the pandemic most helpful in normalizing what they are experiencing. By providing this systemic perspective, we can then move to more individual reactions and thereby deepen our work.

The insights of psychoanalysts can function as good interpretations both on a societal and on a personal level. Now, in light of the pandemic, when our patients need a broader systemic perspective to help them understand their internal experiences, such interpretation is especially important. Moreover, a broader perspective opens up a societal contextual arena informed by an analytic dimension heretofore lacking. Clinically speaking, I have found this enormously useful: patients have a place to go with their healthy outrage beyond the re-experiencing of helplessness and rage owing to familial history. I am not speaking merely of sublimation, but rather of a space for here-and-now self-expression and development. However, in order to go there, we must have a perspective on the system in which we live that allows us to see the transference dimensions to the social order in the context of both parental and societal influence.

We cannot pretend, in the face of the pandemic, that we do not experience a shared sense of trauma from within our own lives. We too confront an inevitable sense of powerlessness and vulnerability. This is hardly something we like to experience. Our own limitations may collude with therapeutic zeal, such that we may be hesitant to appreciate fully the existence of forces that strongly influence us beyond our day-to-day reach. Yet the more we are able to grapple with our own reluctance to knowing/awakening, and with the great vulnerability and interdependent need that lies beneath, the more we can be of help, to others and to ourselves.

There are additional traumas, and multiple factors, determining truth-facing on our own parts. Surely, sadly, we have been victimized ourselves by the neoliberal assault on thought, subjectivity and insight over the last 40 years, as manifested in the EBP mentality and the related denigration of our work. Implicated here is our tolerating the American Psychological Association, which ever increasingly discriminates against therapies of depth, insight and relationship. Meanwhile, the relative comfort of our class position in society may constitute an additional obstacle to bringing an expanded social psychoanalytic level of critique to our societal predicament and, in turn, back into the consulting room. Perhaps this has to do with how hard it is to leave home.

In addition, our privileging of dialog, as in talk therapy, can lead to shortsightedness in the political realm when we do not fully appreciate that real power can and typically does trump discourse and connection in myriad overarching ways. While our ability to offer distinctive insights regarding the play of larger societal forces, economic, political and social, in our own familiar terms can be invaluable, it can also offer us a fantasy of power and control that proves illusory in the face of entrenched and well-funded agendas. We must face the fact that late-stage capitalism, the neoliberal system, is a social and economic reality in which everything we think and feel and do is embedded. It is a complex multifaceted system in and around us that transcends and is ubiquitous in impact, albeit not inevitable.

Psychoanalysis historically and necessarily was a dissident force, subversive toward the status quo, personally and politically. Freud knew this when he spoke of "bringing the plague" to America. He likely believed this more expansively later in life when he realized the potential for psychoanalysis to address social problems in addition to understanding their all too real influences as a source of human distress. This role of psychoanalysis as a dissident voice undoubtedly has played a role in our current marginalization, as the capacity and courage to critique is a threat to the powerful forces being wielded against psychoanalysis and our citizenry more broadly.

The time is ripe for psychoanalysis to strengthen its voice not only as a safeguard of good individual treatment, but as a fulcrum of social change. The protests over racism offer real potential to evolve into structural systemic reforms that address underlying problems related to racism, sexism, classism, childism and ageism, all of which contribute mightily to our societal problems. The mental, physical and socioeconomic well-being of our people, represented by health care for all policies and investment in economic equality, child care, educational opportunity and so on provided in other countries are at issue. Where we go with the current disillusionment is of course the question facing us.

As Freud said in Reflections on War and Death (1918), "Illusions commend themselves to us because they save us pain and allow us to enjoy pleasure instead" (p. 16). However, as French philosopher de Chamfort asserts, "pleasure may come from illusion, but happiness can come only from reality" (p. 1). It is here that psychoanalytic thinking has much to contribute, helping to understand what has been happening both on an external political/historical level as well as what this means to all of us from a personal/internal point of view.

In essence, our work can help people move from disillusionment to empowerment. While we do talk to our patients about politics undoubtedly now more than ever in the wake of Trump as catalyst, it becomes ever more important to engage via consciousness raising or action around current social reality, especially to avoid the danger of blaming the victim (us) for our struggles and recapitulating our trauma by failing to address sufficiently the external forces that terrify and harm us in material and emotional terms.

It is likewise incumbent upon us to go beyond the consulting room to help bring about the larger systemic social change we so desperately need. In this regard, I do not believe that research demonstrating psychoanalytic efficacy will in itself reestablish our place in the mental health world. The research is already there and is ignored. Those who blame our declining status solely or primarily on a lack of "evidence" are themselves blaming the victim (us) of a system that also oppresses us. Of course, we should encourage further research as part of our investment in change, but in the spirit of demonstrating the systemic problems and their human consequences. We have much to contribute in the realm of helping to address the fantasies and illusions involved in perpetuating a sick and sickening system. In doing so, we make ourselves relevant in ways we have not been, yet can and need to be. Now is the time to help set a new course, freer of fantasy and illusion, that meets the real needs of the 99% and not merely those of the 1%.

On a heartening and hopeful note, many of our forebears were courageous dissidents (Fromm, Reich, Fenichel, Horney, Fanon). So too are many currently working in this tradition, including Layton, Hollander, Benjamin and so many more across generations around the world. Our movement is currently being revitalized. The times call upon us not only to think but also to act, as they did during the dawn of our field. Fortunately, the younger generations are standing up in vigorous ways. We can see evidence of this in our conferences, in our journals and in our organizational work. They are speaking passionately about pernicious systemic injustice and exploitation related to sexism, racism, classism ageism, childism and on and on. A proud and much-needed tradition is being revitalized.

Lest I have created undue expectations about what we in psychoanalysis can do to change the world, let me say that our place may best be seen as a profoundly important voice for valuing our subjective experience and all that contributes to it. In an age of "bewilderment" (Bollas, 2018), standing for the worth of clearer sightedness, and, at its best, vision, is offering a great deal. In this sense, we might say that, before the pandemic, the plague was already here. Let us then work to know the ways that can help us find the better path forward. This brings us back to why psychoanalysis arrived on the world stage to begin with. Preserving subjectivity and humanistic values in the face of their being in constant jeopardy under capitalism is no small reason for being.

We might liken where we are to waking from a long sleep in which our dreams can no longer contain the passions and conflicts we have buried. The more we analyze all we have known-but-not-known about our world, the more we can help to address it, and the closer we come to the more painful if ultimately more freeing truths. In our beloved profession, this is, after all, what we are meant to do.

References

American Psychological Association. (1995). Template for Developing Guidelines: Interventions for Mental Disorders and Psychosocial aspects of Physical Disorders. Washington, DC: American Psychological Association.

Brooke, R. (2006). The Return of Expertise in Evidence Based Practice. Psychologist-Psychoanalyst, 26: 23–26.

Bollas, C. (2018). Meaning and Melancholia: Life in the Age of Bewilderment. London: Routledge.

Chamfort, N. www.Pinterest.com.

Chwedyk, R. (2015). Personal Communication.

Cohen, J. (1994). The Earth Is Round. American Psychologist, 49: 997–1003.

Cushman, P. (2019). *Travels with the Self-Interpreting Psychology as Cultural History.* London: Routledge.

Executive Summary. (2014a). Mirror, Mirror on the Wall, 2014 Update: How the U.S. Health Care System Compares Internationally. New York: The Commonwealth Fund.

Executive Summary. (2014b). The Social Progress Index. Washington, DC: The Social Progress Imperative.

Fitz, N. (2015). Economic Inequality: It's Far Worse Than You Think. Scientific American.
Freud, S. (1918). Reflections on War and Death. New York: Moffat, Yard & Company.
Freud, S. (1927). Fetishism. Standard Edition, 21. London: Hogarth Press. 152–159.
Gnaulati, E. (2019). The Woeful Underfunding of Psychotherapy by Health Insurers. Mad in America.
Gorman, D.M. (2017). Has the National Registry of Evidence-Based Programs and Practices (NREPP) Lost Its Way? The International Journal of Drug Policy, 45: 40–41.
Gourguechon, P.L. (2007). The Canary in the Coal Mine: Psychoanalysis and Health. Psychologist-Psychoanalyst Newsletter, Spring: 19–22.
Himmelstein, D. and Woolhandler, S. (2005). Hope and Hype: Predicting the Impact of Electronic Medical Records. Health Affairs, 24: 1121–1123.
Hoffman, I.Z. (2009). Doublethinking Our Way to "Scientific" Legitimacy: The Desiccation of Human Experience. Journal of the American Psychoanalytic Association, 57(5): 1043–1069.
Johnsen, T.J. and Friborg, O. (2015). The Effects of Cognitive Behavioral Therapy as an Anti–Depressive Treatment is Failing: A Meta-analysis. Psychological Bulletin, 141(14): 747–768.
Layton, L. (2006). Attacks on Linking: The Unconscious Pull to Dissociate Individuals from Their Social Context. In Layton, L. Hollander, N.C. and Gutweil, S. (Eds.) Psychoanalysis, Class and Politics: Encounters in the Clinical Setting. London: Routledge.
Layton, L. (2010). Irrational Exuberance: Neoliberal Subjectivity and the Perversion of Truth. Subjectivity, 3(3): 303–322.
Meehl, P.E. (1978). Theoretical Risks and Tabular Asterisks: Sir Karl, Sir Ronald and the Slow Progress of Soft Psychology. Journal of Consulting and Clinical Psychology, 46: 806–834.
Peltz, R. (2005). The Manic Society. Psychoanalytic Dialogues, 15(3): 347–366.
Rampell, C. (2013). Most U.S. Health Spending Is Exploding – But Not for Mental Health. The New York Times.
Sackett, D.L., Strauss, S.E., Richardson, W.S., Rosenberg, W. and Haynes, R.B. (2000). Evidence-Based Medicine: How to Practice and Teach. London: Churchill Livingstone.
Scholom, A. (1998). Managed Care's Assault on Our Hearts and Minds. Psychologist-Psychoanalyst Newsletter, 18(2): 6–12.
Scholom, A. (2013). Challenging the System: American Fantasies and Resistance to Real Reform. American Association for Psychoanalysis in Clinical Social Work Newsletter, Spring (4–9): 18–25.
Scholom, A. (2015). Psychoanalyzing the Affordable Care Act and Its Actors. The Psychoanalytic Activist. Online Newsletter of Section IX of Division 39 of the American Psychological Association. Spring.
Scholom, A. (2017). Trauma in Psychoanalysis and Society and Why There Has Not Been More Activism. Presented at the Division 39 Conference of APA, New York, 2017.
Shean, G.D. (2015). Some Methodological and Epistemic Limitations of Evidence-Based Therapies. Psychoanalytic Psychology, 32(3): 500–516.

Shedler, J. (2010). The Efficacy of Psychodynamic Psychotherapy. American Psychologist, 65(2): 98–109.
Shedler, J. (2015). Where is the Evidence for "Evidence-Based Therapy? The Journal of Psychological Therapies in Primary Care, 4: 49–59.
Snyder, C. and Anderson, G. (2006). Do quality improvement organizations improve the quality of hospital care for Medicare beneficiaries? *JAMA*, Jun 15; 293(23):2900–2907.
Tolleson, J. (2009). Saving the World One Patient at a Time: Psychoanalysis and Social Critique. Psychotherapy and Politics International, 7(3): 190–205.
Walls, G. B. and Scholom, A.H. (1996). APA Practice Guidelines Template Jeopardizes Clinical Autonomy of Practitioners. Psychologist-Psychoanalyst, 16(1): 17–21.
Welch, B. (2008). State of Confusion: Political Manipulation and the Assault on the American Mind. New York: St. Martens Press.
Woolf, S.H. and Aron, L. (2013). U.S. Health in International Perspective: Shorter Lives, Poorer Health. Washington, D.C.: The National Academies Press.
Young, K. and Fairchild, D. (2016). Half of Physician Time Spent on EHR's and Paperwork. NEJM Journal Watch, https://www.jwatch.org/fw111995/2016/09/06/half-physician-time-spent-ehrs-and-paperwork,September 6, 2016.
Young-Breuhl, E. and Schwartz M.H. (2012). Why Psychoanalysis has No History. American Imago, 69(1): 139–159.
Zahra, T. (2015). America, the Not So Promised Land. The New York Times.
Zinn, H. (1980). A People's History of the United States. New York: HarperCollins.

Section II

Therapies of depth, insight, and relationship

7

Relational healing in psychotherapy

Reaching beyond the research

Enrico Gnaulati

Introduction

When psychotherapists are petitioned to decide on the single most important factor contributing to a successful psychotherapy experience, the bulk of them mention "the relationship" (Norcross, 2014). Press the more research savvy ones to "operationalize" what is meant by the relationship and they zero in on characteristics like "the alliance," and "therapist empathy and genuineness." Given the evidence-based politico-scientific climate we are immersed in, the most stalwart spokespersons for the empirical superiority of relational factors undoubtedly would opine that the therapist's alliance-building abilities, empathic responsiveness, and authenticity far outstrip the effectiveness of any technique or method utilized (Laska et al., 2014). Coefficients derived from meta-analyses will likely be enumerated to back up their claims.

What gets lost in the "science wars" is the chasm between the discourse on operationalized definitions of treatment variables and the statistical methods and numerical values that support their effectiveness, on the one hand, and a rather different discourse: prioritizing the need to render scientifically-backed embodied psychotherapeutic attitudes phenomenologically graspable and practically useful. In the case, of empathy, it is one thing to define it as "... the therapist's sensitive ability and willingness to understand clients' thoughts, feelings, and struggles from their point of view" (Rogers, 1957), or report how a meta-analysis of 47 studies uncovered a median *r* of .26 between therapist empathy and psychotherapy outcome (Bohart et al., 2002); it is something entirely different to phenomenologically present and represent therapist empathy so that psychotherapists can incorporate it into their own clinical style in refined and usable ways. This touches upon a frequently overlooked bifurcation in the field: the difference between *declarative knowledge* (factual and definitional information) and *procedural knowledge* (performative abilities). It should come as no surprise to the reader that it is the latter – therapeutic know-how – which practitioners covet to potentiate their work.

What follows is an attempt to reach beyond the empirical interchange and depict certain relational components of effective psychotherapy in descriptive

DOI: 10.4324/9781003325512-10

and evocative terms for pragmatic learning purposes. Obviously, given the intricacies of embodied therapeutic attitudes like alliance-building, empathy, and genuineness, the undertaking will be limited in scope. In ending, I will plead the case for a humanistic revival in the education and training of psychotherapists to equip them to be more relationally adept in their clinical duties and comment on the ramifications of therapist openness and genuineness for notions of professionalism.

Alliance building

The alliance typically refers to the genesis and viability of a collaborative working relationship between client and therapist. It is one of the strongest predictors of successful psychotherapy outcome (Flückiger et al., 2020). Relational-humanistic theorists and practitioners like Bugental (1978) accentuate the growth-promoting features of the alliance: "… a bond between what is best and most dedicated in the therapist and what is most health-seeking and courageous in the client" (p. 72). Not uncommonly, growth is characterized in terms of agreed-upon goals for therapy that are defined *consciously, verbally*, and *explicitly*. Undoubtedly, these have their place, as when client and therapist like-mindedly agree that "less passivity and increased assertiveness would improve the client's chances of getting his needs met, rather than ignored." However, the foundation of a generative alliance pivots more on the salutary subtle intersubjective communications that occur *unconsciously, non-verbally*, and *implicitly* between client and therapist. Paradoxically, during the nascent phase of psychotherapy if there is excessive focus on verbal goal setting and monitoring at a cognitive level, it can foreclose deeper processes of non-verbal affect emergence and resonance leaving the client feeling unrecognized, threatening the formation of a robust alliance. In the words of Wachtel (2018): "We need to explore how to *be with* patients, not just what to say to them" (p. 210).

Most health-promoting interactions in psychotherapy occur at a subliminal or an implicit level (Lyons-Ruth et al., 1998). Moment to moment, the well-attuned psychotherapist is naturally modulating his or her non-verbal behavior to enhance client engagement and recognition. Facial expressivity, eye contact, speech prosody, voice cadence, and physical animation are subliminally coordinated against what clients tacitly need and can tolerate. The well-attuned therapist shows acute awareness of whether his or her expressiveness is too little or too much for the client to assimilate and recalibrates accordingly. It may be a client crossing his legs and averting eye contact indirectly communicating to the therapist she is talking too much, or too loudly. It may be a profoundly uncomfortable silence brought about by the therapist being too non-directive that needs to be broken not by an interpretation that would exacerbate the situation (e.g., *I wonder if the silence is making you uncomfortable?*), but with some lighthearted therapeutic questioning (e.g., *I forgot to ask you how your job interview last week went*).

When psychotherapy is "rolling along" the therapist fluidly tracks and matches the client's shifting emotions with vocal expressions, head nods, well-coordinated facial expressions, and pithy or elaborative verbal statements rooted to the client's level of receptivity. Whether or not the therapist should mute or amplify his or her subjectivity in the room to maximally engender the client's subjectivity is an emotional judgment call. There is a performative dimension to effective psychotherapy. The therapist must be sufficiently skilled at knowing how and when to dampen versus amplify a response, use more words or fewer, prolong or foreshorten an emotional reaction, react animatedly or sedately, make a point loudly or quietly, or make eye contact or avert it. All these micro-decisions must be coordinated as authentic expressions while the therapist rapidly processes verbal and non-verbal in vivo communications. Summing this up, Schore (2003) writes: "Fora working alliance to be created, the therapist must be experienced as being in a state of vitalizing attunement to the patient; that is, the crescendos and decrescendos of the therapist's affective state must be in resonance with similar states of crescendo and decrescendos of the patient" (p. 48).

In the context of this subliminal-transactional conceptualization of the alliance, the client learns to confidently expect full-bodied recognition from the therapist, resulting in more candid self-disclosure. Focal issues that are explicitly referenced as areas of therapeutic aspiration arise situationally and spontaneously out of the client's more transparent confessions and therefore have more personal and emotional meaning than therapy goals arrived at under foreclosed emotional conditions. This might be a client who comes into psychotherapy requesting "tools" to help reduce her anxiety, who when invited to talk more free flowingly about her life situation to a well-enough attuned psychotherapist, realizes she ends romantic relationships prematurely – preemptive action – because she fears men will suddenly abandon her, like her father did to her mother. The client learns she is afflicted with is a form of abandonment anxiety, a realization that has demystifying effects, and that fortifies her in that she knows the past need not repeat itself, both of which help lower her anxiety more resolutely.

Empathic immersion

In the current evidence-based zeitgeist, legions of beginning psychotherapists underappreciate the potency of upholding an empathic stance with clients. Forced to become competent in a smorgasbord of short-term, protocol-driven treatment protocols, they often feel, misguidedly, that they are not being productive enough by simply being *emotionally present*, or identifying with and being moved by clients' subjective experiences in therapeutic ways (Schneider, 2015). Often, there is underexposure to empathy-based models of care (Kahn, 1985; Kaluzeviciute, 2020) that substantiate the need to settle in and become absorbed in the subjective experiential lives of clients; of yielding to and following along with clients' moment-by-moment disclosures; of accepting the free-flowing, non-linear nature of the endeavor; of starting sessions without any conscious agenda, careful to curb one's eagerness to help, confident that something emotionally relevant for the client eventually presents itself.

Empathically immersed psychotherapists give themselves over to the organically unfolding interaction, unconsciously and preconsciously adapting their responses to make them assimilable for a given client. Synchronized, well-timed nods, frowns, grunts, grimaces, leg folds, and chin rubs emotionally lubricate and embolden client disclosures. Optimally, there is abundant barely conscious facial dialoguing that leaves the client feeling the therapist is quietly familiar with what is being revealed, inviting further disclosure.

Sometimes empathic responses by the psychotherapist encompass short phrases or poignant idiomatic offerings inserted into the client's flow of speech to pithily sum up what the client feels. The brevity of the communication reflects a respect for the tempo of the client's speech and a desire to maintain the flow of disclosure, as in the following example:

CLIENT: *Without back-up from my husband I feel I have to go it alone disciplining my kids. It's so unfair since he gets to be the fun parent and I'm the unfun one. You can only imagine how I feel...*
THERAPIST: *Unsupported and underappreciated...*
CLIENT: *Exactly. I don't know how I am going to manage.*

Another form of empathy involves teasing out the implications of clients' word choices and metaphors in ways that draw out disavowed underlying feelings:

CLIENT: *Nothing is going well in my life right now. My friends are avoiding me. My son camps out in his room all day. My husband and I are like ships passing in the night. It's all overwhelming, like there's a big hole in the plane and I'm trying to cover it up...*
THERAPIST: *Planes usually crash when there's a big hole in them.*
CLIENT: (crying) *I know, I'm crashing and burning right now. I feel so defeated and lonely.*

Yet another form of empathy pertains to deep subjective paralleling on the part of the psychotherapist so much so that the synergistic nature of the exchange surrounding the sharing of a troubling life event by a client entails the psychotherapist flitting back and forth from feeling *along with* the client, to *feeling for* the client. The psychotherapist might stand in for the client, supplying a more exact and emphatic communication that simultaneously leaves the client feeling understood and bolsters social and emotional learning by offering an exemplary verbal template:

CLIENT: *I need to learn not to sit back and watch people in my life...* (hesitates)
THERAPIST: *...make a mess of their lives with drugs and alcohol and feel like I have no choice but to sit back and watch...*
CLIENT: *Yes!!*

Real empathic immersion entails emotional engagement and conveyed familiarity with clients' life problems. It is an experiential intermingling of finding oneself in the other while simultaneously discovering the other in oneself. It is not a postured stance resulting in sterile affirmation. It is neither just an applied technique nor "function" the therapist provides. The therapist is emotionally moved by the client's concerns, not removed from them. When psychotherapists give from their humanity, the client not only feels heard, but confirmed. His or her suffering, hopes, aspirations, fears and anxieties, praiseworthy attributes, and personal foibles are not just observed, but authenticated.

Genuine/authentic care

Frank (1999) astutely claims that authenticity as a therapeutic attitude is related to what Rogerian psychotherapists mean by "congruence," a preparedness to be dependably real and respond in a fashion that aligns with one's true thoughts and feelings – to persuasively say what one means and mean what one says. It goes without saying that to practice more authentically as a psychotherapist requires sufficient congruence as a person – display an acquired capacity to act in accordance with one's true intentions. The credible psychotherapist is first a credible person. These personal-psychological achievements get finessed and tailored to the clinical situation – acting naturally and valuing transparency over mystification; directness over indirectness; spontaneity over constraint; tact over tactics; a more egalitarian therapist-client arrangement; and common speech over clinical jargon.

The use of common speech over clinical jargon renders psychotherapy more personal than impersonal, emblematic of a special type of human dialogue than a medical procedure. Using a phrase like, *I wonder if you are unfairly holding your wife responsible for mistakes your mother made*, rather than *perhaps you are displacing your frustration at your mother onto your wife*, is more likely to have de-intellectualizing and emotionally enlivening effects. Verbalized insights modeled after psychotherapist-generated comments such as, *I have trouble holding my ground* and *I exaggerate the danger I'm in ways that worsen my anxiety* are more generalizable to everyday social-communicative situations than, *I'm conflict avoidant and have underdeveloped assertiveness skills*, and *I magnify and need to test the evidence better before making assumptions*. Another form of therapeutic genuineness involves a willingness to engage in what might be called "linguistic authorship" – the use of the first-person pronoun *I* to issue interpretations and therapeutic comments. Psychotherapists are often uneasy about personalized use of language, resorting to second-person and third-person pronouns that are believed to contain an air of objectivity and professionalism: *You say your wife is the one who struggles to manage her anger, but this might be a projection as you yourself seem to struggle to manage your anger* or *Anger is one of those emotions we all have trouble owning and attribute it to others when it is really attributable to the self.*

The comparable statement,... *from what you are telling me I find myself thinking that you, similarly to your wife, might be quick to react with anger*, is languaged whereby it is indisputably authored by the psychotherapist and its potential authoritativeness is predicated on his or her clinical perceptiveness, not on some objective inferential standard.

Prefacing interpretations and clinical comments in personalized ways allows psychotherapists to be authoritative without being authoritarian. They can analyze and deliver therapeutic feedback that derives from their perspective giving clients license to either entertain or reject it based on what seems subjectively applicable or plausible.

Perhaps the most undervalued dimension of practicing with genuineness is the psychotherapist's use of humor (Shearer, 2016). By deploying humor the psychotherapist implicitly establishes him or herself as relatable and approachable and sends a clear message about the likability of the client and the enjoyment of the work together. A humorous remark can shed light on a problem with precision and clarity in non-threatening ways. When clients laugh at the ridiculousness of their beliefs – literally see them as ludicrous – shame is defused, and perspective gained. A clinical example will elucidate.

Joyce, a 27-year-old female, in therapy with me since age 14, was able to extricate herself from a long-term miserable relationship with her first boyfriend but is still susceptible to becoming involved with men who are neither her intellectual equals nor anywhere as adept at pursuing career goals as she. During one of her typical attempts to overlook her 33-year-old boyfriend's poor work ethic and questionable prospects as a mate, and magnify his assets, we had the following exchange:

JOYCE: *I suppose we had a good week and are getting along. We played Monopoly and Scrabble.*

DR. GNAULATI: *So he's good at games involving fake money, but when it comes to the game of life and real money, there are some issues!*

JOYCE: (laughing uproariously) *I know, I know. If he can't even make his share of the rent each month, there's no way I'd ever consider marrying or having kids with him.*

A humorous comment that is on target can also reflect acute empathy, or deep listening and recognition where, simultaneous with an element of surprise, adds up to the client being caught delightfully off-guard. There is immediacy and poignancy to how the client can then absorb the content of what the therapist delivers. Resistances and defenses can be pleasantly by-passed, as reflected in the following clinical vignette:

George, a 45-year-old, hard-edged movie executive was prone to tune me out and ignore my interpretations, conveying superior knowledge on most matters, often hostilely quipping on his way out the door that he did not get his monies worth out of the session. In the midst of complaining that all his efforts to bring contracts into the production company he leads were not being rewarded with an adequate year-end bonus, I offhandedly remarked: *You are the rain maker in your company and you're not getting wet!* George exclaimed: *Exactly!* Jocular quips like this and the reciprocal laugher that ensued, over time, reduced George's aloofness and guardedness and freed him up to heed, rather than dismiss, my therapeutic input.

If clients are to overcome what Sartre (1984) termed "the spirit of seriousness," or their inflexibility and self-righteousness, it necessitates psychotherapists shedding their own professional aloofness, being real, and looking to improvise with humor.

Toward a humanistic revamping of psychotherapy education and training

Despite abundant evidence favoring the need to train early-career psychotherapists in nuanced displays of such humanistic ventures as alliance building, genuineness, and empathy, graduate schools and clinical training sites are awash in non-relational models of care that privilege standardized application and acquisition of techniques – predominantly cognitive behavioral in nature. In clinical psychology doctoral programs, the percentage of faculty aligning themselves with Cognitive Behavior Therapy has risen by about 50% over the past two decades, with an entrenched reconfiguration of psychotherapy as a behavior medicine, technocratic endeavor aimed at reducing psychiatric symptoms (Norcross et al., 2020). In the Veterans Health Administration, the largest mental health training site in the world, short-term, protocol-driven therapies, that require psychotherapists to adhere to formulaic treatment methods, rule the roost (Song et al., 2020).

The education and training of beginning psychotherapists is "science heavy" in ways that are questionably relevant to their future vocational aspirations centering on being demonstrably capable of lessening the emotional suffering of others. Almost 80% of doctoral programs in clinical and counseling psychology require students to take courses on research design, research methods, and advanced statistics (Stein, 2012), even though fewer than 25% of graduates in these domains become university professors or research psychologists (American Psychological Association, 2014). Stein (2012) persuasively argues that research courses deviate from a more intensive focus on clinical training and should be electives for those students bent on becoming academicians or researchers. He draws a comparison to the medical field that is rarely referenced: the education and training of physicians is not tilted in the direction of mandated courses in research methods but direct treatment of identifiable medical problems.

Blanketed by empiricist and data-driven approaches to learning, legions of early-career psychotherapists feel ill-prepared to provide effective care in the regular world of clinical practice (Knafo et al., 2015; McMahon & Hevey, 2017). Construing clinical knowledge as tangential to the personal knowledge used to understand the everyday behavior of real people in the real world deprives newly minted psychotherapists of subjective experiential pathways into clients' sources of anguish (Miller, 2004; Polanyi, 1962). Ready-at-hand citations of studies substantiating the empirical value of therapist empathy as it relates to psychotherapy outcome, or adeptness at supplying an intellectual definition of empathy, are qualitatively different from mastering the procedural knowledge of actually embodying empathy with an in-the-flesh client in the here-and-now. In the words of the innovative psychoanalyst, Peter Lomas (1974): "The forces that have moulded contemporary psychiatry and psychotherapy have, I believe, made it very difficult for two people to meet each other to discuss, in a natural and ordinary way, the problems of one of them" (p. 19). It would not be farfetched to claim that the average psychotherapist educated and trained in sanctioned evidence-based methods faces the peculiar dilemma of having to discard a substantial part of his or her learning simply to ongoingly and thoroughgoingly be emotionally present with clients, uncluttered with internal demands to be directive and productive.

A host of ethical questions emerge related to the under emphasis on clinical relationship-forming skills in graduate school and post-graduate training sites that are beyond the scope of this chapter (Gnaulati, 2019a, 2019b, 2018a). However, a crucial one worthy of consideration pertains to psychotherapy drop-out. Up to 50% of clients who initiate psychotherapy drop-out after the first or second visit, and scarcely 9% attend 20 or more visits (Olfson & Marcus, 2010), even though it is estimated that an effective course of treatment for a typical anxious and depressed client entails at least a year of weekly sessions (Morrison et al., 2003). A key source of premature drop-out is weak treatment alliance (Schoenherr et al., 2019; Sharf et al., 2010). Graduate school courses and training opportunities concentrating on therapeutic alliance-building skills formatted along experiential learning lines are virtually non-existent (Elkins, 2016). This omission in the education and training of beginning psychotherapists is concerning because, conceivably, it contributes to the mental health needs of the public at large being neglected through underpreparing new generations of psychotherapists to maximally engage clients in treatment long enough to reap the benefits.

Allegations of inadequate education and training have also been levied at psychoanalytic institutes. Since its inception, psychoanalysis needed to be rescued from none other than Freud himself lest it become ossified as an arcane, intellectualized pursuit, devoid of spawning true-self experience, emotional enlivenment, and real behavioral change (Gnaulati, 2018b). Even in institutes where relational and intersubjectivity theory have taken hold, the revolutionary implications of these ideas remain stillborn with respect to giving analysts freer license to engage clients with added genuineness, self-disclosure, and personal approachability (Azzone, 2018).

Yet, we remain indebted to the psychoanalytic tradition for its unapologetic endorsement of two core prerequisites that optimally prepare practitioners to embark on their careers: engagement in personal therapy and exposure to case studies. Although psychotherapists' personal therapy has long been considered axiomatic as a quasi-apprenticeship for entering the field and performing meaningful work with clients, some data indicate trainees are shying away from this foundational undertaking (Mix, 2018). One wonders if the evidence-based ethos valorizing fidelity to correct application of techniques has contributed to this downturn by shunting the focus off the salutary effects of psychotherapists' personal adeptness and clinical intuition. If so, this is alarming since the psychotherapist's own therapy remains the single-most important pedagogical platform for performing clinical work (Geller et al., 2005). It is what widens the psychotherapist's emotional thresholds, familiarizing him or her with disavowed darker human tendencies and unmet developmental needs. Plunging into our own therapy primes us to be confidently present and compassionate with clients when they themselves reminisce, grieve, rage, lust, upstage, negate, or access and articulate any number of unformulated experiences that account for their emotional unrest. The more self-awareness and emotional integration derived from their own personal therapy, the stronger the immunity therapists acquire against acting out with clients in ways that bode well for the quality of psychotherapy they offer. Of relevance here is evidence confirming better outcomes and lower drop-out rates in psychotherapy conducted by therapists possessing greater emotional intelligence (Kaplowitz et al., 2011). Psychotherapists' own therapy experience is often the concrete model around which they more confidently construct and enact their own fledgling therapeutic style. This may be why the vast majority of clients prefer seeking treatment from practitioners who have undergone their own psychotherapy (Ivey & Phillips, 2016) and the favorable correlation between psychotherapists' own personal therapy alliance and the successful results of the treatment they provide (Gold et al., 2015).

Case studies, once a potent source of evidentiary knowledge in the field, have been largely sidelined by governing bodies currently approving what constitutes evidence-based psychotherapy practice (McLeod, 2013). Attempts to restore case studies for learning purposes are laudatory since these real-life vignettes often contain rich descriptions of client problems and psychological dynamics in context-sensitive, complexity-preserving ways that serve as templates for beginning psychotherapists to derive a pragmatic understanding of past, present, and future clients (Hoffman, 2009; Miller, 2004). Unlike hypothesis-testing studies – with results written up in abstract and abstruse ways – case study material is more accessible and pragmatically useful, capturing the texture of clients' unique life situation and psychological dynamics, as well as nuanced depictions of therapist interventions. In essence, case studies represent the sort of grounded inquiry and narrative portrayal that avails psychotherapists with direct identification as they compare and contrast depicted dynamics against what they are witnessing in their own client work.

Finally, important voices across the psychoanalytic (Orange, 2016) and existential-humanistic traditions (Elkins, 2009; Krycka et al., 2015; Miller,

2004) are speaking out in favor of would-be psychotherapists receiving a grounding in ethics, or moral philosophy. The rationale here is that psychotherapy is not just a humanistic enterprise, but a *humanitarian* one. Once the discourse on what constitutes psychotherapy is de-medicalized away from techniques aimed at symptom reduction and accentuates the provision of care to alleviate emotional suffering, the good therapist is someone who is ethically responsive to the agonizing problems in living those plague clients. Put differently, the good therapist is someone who cares to care, or suffers along with clients, albeit in a self-differentiated, compassionate way. Not uncommonly, the problems in living clients carry into psychotherapy touch upon virtue ethics and relational ethics: "What is the best version of me that I should strive to become? How can I be more loving? Is it right for me to think I deserve more from my marriage? What is a normal length of time to stay angry over my husband's past infidelities? Will I feel better if I exact revenge, or is better to forgive? If I forgive, am I being masochistic, or magnanimous?" The good therapist makes use of his or her versatile humanity to identify and engage with the client's restricted humanity, or as Van Deurzen (2001) exhorts us: "It is no use occupying the higher moral ground from which we can look down with mere empathy, interpretation, or judgment: we have to struggle with our clients' problems" (p. 108).

Courses on ethics, or moral philosophy, tailored to psychotherapists (Tjeltveit, 1999), would enable trainees to critically ponder a wealth of usable ideas that pertain to the mental wellness goals of clients – What do we mean by the Good Life? Happiness? Love? Virtue? Justice? Loyalty? Forgiveness? Temperance? Courage? Being ethically informed and reflective, trainees would be better equipped to *think their way into* clients' life predicaments. However, if they are to optimally *feel their way into* clients' life predicaments, the clinical training of students will need to incorporate experiential learning opportunities that expand their personal and interpersonal horizons. Graduate schools will need to provide course offerings that augment trainees' own person therapy, encouraging self-disclosure during group activities, and using film, literature, and the arts for experiential learning purposes, thereby emboldening trainees' awareness and expressive mastery of their own personal woundedness and suffering, and how it relates to equivalent experiences shared by clients.

Conclusion: Professionalism reconsidered

Compared to other professions, the personal development of psychotherapists has an unsurpassed role in the effectiveness of the services they offer. If our dentist or accountant seems tactful, discerning, and compassionate, it is a bonus. We employ them for precise application of their technical knowledge, not their human know-how. It is an entirely different matter in the mental health field. The effective psychotherapist somehow must have the presence of mind to become engrossed in a range of vexing client problems without undue doubt or insecurity. Therapists must tolerably suffer what clients find insufferable. We carry clients' unborn grief, sadness, elation, rage, pride, and shame. This capacity requires immense depth and dimensionality of personhood.

Psychotherapists have a professional responsibility to perpetually work on enlarging their self-hood, since this is their therapeutic instrument. Jung's (2003) notion that clients can only discover in themselves emotional potential that has already been attained by their psychotherapist remains germane. It will be difficult for clients to avow aspects of their humanity with a psychotherapist who personally disavows these same inclinations.

In ending, relational modes of care can result in a host of potential boundary violations unless discretion becomes a well-practiced art. The discreet psychotherapist knows how to be friendly, without being the client's friend; bring him or herself to the therapy in self-disclosive ways, without taking over the therapy; be tactfully, rather than tactlessly, honest; know how and when to platonically embrace a client minimizing the potential for seductiveness; and, recognize the client's commendable behavior in non-gratuitous ways, that bolster his or her self-confidence, as opposed to reinforce an other-directed state of mind. This heightened sense of discretion depends greatly on psychotherapists' integrated personhood and degree of self-understanding, psychological achievements that now, more than ever – due to the techno-bureaucratization of psychotherapy – need to be core aspects of ongoing clinical training (Regas et al., 2017).

References

American Psychological Association. (2014). 2010 employment update compiled by center for workforce studies.

Azzone, P. (2018). Understanding the crisis: Five core issues in contemporary psychoanalysis. International Forum of Psychoanalysis, 27(4), 255–265. https://doi.org/10.1080/0803706X.2016.1221134

Bohart, A. C., Elliot, R., Greenberg, L. S., & Watson, J. C. (2002). Empathy. In Norcross, J. C. (Ed.), Psychotherapy relationships that work (pp. 89–107). Oxford University Press.

Bugental, J. F. T. (1978). Psychotherapy and process: The fundamentals of an existential-humanistic approach. McGraw-Hill.

Elkins, D. N. (2009). Humanistic psychology: A clinical manifesto. University of the Rockies Press.

Elkins, D. N. (2016). The human elements of psychotherapy. American Psychological Association.

Flückiger, C., Del Re, A. C., Wlodasch, D., Horvath, A. O., Solomonov, N., & Wampold, B. E. (2020). Assessing the alliance– outcome association adjusted for patient characteristics and treatment processes: A meta-analytic summary of direct comparisons. Journal of Counseling Psychology, 67(6), 706–711. https://doi.org/10.1037/cou0000424

Frank, K. A. (1999). Psychoanalytic participation. The Analytic Press.

Geller, J. D., Norcross, J. C., & Orlinsky, D. E. (Eds.). (2005). The psychotherapist's own psychotherapy: Patient and clinician perspectives. Oxford University Press.

Gnaulati, E. (2018a). Overlooked ethical problems associated with the research and practice of evidence-based treatments. Journal of Humanistic Psychology, 002216781880021. https://doi.org/10.1177/0022167818800219

Gnaulati, E. (2018b). Saving talk therapy: How health insurers, big pharma, and slanted science are ruining good mental health care. Beacon Press.

Gnaulati, E. (2019a). The ethics of neglecting clinical relationship and alliance building in trauma-focused treatments. Ethical Human Psychology and Psychiatry, 21(2), 104–116. https://doi.org/10.1891/EHPP-D-19-00010

Gnaulati, E. (2019b). Potential ethical pitfalls and dilemmas in the promotion and use of American Psychological Association-recommended treatments for posttraumatic stress disorder. Psychotherapy: Theory, Research, Practice, Training, 56(3), 374–382. https://doi.org/10.1037/pst0000235

Gold, S. H., Hilsenroth, M. J., Kuutmann, K., & Owen, J. J. (2015). Therapeutic alliance in the personal therapy of graduate clinicians: Relationship to the alliance and outcomes of their patients. Clinical Psychology & Psychotherapy, 22(4), 304–316. https://doi.org/10.1002/cpp.1888

Hoffman, I. Z. (2009). Doublethinking our way to "scientific" legitimacy: The desiccation of human experience. Journal of the American Psychoanalytic Association, 57(5), 1043–1069. https://doi.org/10.1177/0003065109343925

Ivey, G., & Phillips, L. (2016). Psychotherapy clients' attitudes to personal psychotherapy for psychotherapists. Asia Pacific Journal of Counselling and Psychotherapy, 7(1–2), 101–117. https://doi.org/10.1080/21507686.2016. 1157087

Jung, C. G. (2003). Psychology of the unconscious. Dover Publications.

Kahn, E. (1985). Heinz Kohut and Carl Rogers: A timely comparison. American Psychologist, 40(8), 893–904. https://doi. org/10.1037/0003–066X.40.8.893

Kaluzeviciute, G. (2020). The role of empathy in psychoanalytic psychotherapy: A historical exploration. Cogent Psychology, 7(1), Article 1748792. https://doi.org/10.1080/23311908.2020.1748792

Kaplowitz, M. J., Safran, J. D., & Muran, C. J. (2011). Impact of therapist emotional intelligence on psychotherapy. Journal of Nervous and Mental Disease, 199(2), 74–84. https://doi.org/10.1097/NMD.0b013e3182083efb

Knafo, D., Keisner, R., & Fiammenghi, S. (Eds.). (2015). Becoming a clinical psychologist: Personal stories of doctoral training. Rowman & Littlefield.

Krycka, K. C., Kunz, G., & Sayre, G. G. (2015). Psychotherapy for the other. Duquesne University Press.

Laska, K. M., Gurman, A. S., & Wampold, B. E. (2014). Expanding the lens of evidence-based practice in psychotherapy: A common factors perspective. Psychotherapy, 51(4), 467–481. https://doi.org/10.1037/a0034332

Lomas, P. (1974). True and false experience. Taplinger Publications.

Lyons-Ruth, K., Bruschweiler-Stern, N., Harrison, A. M., Morgan, A. C., Nahum, J. P., Sander, L., Stern, D. N., & Tronick, E. Z. (1998). Implicit relational knowing: Its role in development and psychoanalytic treatment. Infant Mental Health Journal, 19(3), 282–289. https://doi.org/10.1002/(SICI)1097-0355(199823)19:3<282::AID-IMHJ3>3. 0.CO;2-O

McLeod, J. (2013). Increasing the rigor of case study evidence in therapy research. Pragmatic Case Studies in Psychotherapy, 9(4), 382–402. https://doi.org/10.14713/pcsp.v9i4.1832

McMahon, A., & Hevey, D. (2017). "It has taken me a long time to get to this point of quiet confidence": What contributes to therapeutic confidence for clinical psychologists? Clinical Psychologist, 21(3), 195–205. https://doi. org/10.1111/cp.12077

Miller, R. B. (2004). Facing human suffering: Psychology and psychotherapy as moral engagement. American Psychological Association.

Mix, S. A. (2018). Utilization of psychotherapy among doctoral students in clinical and counseling psychology. Dissertation Abstracts International: Section B: The Sciences and Engineering, 79(3–B(E)).

Morrison, K. H., Bradley, R., & Westen, D. (2003). The external validity of controlled clinical trials of psychotherapy fordepression and anxiety: A naturalistic study. Psychology and Psychotherapy: Theory, Research and Practice, 76(2), 109–132. https://doi.org/10.1348/147608303765951168

Norcross, J. C. (2014). The therapeutic relationship. In Duncan, B. L., Miller, S. D., Wampold, B. E., & Hubble, M. A. (Eds.), The heart and soul of change: What works in psychotherapy (pp. 113–141). American Psychological Association.

Norcross, J. C., Sayette, M. A., & Martin-Wagar, C. A. (2020). Doctoral training in counseling psychology: Analyses of 20-year trends, differences across the practice-research continuum, and comparisons with clinical psychology. Training and Education in Professional Psychology. https://doi.org/10.1037/tep0000306

Olfson, M., & Marcus, S. C. (2010). National trends in outpatient psychotherapy. The American Journal of Psychiatry, 167(12), 1456–1463. https://doi.org/10.1176/appi.ajp.2010.10040570

Orange, D. O. (2016). Nourishing the inner life of clinicians and humanitarians: The ethical turn in psychoanalysis. Routledge.

Polanyi, M. (1962). Personal knowledge. University of Chicago Press.

Regas, S. J., Kostick, K. M., Bakaly, J. W., & Doonan, R. L. (2017). Including the self-of-the-therapist in clinical training. Couple and Family Psychology: Research and Practice, 6(1), 18–31. https://doi.org/10.1037/cfp0000073

Rogers, C. R. (1957). The necessary and sufficient conditions of therapeutic personality change. Journal of Consulting Psychology, 21(2), 95–103. https://doi.org/10.1037/h0045357

Sartre, J. P. (1984). Being and nothingness. Washington Square Press.

Schneider, K. (2015). Presence: The core contextual factor of effective psychotherapy. Existential Analysis, 26(2), 304–312.

Schoenherr, D., Paulick, J., Strauss, B. M., Deisenhofer, A.-K., Schwartz, B., Rubel, J. A., Lutz, W., Stangier, U., & Altmann, U. (2019). Nonverbal synchrony predicts premature termination of psychotherapy for social anxiety disorder. Psychotherapy, 56(4), 503–513. https://doi.org/10.1037/pst0000216

Schore, A. N. (2003). Affect regulation and the repair of the self. W.W. Norton.

Sharf, J., Primavera, L. H., & Diener, M. J. (2010). Dropout and therapeutic alliance: A meta-analysis of adult individual psychotherapy. Psychotherapy: Theory, Research, Practice, Training, 47(4), 637–645. https://doi.org/10. 1037/a0021175

Shearer, A. (2016). Why don't psychotherapists laugh? Routledge.

Song, J., Garcia, H. A., Finley, E. P., & Wiltsey Stirman, S. (2020). Graduate training and provider concerns about distress and comprehension in PTSD treatment choice: A mediation analysis. Psychological Services. https://doi.org/10.1037/ser0000429
Stein, D. B. (2012). The psychology industry under the microscope. University Press of America.
Tjeltveit, A. C. (1999). Ethics and values in psychotherapy. Routledge.
Van Deurzen, E. (2001). Paradox and passion in psychotherapy. John Wiley & Sons.
Wachtel, P. L. (2018). Pathways to progress for integrative psychotherapy: Perspectives on practice and research. Journal of Psychotherapy Integration, 28(2), 202–212. https://doi.org/10.1037/int0000089

8

Two perspectives of mental distress

John Thor Cornelius

Introduction

In this chapter, I discuss my work with Whitney to reflect on what I have come to see as a substantial imbalance between two perspectives of mental distress. The Broken Brain perspective understands mental distress from a localized, mechanistic perspective and views it as largely caused by discrete mechanical failures of organic brain function. The Broken Brain perspective is in tension with what I am calling the Symphonic perspective of mind (encompassing, but not limited to, psychodynamic models), which views mental distress as a non-local, wholistic and distributed process spread across the entirety of the mental capacity which results from the impacts of tragic life experience on the normally functioning mind. While these two perspectives overlap in some areas, they most often lead to dramatically different ways of understanding and treating mental distress. And, while the Broken Brain perspective has had preeminence in the last several decades, the increasingly obvious problems regarding its fundamental scientific validity, massive profit-driven biases and problematic long-term, real-world clinical outcomes are of significant concern. While the Symphonic perspective has gone through a period of disrepute, it is increasingly supported both theoretically and clinically by emerging scientific evidence as an efficacious, reasonable and cost-effective treatment approach.

Whitney

Whitney first came to see me after her last provider of mental health services retired. Her only question for me on the phone was whether I was leaving anytime soon. She was relieved when I told her that I had every intention of staying in Sacramento and working for a long time.

During the first meeting, Whitney relayed a disturbing, but all too common, psychiatric history. She had a lifetime of emotional liability including low moods, irritability, insomnia and high anxious energy compounded by periods of unrelenting, forceful crying – so much so that she had been repeatedly hospitalized. She spoke in a rapid, pressured clip that was sometimes hard to follow,

DOI: 10.4324/9781003325512-11

with tears streaming down her face. She let me know she had worked with a variety of mental health professionals over the years and understood her official diagnosis to be bipolar disorder. She took this to mean that her brain was fundamentally broken, and the failure of her various treatments was just confirmation of her terrible genetic condition. Since her feelings were symptoms of her disease, she understood them as problems and felt guilty that she could not "get on with the program" and make her feelings "improve" the way "successful" patients in mental health systems apparently were able to. Whitney denied suicidality even as she was admitted to several inpatient and partial psychiatric hospitalizations for that concern. During one of these hospitalizations, her expressions of distress had been severe enough to prompt a recommendation of electroconvulsive therapy (ECT), which she eventually received. She described the procedure as horrific, made worse by the eerie experience of watching her fellow patients steadily become, in her words, "mindless." She feigned improvement so she could get out of the hospital and escape further ECT treatment. The doctors then encouraged her to have a vagal nerve stimulator surgically implanted in her neck, which she declined.

Physically, she reported she was born with a mild club foot and in midlife experienced a series of disc ruptures in her neck. After a series of repairs that only brought partial relief, her surgeon finally told her she could no longer work full time as a schoolteacher, a job she loved. When Whitney offered to try to work part time, the school district declined and she was put on full-time disability. She also had a history of severe kidney stones and had been hospitalized for their treatment regularly, right up to the time that we first met.

Over decades, she had tried and failed every class of psychotropic medication. She had been on monoamine oxidase inhibitors, tricyclics, serotonergic and noradrenergic antidepressants, mood stabilizers and antipsychotics – I remember being impressed that she had tried most every drug I could think of at the time of the first interview. Her long relationship with medication had begun early; a doctor had prescribed phenobarbital (a barbiturate that is both sedating and life-threatening, currently used in anesthesia, assisted suicide and capital punishment) for night terrors when she was a child. At the time of her intake, she was on a mood stabilizer, a mixed-action antipsychotic, a benzodiazepine, a dual noradrenergic and serotonergic antidepressant and, due to ongoing neck pain, daily methadone, a powerful opioid. I was surprised her body could tolerate the amount of medication in her system. Yet despite all this medication, which left her feeling groggy and "out of it," her symptoms of pain and mental distress were not actually improved, just muffled under a blanket of chronic numbness.

Whitney had no deep friendships, went to an evangelical church despite their distaste for her more liberal beliefs and spent most of her time at home alone. Afraid and completely despondent about her feelings, assuming her brain was broken beyond repair, she had effectively withdrawn from the world. Dreams from this phase of treatment, one where she was sitting far down in a sewer staring into the darkness, and another of a motionless "living room" that contained a freezer with the door open, depicted her withdrawal.

The Broken Brain model of mental distress

The Broken Brain model views mental distress as caused by local, biomechanical breakdowns in organic brain function. The rationale for this model is quite reasonable; it relies upon the same explanatory perspective of mental distress that has been successfully applied in physical medicine for centuries. When someone in physical distress comes to see a doctor, the job of the doctor is to isolate the cause of that distress down to its most rudimentary pathological process, something that is almost always mechanical in nature, with an understandable, scientifically valid etiology. Chest pain, for example, is understood to be a symptom generated by a limited number of discrete causal processes – it may be a fractured rib, pneumonia, a myocardial infarction or referred pain from appendicitis. The doctor uses tests to determine which discrete problem is the cause of the distress, to "localize" the issue down to a specific biomechanical failure, i.e., determine if the problem is either a blockage of the arteries of the heart, a fractured bone, an infection within the lungs or ruptured appendix. Once the discrete problem is identified, different scientifically proven treatments are applied that are uniquely suited for each underlying problem. This reductionistic approach is indisputably effective in physical medicine, garnering justified admiration.

Given its success, it seems logical that the same approach could be applied to mental distress. From this perspective, if someone comes into a mental health provider's office, the job of that provider should then be to trace the complaints down to their most basic and discrete biomechanical causes – "localize" the pathological etiology in the brain. Now there are areas of mental function where this perspective is incredibly effective. For example, if an individual is experiencing seizures, they can be detected using an EEG, and the individual can be given specific medications that decrease their rate or recurrence. There are also a limited set of very clear genetic disorders, such as Huntington's disease, in which a discrete genetic abnormality is passed down, leading to changes in the individual's mental function over time. Again, there are specific tests to detect the genetic code that leads to this pathological protein synthesis and identification of Huntington's disease, thereby optimizing treatment.

Based on the above examples, one might believe that the same approach could apply to *all* psychological complaints. The Broken Brain perspective quietly assumes that such universal application is appropriate and attempts to localize psychological distress down to discrete mechanical brain malfunctions with the hope that isolated mechanical treatments could correct the abnormality, and thus "fix" the "broken brain." It is at this point, however, that the field of mental health runs into a dramatic, and, so far, insurmountable, problem. The problem is that *no generalizable, localized, mechanical etiology of psychological distress has ever been found.* The same can be said for any proposed etiology of any state of mental distress that has been generally described as psychological in nature. Again and again, there are small numbers of cases in which scientists can demonstrate a significant influence by a specific mechanical issue, but any attempt to generalize these etiologies to the larger population of those experiencing psychological distress has failed. To demonstrate this error in thinking here is an example: while it is true that viral infections of the hippocampus cause individuals to experience psychosis, and that antiviral drugs can help dramatically, we can all recognize the error in using that information to claim that *all* psychoses are caused by infections within the hippocampus and then selling antiviral agents as "antipsychotics" to the general population.

Yet those expounding Broken Brain perspectives continue to emphasize such a generalized vision of mental distress. They hypothesize chemical imbalances at the level of the neuronal synapse, abnormally sized and inactive brain regions, and abnormal genetics to be the root cause of psychological distress. Based on these theories, various expressions of mental distress are clustered together and given formal diagnoses. Tests are then given to assess these factors (PET and fMRI scans of the brain, genetic testing, etc.) with the expectation that once these tests are "positive," we'll have "proof" of a causal chain that results in an identifiable pathology within the brain to explain experiences of distress. With a diagnosis and confirmatory testing in hand, the last step is to create a treatment that can "correct" these mechanical brain problems. This is most often a medication, but also includes various other mechanical treatments like ECT, vagal nerve stimulation and transcranial magnetic stimulation (TMS).

The 329 billion ton elephant in the room

The problem with these theories is that they have not been presented merely as interesting hypotheses that need ongoing fundamental research addressing negative evidence and the massive influence of the placebo effect but have instead been fast-tracked and marketed as scientific truth. And while some psychiatrists honestly acknowledge the poor evidence to support them (Pies, 2019), there is so much money in drug treatments (the US spent $329 *billion* dollars on prescription drugs in 2016 alone (Schwartz & Woloshin, 2019)) that pharmaceutical companies can afford to pay billions of dollars every year (approximately $29.6 billion in 2016) marketing the idea that the science supporting their products is solid and that the drugs are effective and safe. Unfortunately, in addition to marketing, these companies have also been repeatedly found to engage in illegal and unethical practices to promote their claims – Abbot, Pfizer, Eli Lilly, Bristol-Myers Squibb, Novartis, Astra Zeneca, Glaxo Smith Klein, Forest Pharmaceuticals, Johnson and Johnson, Merk and more have been found in violation of the Federal False Claims Act for exaggerating drug benefit and minimizing risk, inappropriately expanding who should get their drugs and inappropriately using their financial power to influence physicians and trade groups who prescribe and endorse their products[1] (Field, 2010; Harrington, 2019; violationtracker.org/pharmaceuticals, viewed September 1, 2020).

Simultaneously, drug manufacturers have increasing influence over the science that supports the sale of their products. As any researcher knows, there are many ways to interpret and present data; simple choices around statistical analyses can easily load the dice toward certain outcomes and hide problematic evidence (Preskorn et al., 2015; Rutherford et al., 2009), leading to a reality gap between rosy studies that get FDA approval and the actual outcomes that providers and patients experience in the real world (Zarbin, 2019). To make matters worse, drug companies have been repeatedly caught going so far as directly to bias the evidence base, including flagrant cases of data manipulation and the omission of key findings to make their studies, and therefore their products, look better (Whoriskey, 2012).

Indeed, huge bodies of unpublished negative evidence have been found that would have shown entire drug classes, like antidepressants, to be far less effective than previously claimed (Turner et al., 2008), while key data held by drug companies regarding important side effects like suicidal behavior went unreported or "mis-classified" to the medical community until they were inadvertently discovered (Breggin, 2006). One little-referenced paper regarding the largest antidepressant study ever conducted by the National Institute of Mental Health (*not* a drug company) revealed that despite short-term improvement in mood symptoms, the majority of patients treated with anti-depressants returned to their depressed state within a year of completing the study, most of these within three months (Rush et al., 2008). Along the same lines, a research group at Harvard discovered and was able to force the publication of a huge amount of conveniently unpublished data that demonstrated that antidepressants are far less effective than previously thought and that some studies that had been published as positive were actually negative when the data were independently reviewed (Turner et al., 2008).

Epidemiologic evidence also supports the conclusion that the implementation of antidepressants as a treatment for depression is a failure: despite antidepressant use increasing by almost 400% between 1988–1994 and 2005–2008 (Pratt et al., 2011) culminating with one in eight Americans overage 12 taking an antidepressant (Pratt et al., 2017), the prevalence of depression which was relatively stable, at around 5% between the 1950s and the 1990s (Murphy et al., 2000), showed an increase from 6.6% to 7.3% between 2005 and 2015 (Weinberger et al., 2018). While the CDC reported that the rate of depression did not change between 2007 and 2016, 8.1% of adult Americans experienced a depressive episode between 2013 and 2016 (Brody et al., 2018). For youth, the rate of individuals having a major depressive episode in the last year rose from 8.66 to 13.01% between 2012 and 2017 (Substance Abuse and Mental Health Services Administration (SAMHA), 2018).

Let me state the obvious: given the massive penetration of antidepressants into our society (12.7% of Americans are on a drug class that primarily treats a condition that only 7.3% of us supposedly have), any effective treatment should have decreased the overall prevalence of depression in this country by some amount, yet there is no evidence that this has occurred. Instead, evidence indicates that, at best, antidepressants have done nothing to improve the prevalence of depression in our society, or at worse, that the prevalence of depression has worsened just as antidepressant prescribing has soared.

Suicide rates are also exploding between 1999 and 2020, by a staggering 35%. In 2017, 1.4 million people attempted suicide, with a suicide completed every 11 minutes in 2018 (Hedegaard et al., 2020). Especially concerning is that this increase began at around the time that antidepressants were being introduced to market, while the evidence that antidepressants worsen suicidality in certain populations is substantial (Breggin, 2006; Levin et al., 2018).

Further, a meta-analysis of 17 different studies revealed that simply taking an antidepressant increased an individual's mortality rate by 33% (Brooks, 2017; Maslej et al., 2017). There is also significant evidence that antidepressants independently cause type 2 diabetes (Salvi et al., 2017).

These numbers very much support the conclusion that antidepressants, as a class, are frequently not effective and have significant risks. Yet instead of eliciting a serious, critical and honest scientific debate, antidepressants continue to be promoted as a "first-line" treatment for depression. Unfortunately, many individuals end up like Whitney, on a merry-go-round of revolving and escalating pharmacologic treatments that the evidence shows are not particularly effective for many, if not most, people who take them, especially over the long term.

ECT has a similar history; despite a group of well-funded and vocal proponents, the evidence of ECT providing benefit beyond the placebo effect continues to be controversial and in need of further unbiased exploration. In an intensive re-analysis of ECT, where previous studies were examined on a 24-point quality scale, it was determined that ECT is not effective in the treatment of depression and causes permanent memory impairment (Read et al., 2019). Commenting on the paper, Richard P. Bentall, Professor of Clinical Psychology at the University of Sheffield, described ECT as "a classic failure in evidence-based medicine" (Bentall, 2020).

To find out why these medications and devices are in such widespread use, we need to follow the money. Many physicians, like Marcia Angell MD, a 20-year editor of the *New England Journal of Medicine*, reported with alarm how she witnessed the vast financial power wielded by drug companies being used to alter and influence the medical establishment itself (Angell, 2006). For-profit research companies employ researchers who see themselves more as businesspeople, who are supposed to prioritize profits, than as scientists, who prioritize the truth (Fisher & Kalbaugh, 2012). This re-prioritization of profits was further reinforced when the 1980 Bayh-Dole Act changed federal law to allow universities to patent products and collect revenue on them, removing the shelter academic institutions once provided for impartiality in drug research and scientific inquiry. Unsurprisingly, since that time university professors have also become business people, profiting from their research and, unsurprisingly, have been found to engage in ethical lapses around drug research, from enrolling individuals in studies without their consent, to exaggerating drug results, to downright fraud, all the while taking money from drug companies (Elliott, 2015; Lerner & Moore, 2009).

This influence affects the training of new physicians; outside of a few brave instructors and mentors, the certainty of the Broken Brain perspective was instilled as a basic fact in both my medical school and residency training as a psychiatrist. Many of the academics running these programs, and the institution itself, were receiving large sums of money from drug companies. Methods of critically examining bodies of scientific evidence, including the immense power of the placebo effect (Enck et al., 2011) and the biasing effect of financial influence, were acknowledged but scarcely delved into.

This influence has transformed the entire field: 83% of the panel determining the very definition of psychosis in the Diagnostic and Statistical Manual (DSM)-V had drug company sponsorship (Cosgrove & Krimsky, 2012), over 50% of major medical journal *editors* were receiving money from drug companies (Liu et al., 2017) and government panels that are supposed to review finding and advise the FDA are also regularly staffed by physicians with financial ties to the industry (Piller & You, 2019). How dire is the situation?

> … Similar conflicts of interest and biases exist in virtually every field of medicine, particularly those that rely heavily on drugs or devices. It is simply no longer possible to believe much of the clinical research that is published, or to rely on the judgment of trusted physicians or authoritative medical guidelines. I take no pleasure in this conclusion, which I reached slowly and reluctantly over my two decades as an editor of *The New England Journal of Medicine*. (Angell, 2009)

This behavior has continued unabated for decades and continues to this day; in July 2020, Novartis was fined $678 million for unethical kickbacks to physicians (Vigdor, 2020), its *sixteenth* violation of this type since 2000 (as counted by violationtracker.org, https://violationtracker.goodjobsfirst.org/industry/pharmaceuticals, reviewed August 31, 2020). To give you a sense of scale, there have been 871 violations noted in violationtracker.org since 2000, totaling over 40 billion dollars in fines to the pharmaceutical industry – especially impressive when you realize the violation process regularly includes a long legal battle.

The biasing influence is so widespread that when I present evidence of it in my role as an instructor to future psychiatrists, I don't get surprise or dismay, but merely resigned shrugs and even occasional irritated comments – what are trainees supposed to do when so much of the profession, including those managing medical centers, running universities and in charge of training programs engage in this behavior and are under its influence? Most trainees already know that the real outcomes they see in their clinical rotations don't match the marketing hype manufactured from drug company-sponsored scientific studies. Unfortunately, this cynicism has also led to a disparagement of science in general – if *anything* can be made to look positive in a scientific study, then *everything* is just a marketing ploy.

Yet conversely, despite the evidence of bias that blurs the line between marketing and science, various Broken Brain claims have received so much positive press, commercial support and influence over the years that many news reporters, mental health providers, physicians and the general public have come simply to assume that the scientific bases of these claims are largely settled and that therefore anyone who would say otherwise is simply unscientific. Yet regardless of the marketing and influence, there remains a key difference between the evidence bases for heart attacks vs depression, pneumonia vs bipolar disorder, Huntington's disease vs Schizophrenia: the difference is the gap in scientific validity.

Scientific validity

Scientific validity establishes that an explanation directly mirrors what is happening in the real world and demonstrates that one event directly *causes* the next. It is important to differentiate causation from its close cousin, correlation, which shows merely a temporal relationship between variables. *Correlation does not prove causation, yet the blurring between these two factors occurs again and again and again in the field of mental health.* Do ideas central to the Broken Brain perspective like chemical imbalances, abnormally sized or dysfunctional brain regions and genetics in psychological disorders provide scientifically proven causal chains that establish mental pathology on the order of myocardial infarctions? Does the current diagnostic system itself rest on scientifically validated evidence? Here is just some of the controversy about each of these claims:

Chemical imbalances have been advanced for decades as a central pathological process of mental distress. The idea here is that unlucky individuals have genetic makeups that have led to abnormal levels of neurotransmitters in the chemical synapses of the brain, and that this abnormality is the essential, primary cause of mental distress. This theory was initially proposed because people have varying levels of neurotransmitters in their synapses, and drugs that force alterations in these neurotransmitters are associated with reported mood alterations and psychosis. The leap was then made that altered levels of neurotransmitters were a root cause of not just some individuals' psychological complaints, but of *all* psychological complaints. Meanwhile, scientists had discovered that certain drugs could alter effective neurotransmission in these synapses. These drugs were promptly re-labeled around the symptoms and diagnoses they were marketed to treat ("antipsychotics" and "antidepressants"), implying they somehow "fix" these psychological states.

The problem is that once the marketing and hype is set aside, the evidence supporting these claims is actually quite controversial. In regard to depression, sustained scientific inquiry has been unable to prove a direct causal chain between various levels of serotonin neurotransmission and mood in the majority of people diagnosed as depressed (Lacasse & Leo, 2005; Pies, 2019). Given current knowledge, "Simple biochemical theories that link low levels of serotonin with depressed mood are no longer tenable." (Cowen & Browning, 2015). And while psychoses and an elevation of synaptic dopamine sometimes co-occur, it's again very difficult to prove the process is causal. The complicated and overlapping role of dopamine in the fear response makes the proof of a causal relationship extremely difficult (i.e., that elevated dopamine levels result from being anxious and afraid, which is a *correlated* relationship with psychosis, but not *causal*) (Hardy & Mueser, 2017; Ikegami et al., 2014). Other identified problems include biases present in the current research of psychoses (for example, that most research is conducted on people chronically taking antipsychotics, drugs that independently cause abnormalities in dopamine levels). Thus, the very scientific validity of the dopamine hypothesis itself is still a matter of basic scientific debate (Hengartner & Moncrieff, 2018).

Unfortunately, rather than wrestling with the fundamental problems in these hypotheses (which would necessitate an honest reexamination of the issues and an investment of real money in unbiased basic research while pulling back from many of the claims made in trade journals and commercials), many promoters of chemical imbalances have taken to simply sidestepping acknowledgment of the problems altogether, which has led to the need to read the scientific literature in mental health *very carefully*. For example, one needs to be observant of words like *suggest*, regularly used to make sweeping generalizations that elide controversy. For example, Jeffery Lieberman MD, a university psychiatrist who is affiliated with 14 drug companies and has his own patent on a drug, states, "This pathophysiological model of psychosis is based on many studies that suggest that excess synaptic levels of dopamine and glutamate cause increased postsynaptic stimulation, the downstream effects of which result in psychotic symptoms." (Lieberman & First, 2018).[2] Contrast this with the title of an article by Hengartner and Moncrieff, who are without drug company sponsorship: "Inconclusive Evidence in Support of the Dopamine Hypothesis of Psychosis: Why Neurobiological Research Must Consider Medication Use, Adjust for Important Confounders, Choose Stringent Comparators, and Use Larger Samples" (Hengartner & Moncrieff, 2018). Ronald Pies, a psychiatrist and professor at Tufts University who lectures on bioethics, summarizes: "... The 'chemical imbalance' image has been vigorously promoted by some pharmaceutical companies, often to the detriment of our patients' understanding. In truth, the 'chemical imbalance' notion was always a kind of urban legend – never a theory seriously propounded by well-informed psychiatrists." (Pies, 2011).

Meanwhile, many studies look at the brain scans of individuals who complain of certain psychological phenomena. And indeed, many of these individuals are found to have variations in the *size or activity of different parts of their brains* compared to controls. While this tells us interesting information, it doesn't show that these decreased brain volumes are the *cause* of the mental experience in question, nor that when a brain area is found to be smaller or less active, it's "broken," necessitating mechanical treatments like TMS to provide a "cure." Indeed, the study of neuroplasticity suggests something else entirely: that the size of various brain regions fluctuates in response to use. Rather than changes in brain volumes or activity being the *cause* of various forms of mental activity, including mental distress, they are just as likely to be the *result* of these activities. And again, just because things happen at around the same time, they are not necessarily causal – *correlation does not prove causation.* More accurately, the brain is not actually "broken" in many of these situations but is simply responding to the environment and situations it is exposed to and the various demands placed on it.

For example, a recent article looked at individuals with first episode psychosis and showed that those in its active grip had reduced volumes of their hippocampi, something repeated in multiple studies. However, as some participants demonstrated resolution of their psychotic complaints, an enlargement of their hippocampi occurred right along with it (Lappin et al., 2013). Reinterpreting data from this neuroplastic perspective makes it so much of the current research in this area is actually unexciting in that it's similar to reporting that Olympic sprinters have more muscle mass in their legs than professional boxers and that both have more muscle mass than those who are not exercising altogether. Interpreting the evidence this way supports the theory that the brain is not pathologically malfunctioning in these situations, but instead may be engaging in a natural response to its demand environment and history. It's also important to keep in mind that this means brain volumes and activity are not predictive of future capacities, nor does it tell us anything permanent about an individual. Instead, modern neuroplasticity research demonstrates that brain volume and activity are in constant flux, changing to reflect its use and the demands placed on it. The good news is that most anyone can start training (i.e., start therapy) and reap benefits, and not be catastrophically constrained by their existing state.

In regard to genetics, while a plethora of published papers show associations between psychological states and various lengths and types of chromosomal material, it has become increasingly apparent that much of the research in this area is deeply and fundamentally flawed due to its overreliance on a method called genome-wide association (GWA) in that "... the GWA approach can be problematic because the massive number of statistical tests performed presents an unprecedented potential for false-positive results" (Pearson & Manolio, 2008). For example, literally thousands of papers claim an association between psychosis and variations in specific genes. A single paper in 2016 found 514 new proteins associated with psychosis alone (Ganapathiraju et al., 2016). The error here is that all these statistical *associations* are taken to indicate that Schizophrenia is causally genetic, despite, as the title of one peer-reviewed article states,

"No Evidence That Schizophrenia Candidate Genes Are More Associated With Schizophrenia Than Noncandidate Genes." (Johnson et al., 2017).

After reviewing hundreds of proposed candidate genes, the researchers cited above intensively studied the top 25 with the most evidentiary support and found that *none* of the schizophrenia candidate genes in question were likely to be causative in schizophrenia, and most were no more associated with schizophrenia than would be expected by chance. The authors go so far as to say that this should serve as a cautionary tale for all genetic researchers to prevent future inappropriate implications of genetic causality.[3] Since that time the same critique has been used to overturn similar conclusions made regarding sexual orientation and genetics (Ganna et al., 2019). The journal *Nature* trumpeted, "There is no Gay Gene" (Lambert, 2019). To say this more broadly: in the vast majority of situations, our genes do not determine our minds.

Psychiatric diagnoses

A "revolution" happened in mental health around the development of the DSM-III (Spiegel, 2005). Promising to make the field of mental health "scientific," a group of psychiatrists led by Robert Spitzer revamped the existing diagnostic system based on a psychoanalytic understanding of mind, instead creating the discrete, check-listed criteria with which mental health professionals are so familiar. This update was heralded as a revolutionary advance, but while it was well received by insurance companies and some prescribers, there has always been a dark cloud hanging over it. For example, the DSM-IV was supposed to have been scientifically validated and received a large grant from the MacArthur Foundation for that purpose, yet the data was never published or revealed – those in charge later claimed they ran out of money. Subsequent editions of the DSM have been critiqued even by the creators of the DSM itself (Frances, 2014), to the extent that Thomas Insel, the head of the NIMH, withdrew support for the DSM-V in 2013, stating very clearly that it lacked basic scientific validity (Insel, 2013). Yet the DSM continues to be used in nearly every mental health clinic within the United States and is referenced across the globe.

When I was a chief resident in psychiatry at the University of California, Davis, a speaker from the NIMH, described meeting with one of the DSM's creators, who sheepishly admitted that the two-week criteria for depression were chosen because "it just seemed right, and we had to choose something." Other authors have similarly pointed out that the diagnostic clusters themselves are quite arbitrary – they simply "made sense" to the particular psychiatrists involved in the process, without validated scientific evidence (Frances, 2014). When you realize that people's lives are dependent upon the details of these diagnostic criteria due to reimbursement refusal by insurance companies, the pseudo-scientific and arbitrary nature of these criteria should be extremely disturbing. To save the DSM, the American Psychiatric Association (APA) has tried to focus on reliability (trying to get everyone to say the same thing) and downplay validity, but the absence of scientific validity makes the entire process dubious. This critique is reinforced by my observation of many doctors in many different settings over many years: the attempt to have reliability cover for a lack of validity does not work in real-world practice. Doctors diagnose on the basis of what they think is really going on, so a lack of solid scientific validity means different doctors get different answers. This led to situations in my training where one clinic notoriously diagnosed almost every patient with bipolar disorder or narcissistic personality disorder. In another, one attending was known for diagnosing borderline personality disorder … in nearly everyone. This pseudo-validity has meant that it is more important for trainees to know how a particular clinic or attending wants people to be diagnosed than to know any overarching, scientifically valid diagnostic system. On a larger scale, diagnoses fluctuate throughout the country and over time: there have been periods with unusually high levels of dissociative identity disorder diagnoses followed by backlash periods in which there are almost none. Let me say that the actual patients and their underlying psychological expressions did not change during these fluctuations, nor did the evidence base provide a clarification regarding the underlying science; it was provider and public opinion that charted the course. The APA itself had to put brakes on the diagnosis of childhood bipolar disorder, because the rate was escalating at such a frenetic clip that even psychiatrists became alarmed about the tidal wave of over-diagnosing (Frances, 2010) and over-prescribing (Iordache & Low, 2010) with serious, life-threatening side effects.[4] The critique here, made by a significant number of mental health providers, scientists, participants in the creation of the DSM and even NIMH, is that implicitly assuming scientific validity without actually having it creates a situation that not only impairs further scientific inquiry, but is potentially clinically harmful to patients.

The good news, I believe for everyone, is that once the evidence base for these perspectives is returned to the realm of reality, there is more space to think deeply and creatively about novel and radically different methods of treating people in psychological distress.

The Symphonic perspective of mind

In contrast to the Broken Brain model that asserts the scientific validity of localized biomechanical pathology within the brain, the Symphonic perspective prioritizes the fundamentally interconnected nature of the mind. This distributed processing perspective is relational rather than localized, normalizing rather than pathologizing, humanistic rather than mechanical. Priority is placed on the unique and nuanced quality of the ongoing relationships between processing systems, including the interplay between brain regions, psychic structures within the mind (referred to as mental objects, selves, or parts), different people and groups such as a family, and between therapist and client.

The Symphonic perspective offers a metatheory general enough to encompass various branches of modern psychoanalytic theory, including relational psychoanalysis, object relations, field theory, attachment theory and mentalization based therapy (MBT) as well as a significant number of other contemporary treatments like open dialogue, narrative therapy, family systems theory, and internal family systems theory. And just as it's somewhat nonsensical to ask which individual musician in a symphony is "playing all that music," the Symphonic perspective finds it questionable to the point of nonsense to over-localize and pathologize most mental distress.

Instead, the Symphonic perspective sees emotions and most forms of psychological distress as resulting from the healthy and normal function of the mind. By "normal" here I do not mean happy or pleasant – these are tragic impacts of *experiences of human life* on brains that are functioning and responding normally to extreme, tragic and often chronic human experiences. Whether biomechanical issues are happening or not, the *primary* etiology of the distress is the entirety of the human relational experience; biology is simply responding in supportive and non-pathological ways – ways that may be extremely difficult but were likely evolutionarily compatible with prolonging survival of the species. Offering a case example that contrasts with the case of Whitney can help differentiate these perspectives.

Margaret came in reporting an intractable "low mood" that had started suddenly in her 50s, and which had resisted all attempts at treatment – years of pharmacologic and psychological treatments had been in vain. She had an unremarkable mental health and childhood history but did tell me that in the period before the onset of low mood she had a very distinct and clearly organic event that had led to permanent neurologic impairment at roughly the same time as the mood changes. Closer inspection of the mood complaint also revealed that the woman's "depression" was more accurately described as a dramatic loss of drive, atypical in any previous part of her life. A brain scan revealed a small infarct in a frontal lobe of her brain indicating a small stroke. My course of action was to cross taper her psychotropic regimen to rely increasingly on stimulants, a class found particularly helpful in those struggling with the mental repercussions of strokes (Gall, 2001). While the stimulants didn't return her to her baseline level of function, it was pretty close, and Margaret has had a stable course over the years. While we initially continued psychotherapy, it quickly became clear that our conversations were not really required except around a normal process of grieving about what had happened and the time lost. To me, Margaret's situation best exemplifies a primarily mechanical and localized dysfunction of her organic brain, which necessitates that something "broken" be "fixed."

Whitney's childhood history was very different. Her club foot caused a very strong reaction in her mother – family lore was that her mother did not unwrap Whitney for three days, seeming to "forget" to notice her abnormality. Since that time, Whitney was openly referred to as broken. The mother rarely held

Whitney and interfered with her husband doing so. As Whitney grew older, she was regularly referred to by her parents as a "jinx" and was further differentiated from the rest of the family. When the family played bridge, Whitney was forced to be the "dummy" and was never taught to play. While the mother stayed home to care for the other children, she returned to work during Whitney's childhood, leaving her as an early latchkey child. Her mother accused her of being a drug dealer in seventh grade and assumed she was homosexual – both claims completely inconsistent with Whitney's personality or behaviors. When Whitney had questions about major life events like the onset of menses, she was given a box of tampons and told to read the directions. The only sentence she was told about sex by her mother was to "make sure the guy pulls out." Whitney, desperate for physical contact, would often pretend to be asleep in the car so she had to be carried into the house and reported periods of desperate energy, as demonstrated in a childhood movie of her running frantically in the foreground and biting a garden hose in distress while her family engaged in other activities, oblivious. She was told that her childhood bedroom and toys were not hers and to leave her dolls untouched so she would not "ruin" them. Until late in childhood, Whitney drew herself without arms. She had a period of head banging that stopped when her mother grabbed her head and forcibly slammed it into the floor. Her chronic night terrors were "treated" with phenobarbital, which led to episodes of sleepwalking. She brought me a childhood observation report done at her school in which the observer was surprised to discover that Whitney's father had been in the room during the observation because there appeared to be no relationship between them – Whitney and her father treated each other like strangers. Later, a school nurse noticed Whitney's suffering and made inquiries to the home, but this only resulted in disparaging remarks about the nurse and a complete denial of any problems by the family.

In contrast to Margaret, Whitney's distress was long-standing; she described feeling terrible, fearful, confused and crushingly lonely for much of her childhood. She also let me know she fundamentally agreed with her mother: She was a terrible, broken child who *should* feel bad and likely did not deserve basic care – or even to live. Later in her life, this criticism was carried inside of her – an internal voice constantly criticizing and undermining any hopeful thought she had. Like so many children deeply affected by adversity, she would regularly refer to her childhood as normal, going along with the testaments of her parents and siblings and the fact that her family was solidly middle class and her mother was well appreciated at work. The only place she felt regularly connected to her mother was at church, where they both had an affinity for music and participated in the choir.

Whitney presents a good example of the lack of usefulness of the current diagnostic system, in that various diagnoses were constantly thrown around her and yet none of them mattered in a way that led to clinical improvement. They were not predictive of her course in ways that were illuminating and did not help direct her care in any way that led to true, long-lasting improvement. Of course, after getting a new diagnosis and a new drug, she might say "I *think* I feel better" for a while, but none of it lasted. Just like so many, she received a long run of diagnoses, medications and treatments – mood stabilizers (for bipolar symptoms), antidepressants (for depression symptoms), benzodiazepines (for anxiety) and antipsychotics (because nothing was working and she still couldn't sleep). If anything, the application of various invalid diagnoses by mental health providers caused Whitney additional iatrogenic psycho-logical damage and worsened her psychological state, being quite in line with what her mother had repeatedly told her about being fundamentally broken – a jinx.

Listening, context and dialogue rather than diagnosis and pathologizing

When we approach Whitney from a Symphonic perspective, things change dramatically. This perspective understands that outside of a rare set of organic phenomena, psychological distress is fundamentally a non-local, distributed process of mental function that is not reflective of mechanical brain pathology. It views the various parts of the brain as being different members of the orchestra who have responded to the music they have been given to play. This orchestra has been, and continues to be, directly influenced by its environment. Minds that are surrounded by stable, predictable and benign environments learn to play in distinctly different ways than minds surrounded by unpredictable or harsh environments.[5] This difference in turn leads to the production of very different music. And while the music is, of course, influenced at some level by organic components of the brain, we cannot and should not ignore the primacy of context and environment in understanding mental distress. Here, the actual, real-world context of the individual can replace diagnoses in relatively short order.[6] However, to accomplish this, we need to do something that is becoming increasingly absent from psychiatrists' offices – the need to humbly and sincerely engage with those with whom we work for prolonged periods of time so we can come deeply to understand them – something that simply is impossible in 15-minute medication management appointments that are scheduled months apart. Let's take a look at Whitney and apply this perspective.

This perspective recognizes that Whitney has a normal brain but had parents who chronically struggled in fundamental ways that were not intentional. Her situation was tragically common, as noted by Dr. Nadine Burke Harris, the current Surgeon General of California, who refers to childhood adversity as one of the greatest unrecognized epidemics of our age (Harris, 2014). I listened to how Whitney lived with a chronic underlying sense of terror and confusion as a child. Instead of receiving essential guidance about the fundamental management of feeling states, learning how to cope and think in stressful situations, she was left alone to incorporate intelligent but desperate strategies. And cope she did – she learned to take the bus at a young age, she figured out she had to avoid the stranger who wanted her to enter his car and she got into college and even became a successful member of her university's basketball team – largely self-taught. Yet all these difficult experiences also resulted in the diverse symptomatology she experienced throughout her life. Head banging, night terrors, sleepwalking and biting might be thought of as efforts to express or work off high-energy states – something that in another family would be worked through via parental holding, comfort, understanding and appropriate challenging. Instead, Whitney's early attachments and experiences explain why her interactions with others were such an anxiety-producing struggle throughout the rest of her life. Given her parent's chronic criticism, lack of physical holding and her "latchkey kid" status, it makes sense that she struggled to interpret other people's intentions; it should come as no surprise that her first marriage was to a clever and manipulative drug addict, which she didn't recognize at the time despite evidence in hindsight.

Similarly, we should recognize the way that Whitney's second marriage to a much more stable man was truly a blessing for her. When this man was diagnosed with terminal cancer at a young age it was extraordinarily hard on Whitney, probably harder than a similar tragedy would be on others without her childhood difficulties. With family stories of her being a jinx, it made tragic sense that she felt deeply responsible for that man's death, further magnifying her grief, to the point of being convinced she should die instead of her husband. Given her experience of being misunderstood and having limited help metabolizing her grief after his death, it's easy to understand why her despair escalated to the point of hospitalizations.[7] If you thought your existence jinxed the ones you love, you would feel horrible as well.

In this light, Whitney's responses stop seeming bizarre or arbitrary or biomechanically "pathological" and instead become understandable and reasonable in a tragic way. Many, if not most, people growing up with Whitney's level of adversity would respond with struggles on a similar level.[8] Through this lens we can recognize that her tragedy is not localized inside Whitney's synapses or determined by her genes, but within her life experience itself. It should also then make sense why medications, ECT and vagal nerve stimulation would be at best an indirect treatment of Whitney's psychological distress. It's the deep and ongoing music of mind, reflecting the past and the present, that is primary in the Symphonic perspective – an idea consistent with the current understanding of memory integration (Schlichting & Preston, 2015). I would no more expect a French speaker to spontaneously speak Chinese than I would expect someone with Whitney's level of adversity to experience lasting change in a short time period – it's frankly bizarre when this expectation is implied in some scientific literature, the media or commercials for pharmaceutical companies. Whitney was formed in a world that offered dramatic shortages of attention, coordinated familial cooperation, understanding and attachment. Given the chronicity of Whitney's course, then, any thought of sustained improvement through the application of a short-term treatment is simply not in keeping with clinical observation, childhood adversity research, the attachment literature, modern learning theory, or even brain research's fundamental assumptions of neuroplasticity and the neuroscience of memory.

Given the concerns about Broken Brain evidence, while we can appreciate the anecdotal evidence of Whitney's recovery, we might wonder: is there is any scientific validity regarding Symphonic treatments? The answer is a resounding yes (Barsness, 2018; Cornelius, 2014; Shedler, 2011; Steinert et al., 2017). Many studies, both individual and meta-analyses, by impartial research teams like the Cochrane Library, demonstrate the long-term benefit of these forms of treatment (Abbass et al., 2006). In addition, a key benefit is that in contrast to other treatments, many of the Symphonic studies demonstrate the continuation of their effects long after formal treatments end (Bateman & Fonagy, 2008; Bergström et al., 2018; Leichsenring et al., 2013). Even more impressive is that these treatments have shown effectiveness in individuals struggling with a whole range of symptom clusters that traditional psychiatry has found difficult to treat – not just depression and anxiety (Leichsenring et al., 2013), but also psychoses (Bergström et al., 2018) and the complex struggles conventionally leading to a diagnosis of Borderline Personality Disorder (Bateman & Fonagy, 2008). The biggest difference in the impact of these studies compared to studies from a Broken Brain perspective is their lack of penetration into the marketplace, an absence of financial and political backing, and an unwillingness on the part of the mental healthcare industry to face decidedly difficult truths about the role that marketing has had in shaping healthcare.

Beginning symphonic treatment and deprescribing

Consistent with a Symphonic understanding of mental function, work with Whitney was slow.[9] We met multiple times a week, in which she laid down on my couch and mostly cried. Symphonic work involves joining the suffering individual, engaging in a deep and painful dialogue, maintaining empathy and metabolizing terrible experiences. It is guided by ideas like truth, suffering and purpose. And given its depth, I struggled right along with Whitney. It was a hard, painful journey, but as is often the case in deep ongoing therapy, it began to work. Whitney's dreams began to shift, first reflecting the tragic depth of her distress, then gradually including the existence of benign figures, and finally incorporating surprisingly hopeful themes, including one of winning the lottery. Her capacity to cope with her life improved and she became more active. Her disorganization around her distress decreased and her periods of panic around people became more manageable. With a renewed sense of purpose, Whitney switched to a different church that was more accepting of her, and she began to tutor children. She began to develop friendships, got a dog and went on trips. Several years into our work, I asked her if she felt she needed to be on all those drugs.[10] While she had clearly recognized that the medications were not helpful, my question surprised her – she had not really imagined that she could live without them. Yet once she realized that I honestly believed deprescribing was a reasonable thing for us to try, she took on the process with vigor.

Unfortunately, deprescribing is not without significant risks (Gupta & Cahill, 2016). Mood fluctuations, agitation and even suicidal thoughts can increase when these drugs are decreased and withdrawn, especially if done too quickly (Fava & Belaise, 2018). And worse, in contrast to the process of mental distress itself, in which brain changes have generally been shown to return to previous levels of function (Wiswede et al., 2014), some of the effects of drugs and ECT have been found to be permanent (Read et al., 2019; Stroup & Gray, 2018). For Whitney however, the realization that her brain was not *inherently* broken was incredibly valuable to her. Maybe she wasn't a jinx after all. The tapering of medications took years. But she did indeed stop them all; the benzodiazepine, the antidepressant, the mood stabilizer and the antipsychotic. She reported that a fog was lifting from her mind and her emotional range improved and normalized. Rather than feeling chronically numb, her ability to feel her full and authentic range of feelings began to return. Her cognition improved. She then recognized how her physical pain was also influenced by what she had been through, and with incredible courage, she slowly but completely tapered off her methadone as well. She has been off all mind-altering medication for the last seven years, and while she struggles, she reports that these symptoms are now, at their worst, the same as they were when she was taking the medications, just without all the horrible side effects.

There have been no hospitalizations, no suicide threats, no need for ECT, and the clarity of her thinking has improved while her level of incapacitation has dramatically decreased. She now works, runs her church choir, vacations with friends and is looking into dating. Interestingly, her medical conditions have improved as well – her kidney stones, which were so severe that they regularly necessitated ER visits and hospitalization, have become only an intermittent inconvenience. Whether it was a change in diet, an interaction between some of her medications, a decrease in her baseline stress level as a result of the therapy or an additional unknown factor is unclear. Yet given the overwhelming incidence of physical illness associated with childhood adversity, it makes sense that effective psychological treatments can affect the occurrence and severity of physical illnesses (Harris, 2018).

Costs

Broken Brain advocates tend to advance their arguments in a typical manner. They begin by asserting superior scientific validity, then offer a general exaggeration and generalization of benefits associated with drugs like antidepressants and treatments like ECT (or TMS, or vagal nerve stimulators, or ketamine, or psilocybin). However, after those arguments are exhausted, they finally assert that psychological treatments are *more* expensive than Broken Brain treatments. It must be expensive to have trained professionals see people for such intensive, long periods of time, right? The idea of cost *saving* is then used to support the use of the Broken Brain perspective.

It's difficult to generalize costs, since they vary by region, and data is frequently obfuscated by profiting organizations so a full evaluation is outside the scope of this paper. But to get a ballpark range, I will engage in a decidedly unscientific, back-of-the-envelope calculation of the treatment costs for someone like Whitney, an individual in severe and chronic distress and a history of repeated hospitalizations and medical comorbidities, using numbers from the Sacramento area determined through an informal polling of colleagues. If we factor in the medicines, Whitney was on when we first met and imagine she was taking the same medicines today, their current out-of-pocket would be around $4,000 per year on GoodRx.com. A psychiatrist, who would ideally see Whitney monthly, typically charges at least $2,000 per year at that frequency. The costs for psychiatric hospitalization vary dramatically, with negotiated costs estimated at about $9,000 nationally in 2017 (Unger, 2019), while uninsured individuals report costs of up to $3,500 *per day*, with most hospitalizations in the 5–10-day range (Chatel, 2019; Unger, 2019). In Sacramento, individuals move from the inpatient hospital to a 10-day partial hospitalization program (PHP) (estimated at $13,000 including doctors' fees) and then an intensive outpatient (IOP) program costing $11,000, together totaling around $24,000 for 6 weeks (N. Pardo, personal communication, August 19, 2020). ECT costs around $2,400 per treatment, not including doctor's fees (J. Sidley, personal communication, August 26, 2020) and a single course of ECT consists of at least 10–15 treatments (Ross et al., 2018). Methadone treatment is about $6,000 per year (NIDA, 2020). We also have to add ER visits that cost $1,300 per visit on average (Alltucker, 2019), since those in severe distress have a significantly increased and regular use of both ERs and hospitalization (Chow et al., 2019). It is also well known that psychotropic medications cause a whole host of severe and chronic medical illnesses, including a dramatic increase in the occurrence of diabetes directly related to the drugs (Holt, 2019; Salvi et al., 2017), which adds approximately $16,000 per person per year in treatment costs (Riddle & Herman, 2018). Each hospital stay for Whitney's kidney stones cost roughly $15,000 dollars (CALPIRG Education Fund, 2012). Additionally, the indirect costs of severe depression have been estimated at $15,000 per year, not including the costs of lost income (Chow et al., 2019). Finally, there is the cost of the increased morbidity caused by the antidepressants and antipsychotics themselves, which significantly increase the occurrence of heart disease, strokes, falls, cognitive impairments and a host of other ailments that affect specific populations like the elderly. While yearly expenses would fluctuate for someone like Whitney, we are talking about costs ranging from $40,000 to far over $100,000 per year – not including the intangible, human cost of missing out on all the things they would have done if they had not been incapacitated. Whitney spent decades without the satisfactions of work, productivity, creative interests, social relationships and travel. Instead, she was isolated at home, feeling miserable and alone. And to make this list complete, I should add that the financial cost of one person completing suicide is estimated at $1,329,553 (Shepard et al., 2015).

In contrast, someone in Whitney's level of distress usually comes to see me between two and five times a week, at a cost of between $18,000 and $50,000 per year. Make no mistake; this is an intensive, serious and expensive treatment. Yet these numbers are reasonable in the context of potential benefits (decreases in drugs and their side effects, psychiatric and medical hospitalizations, ER visits, ECT and its permanent memory damage, opioids, suicidality and other ancillary medical costs) and increases in the ability and desire to return to work, life satisfaction, friends, accomplishments. And most important, given the transformative power of Symphonic therapies, these expenses, while extensive, are also time-limited as evidence shows people get better, for life. This is not wishful thinking or cherry-picking; these ongoing changes in lifestyle and medical utilization through Symphonic treatments such as mentalization and open dialogue interventions for severely disturbed and even psychotic patients are born out in research (Bateman & Fonagy, 2008; Bergström et al., 2018; Seikkula et al., 2006). Not only did these therapy programs have high and long-lasting recovery rates from severe forms of distress but showed markedly less service utilization and increased social and economic recovery over the long term. The Finnish district that piloted open dialogue reduced their mental health services costs by a third during the initial five years of study, while outcomes simultaneously improved. For individuals and society as a whole, Symphonic psychotherapy, even though intensive, is cost-effective over the long term – especially relative to other options for those in serious and chronic psychological distress.

What's left

Whitney continues to face an ongoing mountain of grief, sadness and anxiety about how to be intimate with other people. She recently let me know it was the 25th anniversary of her second husband's death. We both sensed that marking the date was important, so we decided to meet at the gravesite. It was a beautiful spring day at the community cemetery, and children rode their bikes on the hilly road weaving through the grounds. After a brief hug, Whitney told me that her husband hated water spots, so she pays an annual fee to have them removed from his headstone even though she knows she really doesn't have to. Then we fell quiet for a while. Whitney idly knelt and rubbed an empty spot next to her husband's name. "This is where I was going to be… I am so glad I didn't do that now… but I still wonder if it would have been better if I had died and not him. I still think he was a lot better at living than me… but it was 25 years ago! It's been a long time… and I was just out of it for so much of that. I really only think I have come out of it in the last five years or so." Then she looked up, and our eyes filled with tears. "… but I have like, what, 25 years left? Maybe 20. I can do something with that."

Notes

1 For example, it was revealed in 2009 that the National Alliance for Mental Illness (NAMI) received the vast majority of its drug funding from drug companies (Harris, 2009).
2 The writers of this review article go on exclusively to describe the process of psychosis from a Broken Brain perspective, completely leaving out negative evidence and other theories that also have scientific support. This is in contradiction to the spirit of review articles, which are supposed to offer balanced and thorough overviews of a subject. At the very end of the article, Dr. Lieberman discloses he is affiliated with 15 different drug companies. This is even more breathtaking when you realize this article was published in the New England Journal of Medicine, a premier medical journal of the United States.
3 Another often repeated claim is that twin studies of those with schizophrenia supposedly showed a high rate of heredity. Another look at that data has revealed that the authors of these series of papers engaged in a series of statistical inflation techniques to achieve these numbers. If you remove those statistical inflators and use the regularly accepted method of determining heredity, the results are much, much lower – very much in keeping with the argument I have presented here (Ross & Ross, 2018).
4 For example, a study from 2019 found an increase in the rate of unexplained death in children prescribed antipsychotics, a class of drug regularly prescribed to children with these diagnoses (Ray et al., 2019).
5 This is entirely in keeping with our understanding of other lasting mental phenomena like language. Those who learn English early keep speaking English, those who learned Greek early keep speaking Greek, etc. Changing primary language, including emotional language, is a difficult thing.
6 I have found that I can write a short paragraph describing an individual's history and expressions of distress integrated with my understanding of the problem that is far more helpful to myself, the individual, the family and other professionals than ever using the DSM.
7 It was at this point that Whitney's parents finally began to recognize their role in their daughter's distress. With great courage, they approached Whitney and began acknowledging their treatment of her. This began a positive transformation for Whitney. I believe it was this capacity for change, as exhibited by her parents, that saved Whitney's life.
8 Broken Brain scientists have difficulty understanding why some people clearly struggle with certain events more than others, and look toward genetics, chemical imbalances, etc. for answers. However, given the mounting evidence around the shockingly high rates of childhood adversity, it is increasingly obvious that this confusion can be more straightforwardly explained through an understanding of childhood and familial trauma (Harris, 2018).
9 I work in a way informed primarily by Donald Winnicott, Wilfred Bion and contemporary field theorists like Antonino Ferro and Guiseppe Civitaresse, combined with ideas derived from the Open Dialogue techniques developed in Finland.
10 Approximately 20% of those with whom I work continue to take some form of psychotropic medication on a regular basis. While I intend psychotropic drugs to be used for short durations during times of extreme distress and only after an extensive review of their significant risks and limited benefits, there are still occasions in which I believe medications are the best course of action – just far less often than is promoted in the psychiatric literature.

References

Abbass, A., Hancock, J., Henderson, J., & Kisely, S. (2006). Short-term psychoanalytic psychotherapies for common mental disorders. *Protocols Cochrane Database of Systematic Reviews*. https://doi.org/10.1002/14651858.cd004687.pub2

Alltucker, K. (2019, June 4). 'Really astonishing': Average cost of hospital ER visit surges 176% in a decade, report says. *USA Today*. Retrieved August 17, 2020, from https://www.usatoday.com/story/news/health/2019/06/04/hospital-billing-code-changes-help-explain-176-surge-er-costs/1336321001/

Angell, M. (2006). *The truth about the drug companies: How they deceive us and what to do about it*. Scribe.

Angell, M. (2009, August 30). *Drug companies & doctors: A story of corruption*. The New York Review of Books.

Barsness, R. E. (2018). *Core competencies of relational psychoanalysis: A guide to practice, study and research*. Routledge.

Bateman, A., & Fonagy, P. (2008). 8-Year follow-up of patients treated for borderline personality disorder: Mentalization-based treatment versus treatment as usual. *American Journal of Psychiatry AJP*, *165*(5), 631–638. https:// doi.org/10.1176/appi.ajp.2007.07040636

Bentall, R. (2020, June 4). *Guest blog by Richard P. Bentall: ECT is a classic failure of evidence-based medicine*. Council for Evidenced Based Psychiatry. http://cepuk.org/2020/06/04/guest-blog-by-richard-bentall-ect-is-a-classic-failure-of-evidence-based-medicine/

Bergström, T., Seikkula, J., Alakare, B., Mäki, P., Köngäs-Saviaro, P., Taskila, J. J.,... Aaltonen, J. (2018). The family-oriented open dialogue approach in the treatment of first-episode psychosis: Nineteen–year outcomes. *Psychiatry Research*, *270*, 168–175. https://doi.org/10.1016/j.psychres.2018.09.039

Breggin, P. R. (2006). Court filing makes public my previously suppressed analysis of paxil's effects. *Ethical Human Psychology and Psychiatry*, *8*(1), 77–84. https://doi.org/10.1891/ehpp.8.1.77

Brody, D. J., Pratt, L. A., & Hughes, J. (2018). *Prevalence of depression among adults aged 20 and over: United States, 2013–2016*. NCHS Data Brief, no 303. National Center for Health Statistics.

Brooks, M. (2017, September 21). *Antidepressants tied to a significantly increased risk for death*. Medscape Psychiatry. Retrieved July 31, 2020, from https://www.medscape.com/viewarticle/886015

CALPIRG Education Fund. (2012, Summer). *Your Price May Vary - Geographic Variation in Hospital Charges in California*. Retrieved August 17, 2020, from https://calpirg.org/sites/pirg/files/reports/Your%20Price%20May% 20Vary%20web.pdf

Chatel, A. (2019, February 7). *The cost of mental health hospitalization is part of what makes mental healthcare inaccessible*. Bustle. Retrieved August 25, 2020, from https://www.bustle.com/p/the-cost-of-mental-health-hospitalization-is-part-of-what-makes-mental-health-care-inaccessible-15919218

Chow, W., Doane, M., Sheehan, J., Alphs, L., & Le, H. (2019, February). Economic burden among patients with major depressive disorder: An analysis of healthcare resource use, work productivity, and direct and indirect costs by depression severity. *American Journal of Managed Care*. Retrieved August 30, 2020, from https://www.ajmc.com/ view/economic-burden-mdd

Cornelius, J. (2014, October). *The case for psychoanalysis, version 4 {Video file}*. John Cornelius, M.D. https://www. youtube.com/watch?v=IQBx5TONHac

Cosgrove, L., & Krimsky, S. (2012). A Comparison of DSM-IV and DSM-5 panel members' financial associations with industry: A pernicious problem persists. *PLoS Medicine*, *9*(3): 1–4. https://doi.org/10.1371/journal.pmed.1001190

Cowen, P. J., & Browning, M. (2015). What has serotonin to do with depression?. *World Psychiatry*, *14*(2), 158–160. https://doi.org/10.1002/wps.20229

Elliott, C. (2015, May 26). The University of Minnesota's medical research mess. *New York Times*. Retrieved September 02, 2020, from https://www.nytimes.com/2015/05/26/opinion/the-university-of-minnesotas-medical-research-mess.html

Enck, P., Klosterhalfen, S., Weimer, K., Horing, B., & Zipfel, S. (2011). The placebo response in clinical trials: More questions than answers. *Philosophical Transactions of the Royal Society B: Biological Sciences*, *366*(1572), 1889–1895. https://doi.org/ 10.1098/rstb.2010.0384

Fava, G., & Belaise, C. (2018). Discontinuing antidepressant drugs: Lesson from a failed trial and extensive clinical experience. *Psychotherapy and Psychosomatics*, *87*(5), 257–267. https://doi.org/10.1159/000492693

Field, R. I. (2010). Antipsychotic medications are spelling legal trouble for drug makers. *P & T: A Peer-reviewed Journal for Formulary Management*, *35*(11), 621–622. PMID:21139818

Fisher, J. A., & Kalbaugh, C. A. (2012). United States private-sector physicians and pharmaceutical contract research: A qualitative study. *PLoS Medicine*, *9*(7), e1001271. https://doi.org/10.1371/journal.pmed.1001271

Frances, A. (2010, April 8). Psychiatric diagnosis gone wild: The "epidemic" of childhood bipolar disorder. *Psychiatric Times*. Retrieved July 25, 2020, from https://www.psychiatrictimes.com/view/psychiatric-diagnosis-gone-wild-epidemic-childhood-bipolar-disorder

Frances, A. (2014). *Saving normal: An insider's revolt against out-of-control psychiatric diagnosis, DSM-5, big pharma, and the medicalization of ordinary life*. William Morrow.

Gall, A. (2001). Post-stroke depression. *British Journal of Therapy and Rehabilitation*, *8*(7), 252–257. https://doi.org/10.12968/bjtr.2001.8.7.13779

Ganapathiraju, M. K., Thahir, M., Handen, A., Sarkar, S. N., Sweet, R. A., Nimgaonkar, V. L.,... Chaparala, S. (2016). Schizophrenia interactome with 504 novel protein-protein interactions. *NPJ Schizophrenia*, *2*(1), 16012. https://doi. org/10.1038/npjschz.2016.12

Ganna, A., Verweij, K. J., Nivard, M. G., Maier, R., Wedow, R., Busch, A. S.,... Zietsch, B. P. (2019). Large-scale GWAS reveals insights into the genetic architecture of same-sex sexual behavior. *Science*, *365*(6456), 6456. https://doi.org/10.1126/science. aat7693

Gupta, S., & Cahill, J. D. (2016). A prescription for "deprescribing" in psychiatry. *Psychiatric Services*, *67*(8), 904–907. https:// doi.org/10.1176/appi.ps.201500359

Hardy, K. V., & Mueser, K. T. (2017). Editorial: Trauma, psychosis and posttraumatic stress disorder. *Frontiers in Psychiatry*, *8*, 220. https://doi.org/10.3389/fpsyt.2017.00220

Harrington, A. (2019). Chapter 8. In *Mind fixers: Psychiatry's troubled search for the biology of mental illness* (pp. 247–270). W.W. Norton & Company.

Harris, G. (2009, October 21). Drug makers are advocacy group's biggest donors. *The New York Times*.

Harris, N. (Director). (2014). *{Video file}*. TED. Retrieved July 17, 2020, from https://www.ted.com/talks/nadine_burke_harris_how_childhood_trauma_affects_health_across_a_lifetime

Harris, N. B. (2018). *DEEPEST WELL: Healing the long-term effects of childhood adversity*. Houghton, Mifflin, Harcourt.

Hedegaard, H., Sc, C., & Warner, M. (2020). *Increase in suicide mortality in the United States, 1999–2018*. NCHS Data Brief, no 362. National Center for Health Statistics.

Hengartner, M. P., & Moncrieff, J. (2018). Inconclusive evidence in support of the dopamine hypothesis of psychosis: Why neurobiological research must consider medication use, adjust for important confounders, choose stringent comparators, and use larger samples. *Frontiers in Psychiatry*, *9*. https://doi.org/10.3389/fpsyt.2018.00174

Holt, R. I. (2019). Association between antipsychotic medication use and diabetes. *Current Diabetes Reports*, *19*(10), 96. https://doi.org/10.1007/s11892-019-1220-8

Ikegami, M., Uemura, T., Kishioka, A., Sakimura, K., & Mishina, M. (2014). Striatal dopamine D1 receptor is essential for contextual fear conditioning. *Scientific Reports*, *4*(1): 1–10. https://doi.org/10.1038/srep03976

Insel, T. (2013, April 29). *Post by former NIMH director Thomas Insel: Transforming diagnosis*. NIMH. Retrieved July 25, 2020, from https://www.nimh.nih.gov/about/directors/thomas-insel/blog/2013/transforming-diagnosis.shtml

Iordache, I., & Low, N. C. (2010). The overdiagnosis of bipolar disorder. *Journal of Psychiatry & Neuroscience: JPN*, *35*(3), E3–E4. https://doi.org/10.1503/jpn.100032

Johnson, E. C., Border, R., Melroy-Greif, W. E., Leeuw, C. A., Ehringer, M. A., & Keller, M. C. (2017). No evidence that schizophrenia candidate genes are more associated with schizophrenia than noncandidate genes. *Biological Psychiatry*, *82* (10), 702–708. https://doi.org/10.1016/j.biopsych.2017.06.033

Lacasse, J. R., & Leo, J. (2005). Serotonin and depression: A disconnect between the advertisements and the scientific literature. *PLoS Medicine*, *2*(12), e392. https://doi.org/10.1371/journal.pmed.0020392

Lambert, J. (2019, August 29). No 'gay gene': Massive study homes in on genetic basis of human sexuality. *Nature*. Retrieved August 30, 2020, from https://www.nature.com/articles/d41586-019-02585-6

Lappin, J. M., Morgan, C., Chalavi, S., Morgan, K. D., Reinders, A. A., Fearon, P.,... Dazzan, P. (2013). Bilateral hippocampal increase following first-episode psychosis is associated with good clinical, functional and cognitive outcomes. *Psychological Medicine*, *44*(6), 1279–1291. https://doi.org/10.1017/s0033291713001712

Leichsenring, F., Abbass, A., Luyten, P., Hilsenroth, M., & Rabung, S. (2013). The emerging evidence for long-term psychodynamic therapy. *Psychodynamic Psychiatry*, *41*(3), 361–384. https://doi.org/10.1521/pdps.2013.41.3.361

Lerner, M., & Moore, J. (2009, March 19). Once-secret drug-company records put U on the spot. *Star Tribune*. Retrieved September 02, 2020, from https://www.startribune.com/once-secret-drug-company-records-put-u-on-the-spot/41470522/?refresh=true

Levin, M., Jury, N., Mohseni, K., & Srinivasan, V. (2018, November 7). *Do antidepressants increase suicide attempts? Do they have other risks?* National Center for Health Research. Retrieved August 29, 2020, from http://www.center4research.org/antidepressants-increase-suicide-attempts-risks/

Lieberman, J. A., & First, M. B. (2018). Psychotic disorders. *New England Journal of Medicine*, *379*(3), 270–280. https://doi.org/ 10.1056/nejmra1801490

Liu, J. J., Bell, C. M., Matelski, J. J., Detsky, A. S., & Cram, P. (2017). Payments by US pharmaceutical and medical device manufacturers to US medical journal editors: Retrospective observational study. *BMJ*, j4619. https://doi.org/ 10.1136/bmj.j4619

Maslej, M. M., Bolker, B. M., Russell, M. J., Eaton, K., Durisko, Z., Hollon, S. D.,... Andrews, P. W. (2017). The mortality and myocardial effects of antidepressants are moderated by preexisting cardiovascular disease: A meta-analysis. *Psychotherapy and Psychosomatics*, *86*(5), 268–282. https://doi.org/10.1159/000477940

Murphy, J. M., Laird, N. M., Monson, R. R., Sobol, A. M., & Leighton, A. H. (2000). A 40-year perspective on the prevalence of depression. *Archives of General Psychiatry*, *57*(3), 209. https://doi.org/10.1001/archpsyc.57.3.209

NIDA. (2020, June 14). *How much does opioid treatment cost?*. Retrieved 2020, August 16 from https://www.drugabuse.gov/publications/research-reports/medications-to-treat-opioid-addiction/how-much-does-opioid-treatment-cost

Pearson, T. A., & Manolio, T. A. (2008, March). How to interpret a genome-wide association study. *JAMA*, *299*(11), 1335–1344. https://doi.org/10.1001/jama.299.11.1335

Pies, R. (2011, July 11). Psychiatry's new brain-mind and the legend of the 'chemical imbalance.' *Psychiatric Times*. Retrieved July 24, 2020, from http://www.psychiatrictimes.com/blogs/couch-crisis/psychiatry-new-brain-mind-and-legend-chemical-imbalance

Pies, R. (2019, August 2). Debunking the two chemical imbalance myths, again. *Psychiatric Times*. Retrieved July 24, 2020, from https://www.psychiatrictimes.com/view/debunking-two-chemical-imbalance-myths-again

Piller, C., & You, J. (2019, February 27). Hidden conflicts? Pharma payments to FDA advisers after drug approvals spark ethical concerns. *Science*. Retrieved August 29, 2020, from https://www.sciencemag.org/news/2018/07/hidden-conflicts-pharma-payments-fda-advisers-after-drug-approvals-spark-ethical

Pratt, L. A., Brody, D. J., & Gu, Q. (2011). *Antidepressant use in persons aged 12 and over: United States, 2005–2008*. NCHS data brief, no 76. National Center for Health Statistics.

Pratt, L. A., Brody, D. J., & Gu, Q. (2017). *Antidepressant use among persons aged 12 and over: United States, 2011– 2014*. NCHS Data Brief, no. 283. National Center for Health Statistics.

Preskorn, S. H., Macaluso, M., & Trivedi, M. (2015). How commonly used inclusion and exclusion criteria in antidepressant registration trials affect study enrollment. *Journal of Psychiatric Practice*, *21*(4), 267–274. https://doi.org/10.1097/pra.0000000000000082

Ray, W. A., Stein, C. M., Murray, K. T., Fuchs, D. C., Patrick, S. W., Daugherty, J.,... Cooper, W. O. (2019). Association of antipsychotic treatment with risk of unexpected death among children and youths. *JAMA Psychiatry*, *76*(2), 162. https:// doi.org/10.1001/jamapsychiatry.2018.3421

Read, J., Kirsch, I., & Mcgrath, L. (2019). Electroconvulsive therapy for depression: A review of the quality of ECT versus sham ECT trials and meta-analyses. *Ethical Human Psychology and Psychiatry*, *21*(2), 64–103. https://doi.org/ 10.1891/ehpp-d-19-00014

Riddle, M. C., & Herman, W. H. (2018). The cost of diabetes care—An elephant in the room. *Diabetes Care*, *41*(5), 929–932. https://doi.org/10.2337/dci18-0012

Ross, C. A., & Ross, A. W. (2018). Misleading use of heritability estimates in schizophrenia genetics. *Psychosis*, *11*(1), 90–91. https://doi.org/10.1080/17522439.2018.1545862

Ross, E. L., Zivin, K., & Maixner, D. F. (2018). Cost-effectiveness of electroconvulsive therapy vs pharmacotherapy/ psychotherapy for treatment resistant depression in the United States. *JAMA Psychiatry*, *75*(7), 713. https://doi.org/ 10.1001/ jamapsychiatry.2018.0768

Rush, A. J., Trivedi, M. H., Wisniewski, S. R., Nierenberg, A. A., Stewart, J. W., Warden, D., & Fava, M. (2008). Acute and longer-term outcomes in depressed outpatients requiring one or several treatment steps: A STAR*D report. *Focus*, *6*(1), 128–142. https://doi.org/10.1176/foc.6.1.foc128

Rutherford, B. R., Sneed, J. R., & Roose, S. P. (2009). Does study design influence outcome?. The effects of placebo control and treatment duration in antidepressant trials. *Psychotherapy and Psychosomatics*, *78*(3), 172–181. https://doi.org/10.1159/000209348

Salvi, V., Grua, I., Cerveri, G., Mencacci, C., & Barone-Adesi, F. (2017). The risk of new-onset diabetes in anti-depressant users – A systematic review and meta-analysis. *PLos One*, *12*(7): 1–14. https://doi.org/10.1371/journal. pone.0182088

Schlichting, M. L., & Preston, A. R. (2015). Memory integration: Neural mechanisms and implications for behavior. *Current Opinion in Behavioral Sciences*, *1*, 1–8. https:// doi.org/10.1016/j.cobeha.2014.07.005

Schwartz, L. M., & Woloshin, S. (2019). Medical marketing in the United States, 1997-2016. *JAMA*, *321*(1), 80. https://doi.org/ 10.1001/jama.2018.19320

Seikkula, J., Alakare, B., Aaltonen, J., Haarakangas, K., Keränen, J., & Lehtinen, K. (2006). Five years experiences of first-episode non-affective psychosis in open dialogue approach: Treatment principles, follow-up outcomes and two case analyses. *Psychotherapy Research*, *16*, 214–228. https://doi.org/10.1080/10503300500268490

Shedler, J. (2011). The efficacy of psychodynamic psychotherapy. *Psychodynamic Psychotherapy Research*, *9–25*. https://doi. org/10.1007/978-1-60761-792-1_2

Shepard, D. S., Gurewich, D., Lwin, A. K., Reed, G. A., Jr., & Silverman, M. M. (2015). *Suicide and suicidal attempts in the United States: Costs and policy implications*. Suicide and Life-Threatening Behavior.

Spiegel, A. (2005, January 3). The dictionary of disorder: How one man revolutionized psychiatry. *The New Yorker.*

Steinert, C., Munder, T., Rabung, S., Hoyer, J., & Leichsenring, F. (2017). Psychodynamic therapy: As efficacious as other empirically supported treatments? A meta-analysis testing equivalence of outcomes. *American Journal of Psychiatry*, *174* (10), 943–953. https://doi.org/10.1176/appi.ajp.2017.17010057

Stroup, T. S., & Gray, N. (2018). Management of common adverse effects of antipsychotic medications. *World Psychiatry*, *17*(3), 341–356. https://doi.org/10.1002/ wps.20567

Substance Abuse and Mental Health Services Administration. (2018). *Key substance use and mental health indicators in the United States: Results from the 2017 national survey on drug use and health* (HHS Publication No. SMA 18-5068, NSDUH Series H-53). https://www.samhsa.gov/data/

Turner, E. H., Matthews, A. M., Linardatos, E., Tell, R. A., & Rosenthal, R. (2008). Selective publication of antidepressant trials and its influence on apparent efficacy. *New England Journal of Medicine*, *358*(3), 252–260. https://doi.org/10.1056/ nejmsa065779

Unger, L. (2019, October 31). *Grief grew into a mental health crisis and A $21,634 hospital bill.* KHN. Retrieved August 25, 2020, from https://khn.org/news/grief-grew-into-a-mental-health-crisis-and-a-21634-hospital-bill/

Vigdor, N. (2020, July 2). It paid doctors kickbacks. Now, Novartis will pay a $678 million settlement. *New York Times*. Retrieved August 27, 2020, from https://www.nytimes.com/2020/07/01/business/Novartis-kickbacks-diabetes-heart-drugs.html

Weinberger, A., Gbedemah, M., Martinez, A., Nash, D., Galea, S., & Goodwin, R. (2018). Trends in depression prevalence in the USA from 2005 to 2015: Widening disparities in vulnerable groups. *Psychological Medicine*, *48*(8), 1308–1315. https://doi.org/10.1017/S0033291717002781

Whoriskey, P. (2012, November 24). As drug industry's influence over research grows, so does the potential for bias.*Washington Post*. Retrieved August 29, 2020, from https://www.washingtonpost.com/business/economy/as-drug-industrys-influence-over-research-grows-so-does-the-potential-for-bias/2012/11/24/bb64d596-1264-11e2-be82-c3411b7680a9_story.html

Wiswede, D., Taubner, S., Buchheim, A., Münte, T. F., Stasch, M., Cierpka, M.,… Kessler, H. (2014). Tracking functional brain changes in patients with depression under psychodynamic psychotherapy using individualized stimuli. *PLoS One*, *9*(10), e109037. https://doi.org/10.1371/journal.pone.0109037

Zarbin, M. (2019). Real life outcomes vs. clinical trial results. *Journal of Ophthalmic & Vision Research*, *14*(1), 88–92. https://doi.org/10.4103/jovr.jovr_279_18

9

Diagnosis and its discontents

Reflections on our current dilemma

Nancy McWilliams

Introduction

In this essay, I explore the social construction of psychopathology and the unintended consequences of our currently dominant psychiatric taxonomies. In that context, I review the development of both editions of the *Psychodynamic Diagnostic Manual* (PDM; Lingiardi & McWilliams, 2017; PDM Task Force, 2006), an endeavor intended to preserve clinically meaningful diagnostic practices and to bridge the gap between, on one hand, the categorical, "neo-Kraepelinian" diagnosis exemplified in the classifications of the *Diagnostic and Statistical Manual* (DSM) of the American Psychiatric Association and the *International Classification of Diseases* (ICD) and, on the other, the traditional "biopsychosocial" clinical practice of diagnostic formulation. Contributors to the PDM effort tried to preserve a diagnostic sensibility that is not simply categorical but also dimensional, inferential, contextual, and integrative.

The term "diagnosis" comes from Greek root words meaning "understanding" and "through," a combination that implies an in-depth, focused meaning-making. In that original sense, all clinicians who struggle to understand the suffering of their patients engage in a diagnostic process. Currently, putatively in the service of such efforts, therapists are pressed from many directions to match patient data to preexisting categories that have been arrived at by expert consensus. This process has some value, but as Ludwig Wittgenstein famously observed, the language in which we speak about something determines our ability to think about it. Although there are ample and erudite critiques of the categorical, descriptive, symptom-based taxonomies that predominate in our era (e.g., Frances, 2013; Sadler, 2005), clinicians all nevertheless feel the effects of being required to speak in a language that constricts how we can think and what we can imagine.

Our overall challenge in the area of clinically meaningful diagnosis seems to me to be a piece of a larger problem endemic to large democratic societies: When decisions are made on the basis of statistical averages and mass impact, bureaucracy thrives, but thoughtful attention to individuality declines, along with sensitive consideration of the needs of distinct sub-groups. In bureaucratized

DOI: 10.4324/9781003325512-12

cultures, people easily find themselves feeling like nameless, faceless cogs in some huge machine, or, if still animate, like Kafka's cockroach. This dehumanizing effect can be particularly problematic when individual and group differences matter greatly, as they do in psychology and psychotherapy. Depending on someone's current situation, personality, life stage, gender experience, economic position, ethnic and racial identity, and many other factors, one person's sanity can be another person's craziness. For an overly controlled woman, to act impulsively may be an achievement, whereas impulsivity would be more-of-the-same pathology for her chronically out-of-control friend. A Hindu man's respect for astrology has a different meaning from an appeal to the stars for guidance by a woman who was raised as a Lutheran.

Within the lifetimes of many of us, the mental health field has undergone a gradual but profound shift, away from trying to understand the unique patient and toward assigning labels based on categories of psychological suffering about which academic experts concur. Within recent memory, therapists were trained to develop for each client a "case formulation" that attempted to capture what was unique to that person. Such a formulation included observations about the individual's temperament, maturational issues, defenses, emotional tendencies, identifications, relationship patterns, underlying beliefs and conflicts, and sources of self-esteem, among other factors. Contemporary therapists who value case formulation also consider attachment styles, experiences of trauma, and issues of privilege and diversity when conceptualizing individuality.

Currently, therapists are expected instead to formulate patients' suffering in terms of agreed-upon, nameable "disorders." In the DSM and ICD, psychological problems have been grouped together based on whether they share certain externally observable symptoms. Rather than developing and testing hypotheses about the ultimate nature of each person's problem (the "local clinical scientist" model long advocated by George Stricker (Stricker & Trierwelier, 1995), one matches the patient's report to pre-formulated criteria for each category. Along with this shift have come powerful pressures to restrict the client's treatment to specific procedures that have been shown, in research that depends on artificial conditions and statistical averages, to reduce measurable symptoms that define those reified disorder categories. As with most top-down change, certain efficiencies have resulted, but at a heavy hidden price.

Psychiatry has developed differently in this respect from other areas of medicine, in which we do not find problems categorized as, for example, "fever disorders" or "skin rash disorders," or "tremor disorders." Instead, physical illnesses are grouped by the underlying systemic causes of their symptoms, as inferred from the patient's history, current circumstances, and description of the intensity and severity of the person's experience. But because psychiatry is a young science, and there are few mental health problems for which experts agree about causes, the American Psychiatric Association has classified them by their manifest symptoms. And that poses a big problem for therapists.

The legacy of changes in diagnostic conventions

In the 1970s, there was a concerted professional push to change psychiatric classification from more *inferential, dimensional, contextual* diagnosis to *descriptive* and *categorical* ways of characterizing mental suffering. Inferential diagnosis involves the assumption that a symptom is expressing something, that it has origins and meaning. Dimensional diagnosis assumes that most people have elements of any notable psychological condition, and that whether it should be considered a problem is a matter of *degree*, not *kind* (as in Harry Stack Sullivan's famous comment, "We are all more simply human than otherwise" – Sullivan, 1973). Contextual diagnosis means that a person with, for example, observable "paranoid" tendencies who is being realistically persecuted must be understood differently from a person who has become paranoid in a benign environment. In contrast, descriptive diagnosis deliberately avoids assumptions about meaning or cause, and categorical diagnosis assumes that psychopathology is best understood in terms of distinct disorders that are either present or absent rather than in terms of a spectrum that runs from, say, normal obsessional tendencies to diagnosable obsessive-compulsive disorders, in which one infers pathology only toward the end point of a long continuum.

This "neo-Kraepelinian" movement (that is, a movement back toward the assumptions of the great 19th-century psychiatric observer, Emil Kraepelin – See, e.g., Clegg, 2012; Klerman, 1978; Spitzer, 1991) was the product of at least two challenges that mental health professionals were facing in the second half of the 20th century. First, they were trying to reduce the difficulties facing mental health researchers, whose work was burdened by the fact that different professional communities observed different diagnostic practices. In the United Kingdom, for example, a constellation of symptoms that in the United States would be diagnosed as schizophrenia was more likely to be diagnosed as manic-depressive psychosis. Behavioral scientists were frustrated with these divergences and wanted uniformity so that their findings could be applied across societies and groups with somewhat different mental health conventions.

Researchers were stymied also by the belief of many therapists that one cannot make a reliable diagnosis until a client has been in treatment long enough for his or her psychological patterns to have become visible *within the therapeutic relationship*. Empirical investigators wanted agreed-upon, present-versus-absent criteria that they could employ without having to undergo extensive clinical training or see patients for weeks before choosing research subjects. Some researchers reported, for example, having asked clinicians for their criteria for diagnosing narcissistic personality disorder and having been told something like "You take the person into treatment, and if a self-object transference develops, that's evidence of a narcissistic organization."

Second, the diagnostic syndromes described in the first two editions of the DSM of the American Psychiatric Association were heavily infused with the assumptions of psychoanalysis, the prevailing explanatory psychiatric paradigm of the first half of the 20th century. By the late 1960s, there were other models accounting for psychopathology, including biological psychiatry, a wide range of humanistic approaches, family systems models, behavioral analyses, and the nascent cognitive psychology movement. There was a clear need for nomenclature that did not privilege one theoretical preference over others.

With the publication in 1980 of the third edition of the DSM, these problems were addressed by a manual intended to meet the needs of researchers and nonpsychoanalytic therapists, as well as those of billing organizations, funding entities, and demographic record-keepers. It was descriptive rather than inferential and depicted discrete disorders rather than ranges and variations on themes. One of my first epiphanies about the downside of this change occurred in the 1990s, when I was invited to speak at a well-respected psychiatric hospital. I was asked to interview, in front of the medical residents, two patients who presented confusing diagnostic pictures. Like most competent therapists, I was able to make a relationship with each individual, and both patients revealed to me vital information that the staff had not known. As I was leaving, I heard one resident remark, "That's a great line she uses. I'm going to use that line when I interview patients." I got curious and asked him which "line" of mine he was referring to. His answer was "Can you say more about that?"!

This young doctor, a bright and highly compassionate young man, had been trained on DSM-III and was poised to ask questions such as, "Has the problem bothered you for more than two weeks or less than two weeks?"– questions for which there are yes or no answers, questions that do not invite unexpected disclosures. He knew how to fit the patient into preexisting categories but not how to learn from the patient something about what it is like to be in that person's shoes. A friend who trains psychiatric residents reports asking them questions like, "How do you understand the patient's anxiety?" and sometimes receiving puzzled looks and the "explanation" that "The patient has an anxiety disorder." The idea that one is anxious (or depressed or obsessive) *about* something that has meaning is being lost. Fitting an individual into a category tends to foreclose exploration of what is unique to a patient; it especially prevents insights into unexpected aspects of a person's psychology or exploration of areas that are felt as shameful – the very areas that are of particular value in planning and carrying out psychotherapy.

Since that time, things have only gotten worse for those of us who want to understand individuals in all their complexity. Students in many helping professions, not just psychiatry, are trained on the DSM as a kind of "bible" of available mental health problems and are not asked to listen with curiosity and humility to a person's idiosyncratic subjective experience. Unless one equates symptom removal with overall mental health, the DSM has no implicit concept of psychological wellness. As with any committee product, the manual is a political compromise reflecting diverse influences (See Pilecki et al., 2011) and, as its authors explicitly stated until its most recent incarnation (DSM-5), was not designed to substitute for clinical inference. As many have pointed out, the current DSM is a poor reflection of the range and depth of human suffering, and its uncritical use has contributed to the over-medication and misunderstanding of many conditions.

The unintended consequences of efforts at cost containment

There is impressive, long-standing evidence that traditional psychotherapy not only reduces psychopathology (e.g., Lambert et al., 2001; Morrison et al., 2003; Seligman, 1995) but also prevents or mitigates problems that create significant long-term social costs, such as physical illness, addiction, crime, incarceration, and loss of productivity (Lazar, 2010). On a sheerly rational basis, one would think that, in a rapidly changing world in which stress and trauma are constantly creating psychological difficulties, societies would put resources into supporting psychotherapy, that despite the expense of training and compensating skillful therapists, this investment would be seen as cost-effective in the long run.

Even if it is cost-effective over time, however, all the incentives to funding organizations (insurance companies, governments) are short term: How much did you save us *this year*? When cost-cutters try to save taxpayers money, among the first programs they tend to eliminate are those that prevent future psychopathology. The value of such programs is not immediately obvious, and long-term studies of effectiveness are expensive to conduct. Politically, it can be hard to sell prevention to taxpayers, especially in the United States. Even with respect to predicted physical illness, we have witnessed Donald Trump's elimination, two years before the COVID-19 outbreak, of the part of the US Center for Disease Control that concerned itself with future pandemics. We tend to spend money only on what is manifestly present rather than what is preventable – at an enormous ultimate price. It is clearly cost-effective *in the short term* to frame mental health services as the quickest reduction of the most disabling symptoms of certain agreed-upon, isolated disorders. In the long term, we pay for this short-sightedness in high costs for increased homelessness, crime, addiction, and other social woes.

One interesting (and, to a therapist, somewhat disconcerting) side effect of the 1980 change toward descriptive and categorical psychiatric diagnosis involves the ways people in Western cultures have begun talking about themselves since the DSM-III paradigm shift. It used to be that a socially avoidant woman would come for therapy saying something like, "I'm a painfully shy person, and I need help learning how to deal better with people in social situations." Now a person with that concern is likely to tell me that she "has" social phobia – as if an alien affliction has invaded her otherwise problem-free subjective life. People talk about themselves in acronyms oddly dissociated from their lived experience: "my OCD," "my eating disorder," "my bipolar." There is an odd estrangement from one's sense of an agentic self, including one's own behavior, body, emotional and spiritual life, and felt suffering, and consequently one's possibilities for solving a problem. There is a passive quality in many individuals currently seeking therapy, as if they feel that the prototype for making an internal psychological change is to describe their symptoms to an expert and wait to be told what medicine to take, what exercises to do, or what self-help manual to read.

Mental health problems are listed in the DSM and similar classifications as if there is no narrative that holds together the kinds of difficulties a person reports. Experienced therapists tend to see connections between someone's "having," simultaneously, a personality disorder, a depression, an addiction, a post-traumatic symptom, and a self-harming behavior. Since we know from clinical experience and research on self-reflective function (e.g., Fonagy et al., 1991; Gabbard, 2005; Jurist & Slade, 2008; Müller et al., 2006) that the development of a personal narrative about the connections between one's unique life experiences and one's idiosyncratic psychology is a key element of mental health – so evident in its absence from the shattered mental life of many survivors of trauma – it is not hard to view our current psychiatric nomenclature as contributing to self-fragmentation rather than providing a means to heal it.

The assumption that complex human miseries are describable by *measurable, free-standing symptomatic entities* has been critiqued by some clinicians as reflecting a primitive, either-or mentation that one sees in young children, before they have emotionally integrated the complexity of life, or in people under stress who want to attribute blame unambivalently to a one-dimensional other. One of my crankier colleagues, a psychoanalytic theorist who is fond of Melanie Klein's (1946) differentiation between the paranoid-schizoid idea of categorically good or bad entities and the depressive appreciation of nuance and continuity, quipped that the DSM "IS the paranoid-schizoid position."

Unintended consequences of the interests of pharmaceutical corporations

Drug companies have a natural interest in defining mental suffering in terms of discrete disorders: Once there is a "disease," a drug can be marketed to treat it. There is nothing inherently cynical about this process; this is how the pharmaceutical corporations play their role in the overall mental health scene. In their defense, it is reasonable to think of some kinds of mental suffering (e.g., bipolar disorders, autism) as specific conditions or illnesses. Without chemical treatment of some depressive, manic, and psychotic states, psychotherapy would be impossible: In the absence of medication, the patient's level of terror or self-hatred or agitation would overwhelm any other focus of attention.

Most clinicians are consequently grateful to the pharmaceutical industry for developing medications that reduce psychological suffering. Yet it is the role of therapists and patients in therapy to deal not simply with the isolated symptoms of psychological miseries but also with the larger issues that have converged in the person's presenting complaints. Whether we approach our understanding from a family systems perspective, or from a cognitive angle of vision, or with a psychoanalytic ear, we need to make inferences that guide treatment. Why is the perspective of drug companies overtaking our capacity to look at the bigger picture?

One answer may be that viewing psychological suffering as a set of disorders that can be *fixed or improved* chemically can easily invite the obverse assumption that those painful experiences are ultimately *caused* by random or genetically based chemical differences among individuals. This is a false conclusion, of course, something like saying that because marijuana improves appetite, the cause of low appetite is lack of marijuana. But it is nevertheless a frequent leap of illogic – in the thinking of nonprofessionals and of some professionals as well – to ascribe much severe psychological suffering to a "chemical imbalance." Such a construction tempts us to ignore all the painful other sources of psychological suffering, such as poverty, neglect, trauma, and the myriad ways in which human beings can injure each other psychologically.

I remember when that construction began. In the 1960s, when the new neuroleptics began to be widely prescribed for psychotic symptoms, their effects could be so remarkable in reducing the psychic hell in which many patients had lived for months or even years, that mental health professionals felt the best thing they could do for individuals diagnosed with schizophrenia was to convince them that they needed to take this medication – and keep taking it interminably. A false but convenient analogy was made between antipsychotic medicines for people with schizophrenic illnesses and insulin for people with diabetes. Patients were told that they simply had a chemical imbalance that Thorazine would correct, and that if they took it regularly, their problems would be drastically mitigated, now and in the long term, just as they were for medication-compliant diabetics. It is not surprising that this formulation became popular. Viewing mental struggles as afflictions that simply "happen" to us (much as one catches the flu from a random virus or develops Huntington's disease for purely genetic reasons) exonerates ourselves and the people we love.

There is no shame in an accidental or genetically explained disorder, and no one can be blamed for our suffering. There is something profoundly appealing about this relief from culpability, especially in the realm of problems that carry as much stigma as mental health difficulties historically have borne. But at best, it is only a partial truth to view psychological misery this way. Furthermore, it is important to note that having a more comprehensive understanding of the origins of mental distress does not equate with "blame"; most of those whose behavior has contributed to problems in others usually acted out of the limitations of their own psychologies and not with conscious or voluntary intent to harm.

There have been many unintended negative consequences of the efforts of Big Pharma to define their products as "the" treatment for particular mental problems. When sweeping advertising claims were being made for the value of anti-anxiety and anti-depressant medications in the second half of the 20th century, a number of psychological researchers (See, e.g., Barlow, 2011), suspecting that such conditions may respond just as quickly to psychotherapy alone, became involved in the scientific comparison of medications and talk therapies. In these investigations, despite the long tradition in academic psychology of critiquing the "medical model" of psychopathology, the researchers adopted the DSM definitions of disorders in order to test whether structured, short-term psychotherapies were as effective for them as the medications being touted as the treatments of choice.

In general, the talk therapies relieved symptoms of depression and anxiety as effectively as the medications (and without side effects). Most therapists appreciate these studies by our academic colleagues; they gave scientific support to what we feel we know from clinical experience (though clinical experience has also attested to wide individual differences in responsiveness to both therapy and medication; again, statistical averages show them coming out about even, but for any given individual, pharmaceutical treatments might work better, or talk therapy, or both). In the service of doing efficient, manageable research on psychotherapy versus medication, however, the scientists had to adopt the drug companies' favored paradigm of construing mental health problems as discrete disorder categories; thus, their work inadvertently contributed to supporting an artificial, medicalized paradigm.

University professors, and then their students, began to think in those terms about the very nature of psychotherapy. Framed as discrete disorder categories, psychological suffering is much easier to research than the murkier, more vexed issues that real patients and therapists face together, such as whether to come out as gay to one's Christian fundamentalist family, how to deal with one's infertility, whether and when to retire if our personality is defined by work, or how to accept and enjoy one's actual body in a culture that bombards us with Barbie-doll images of beauty. In other words, what is easily researchable came to define what is important to understand, in defiance of the real world of psychotherapy practice.

In the general sensibility that emerged from such interests, psychologists and social workers who had previously resisted reductionistic categories slowly joined their medical colleagues in representing mental suffering by acronyms such as BPD, OCD, ODD, and ADHD. This acceptance of the definitions favored by pharmaceutical corporations and some researchers has fostered a general assumption that individuals suffer from discrete illnesses, and that when they report more than one problematic behavior or experience, their situation is best characterized in terms of their having two or more "comorbid" disorders.

Sometimes, just as one could have two unrelated medical conditions such as a broken toe and colitis, one *can* have two coexisting kinds of psychological suffering that are genuinely unrelated. One might, for example, suffer from a long-standing addiction to gambling and an acute "adjustment disorder" related to a loss. But much more commonly, a person's psychological problems are complexly interwoven and not conceptually separable. Our getting into the habit of thinking of them as distinct conditions that one "has" has distracted us from looking at what kinds of psychological capacities, integrations, and continuities characterize overall mental health, and how therapists can better help patients to develop them.

Unintended consequences of changes in academia

In recent years, we have witnessed an increasing estrangement between scientific researchers and practicing therapists. Professors in universities and medical schools are understandably frustrated when therapists do not use techniques they have studied and validated, and therapists are understandably exasperated when academics talk down to them about an art they have been practicing for years. Some amount of this tension is healthy. But contemporarily, therapists are finding the growing estrangement between practitioners and academics potentially dangerous, as our university colleagues complain to media outlets that we are not using the "best, evidence-based techniques" (approaches typically developed in laboratory settings that may or may not apply to complexly troubled individuals) or that we are ignoring "demonstrated best practices" (recommendations based on statistical averages from which any individual in the real world of clinical practice may deviate – the average of 2 and 10 is 6, but both numbers are quite far from 6). Some have even argued that if we are not applying a laboratory-derived treatment to a disorder for which such a treatment has been studied, then we are "practicing unethically."

Such public laments by researchers have painful implications for practice: Insurance companies and governments have been eager to adopt the common attitude in academic psychology and medicine to the effect that there are quicker, easier, more empirically justified – and less expensive – ways of helping people than the long slog so often required in traditional therapies. They then dictate to therapists what makes sense to them to support financially, and not surprisingly, it is always the interpretation of the research that would support the least expensive outlays.

There have always been temperamental differences between academics and therapists. The motive to critique and improve existing knowledge and the motive to reduce and prevent mental suffering are somewhat disparate callings, similar to the difference between the pure scientist and the applied scientist, the theoretical physicist or mathematician and the engineer. Researchers and therapists (as well as administrators of mental health delivery systems) also inhabit different roles, work under different pressures, and face different incentives (See Boswell et al., 2014). But developments in academic life over the past few decades have increased the gulf between the two groups. As someone on an academic faculty who is also in the clinical trenches, I have had more opportunity to see these changes close-up than most of my therapist colleagues.

When I was originally studying to be a therapist, most professors of clinical psychology had a fair amount of clinical experience, and often continued to maintain a therapeutic practice. These days, it would be professional suicide to do so, however, as it has become so consuming to pursue promotion and tenure in universities and medical schools that one must put all one's energy into developing research projects, pursuing grants, dealing with academic internal review boards, and writing for professional publication. A consequence of that reality is that few academics now have an experiential basis for empathy with psychotherapists and the world of actual clinical practice. How would they know that the problems for which most people seek treatment are not well captured by the DSM categories? How would they know that the quickest way to reduce a specific symptom is not necessarily the same thing as moving toward psychological health?

Like all of us, academic researchers generalize from the experiences that organize their lives. To do outcome studies that compare the effectiveness of different kinds of therapy or that compare talk therapy to medication, one has to take several methodological safeguards: (1) The condition to be studied must be defined as narrowly as possible, so that results will not be contaminated by extrinsic factors; (2) there must be objective assessment of reportable symptoms when a treatment begins; (3) all individuals carrying out a particular approach must follow the same protocol; (4) at the end of treatment, one must evaluate the status of the symptoms assessed at the beginning of the study. In addition, given the time limitations of grants and the pressures on professors to amass publications, these studies typically need to be done in limited time periods. These components – cherry-picking and elimination of comorbidities, baseline measurements, manualization, outcome measures, and required termination of treatment – constitute a reasonable research paradigm, and studies done this way have made valuable contributions to the practice of therapy in the world outside academia.

But when therapists find that academics expect them to (1) define problems narrowly, (2) take objective measures of symptoms at the beginning of treatment, (3) adhere closely to a manual developed for a specific disorder, (4) judge outcome by changes in symptoms rather than improvement in overall psychological functioning, and (5) offer only short-term psychotherapies, we feel we are being asked to apply a research paradigm to a clinical situation with very different properties. Taking each of these in order, let me explain why this research paradigm is a bad fit for clinical practice. Patients may come to therapists complaining that they suffer from a particular disorder, but it rarely turns out that the initially reported disorder is the only focus of clinical attention. A man may come for "anger management," for example, and be found to have an addiction that disinhibits his anger. The addiction is thus the most important object of intervention, not the skill training about managing anger. A woman with an "anxiety disorder" may turn out to have a complex set of post-traumatic problems. Reducing her current anxiety symptoms will not change her ongoing maladaptive responses to her traumatic history, which must be addressed as the main issue. A transgender adolescent with "depression" needs a lot more in the way of therapeutic conversation than a preformulated approach to symptoms. Objective measurement of observable symptoms is valuable in research, but in therapy, it can be the more subjective, implicit suffering that matters most. Manualization makes patients feel as if the therapist is simply following a cookbook (and in fact, some empirical literature suggests that carefully following a treatment manual correlates *inversely* with therapeutic progress – See Truijens et al., 2019).

Symptoms come and go in therapy, and sometimes get worse in the service of overall improvement. In the short term, their presence or absence, improvement or amelioration, are often not the best indicators of important psychological change. Individuals may test as *more* anxious when they are trying out new, more effective but unfamiliar behaviors; they may show *more* depressive symptoms when they are finally letting themselves grieve a loss that they have handled for years by maladaptive defenses such as dissociation and denial. Even within the limits of the so-called medical model, we note that no self-respecting physician would equate the removal of a fever or skin rash with the cure of the disease behind the elevated temperature or dermatitis. Nor should therapists equate symptom-reduction with overall psychological healing.

The philosopher Gilbert Ryle famously called the misapplication of the concepts of one field to the needs of another a "category mistake." I think this has happened between academic research and the practice of therapy. I know of no clinician who thinks that psychotherapy should not be strongly influenced by research, but being *informed by* research is a different matter from being *like* research.

What price are we paying?

Treating all superficially similar psychological suffering as the same phenomenon, and then determining therapies for people in that category based on statistical averages, is a recipe for therapeutic malfeasance. We can define a depression by certain externally observable signs, but if we do not understand its meaning, its level of severity, or its context, we will likely fail the patient. Given differences in personality, culture, belief systems, and circumstances, one depressed person will do better with medication, another with therapy characterized by compassionate concern, another with encouragement of exercise and sleep hygiene, another with a treatment that explicitly challenges implicit self-hating beliefs. Making these distinctions is the proper role of the therapist, and research on such distinctions among patients would provide therapists with more valuable understandings than being told what works in the psych lab with self-identified sufferers of a single disorder "with no comorbidities."

A depression is an illness of sorts, but as a medical condition, it is more like a limp than a disease process. A limp is a definable, describable result of certain kinds of damage. That damage may result from many possible causes and influences, and it may have affected the leg from any one of several possible bodily directions (damage to the foot, the thigh, the hip, the shoulder). We can easily describe a limp, and we can all agree on present-versus-absent criteria for "diagnosing" it, but when we want to help someone who limps, we need to know how the distorted gait developed, how much pain is involved, what it prevents the person from doing, whether it serves some purpose we should take into account in making recommendations, whether our proper job is to help the limping person to walk normally or to encourage the individual's grieving process in the face of a painful fact of life that cannot be changed.

If some of my zealous research colleagues with limited experience as therapists persuade the funders of psychotherapy treatments that all cases of DSM-diagnosed OCD should be treated by "evidence-based" exposure therapy (an excellent, effective treatment for many obsessive-compulsive problems), am I at risk of being charged with malpractice when I try to help the person who wants to work another way – even if I think this person's individual version of obsessive symptoms warrants a different approach, and even if I have experience with reducing obsessive-compulsive symptoms through other methods?

For example, consider patients at the extreme end of the obsessive-compulsive continuum, whose obsessions border on delusional beliefs, who suffer profound annihilation anxiety, who whole-heartedly believe they will die if they fail to carry out their rituals, and who regard the therapist with suspicion for not sharing their conviction – in other words, the subgroup of obsessive patients that Kernberg (1984) would consider as psychologically organized at the low borderline or psychotic level. My experience suggests that with this group exposure therapy not only fails, it demoralizes the patients, makes them feel like failures personally, and kills any hope they may have that psychotherapy can help. It also demoralizes therapists, who have been told again and again that exposure therapy is the treatment of choice for OCD. If they believe their teachers, such clinicians can easily conclude they are simply not good enough therapists.

Laboratory studies of treatments for specific disorders typically eliminate patients at the most disturbed end of any spectrum, who almost always have "comorbidities" such as personality disorders and addictions. An influential study by Edna Foa and her colleagues, for example, excluded more than half of potential patients with PTSD because they had comorbid problems (See Huppert et al., 2002). (Patients with real-world complex trauma also tend to be less reliable and cooperative research subjects than those with mild, ego-dystonic symptoms, making them more attractive to researchers but not at all representative of the traumatized patients regularly seen by therapists.) Concerns with such disconnects between what can be easily researched and what is prescribed prompted the American Psychological Association (See Campbell et al., 2013) to issue a press release emphasizing (1) the empirically established power of the therapy *relationship* over the type of intervention and (2) the importance of taking into consideration the patient's values and sensibilities when planning treatment. Unfortunately, APA's position is often honored, even by APA itself, only in the breach, as exemplified by what Norcross and Wampold (2019) have understandably depicted as the "tragedy" of the recently adopted APA guidelines on the treatment of trauma.

When we define common psychiatric symptom constellations as reified "disorders" and then assume a "one-size-fits-all" approach to psychotherapy, we are at particular risk of mistreating people in minority populations. For example, some treatments developed for autistic children emphasize systematically training them to make sustained eye contact. These approaches can be very helpful. But they assume a milieu in which looking others in the eye is normative. In some cultures, such behavior is rude. A sensitive therapist would not insist on eye contact with an autistic child from a culture that construes a direct gaze as aggressive. If a therapist cannot adapt a treatment with respect for the patient's context and background, the treatment is probably doomed.

It took decades for people of minority sexual orientation to persuade therapists who identified with the heterosexual majority that there is nothing pathological about their version of love. It would have taken even longer if some of the "treatments" for atypical gender expression developed by psychologists in the 1970s (e.g., Rekers & Lovaas, 1974) had been required for therapists to practice on the grounds of their being "evidence-based." They had indeed been developed via stringent methodologies, and they showed effectiveness at reducing "feminine" behavior in boys. But there were much bigger questions that that focus would have foreclosed, and those questions included some vision of what would make for a satisfying life for someone in a sexual minority.

There are many ways to help people. In all of them, psychotherapy is ideally a two-way process in which clinicians learn as much from their patients as vice versa. I became a therapist to try to be a healing influence for people who suffer psychologically, and to learn from them as much as I could about the immense complexity of the human condition. I like thinking of myself as a healer. I feel my patients confer upon me a sacred trust, and it is central to my self-esteem to try to justify their faith. There is nothing ennobling or sacred, however, about seeing oneself as a technician. And for patients, there is often nothing developmentally gratifying, nothing that fosters a sense of personal growth and accomplishment, about targeting and reducing a particular symptom. It does feel better not to be symptomatic, and that is no small thing. But reduction of observable, reportable symptoms such as anxiety, depression, phobia, compulsion, eating habits, and so on, is far from the whole picture of what we hope to accomplish in a meaningful therapy relationship. We hope to help people toward a more authentic, satisfying, livable life.

In the professional trenches these days, therapists are under constant pressure to redefine themselves as skillful deliverers of commodities (medications, manualized techniques) rather than as providers of an overall healing relationship (within which many technical interventions may be useful). As David Mintz has noted (personal communication, August 10, 2016), we have become "mental illness professionals" rather than "mental health professionals." The current emphasis on simply reducing the symptoms of observable, measurable suffering is obscuring the more important question of how we want to define mental health or maturity or emotional wisdom or psychological wellness.

The PDM project: An effort to address unintended effects of current taxonomies

The following account describes one effort to counteract some of the forces I summarized in the previous section. In case readers worry that Vittorio Lingiardi and I have a conflict of interest, let me mention at the outset that royalties from the PDM do not go to editors and authors; instead, they go into a fund that supports research that clinicians may find more relevant to their work than short-term laboratory trials of treatments for DSM-defined disorders. In 2019, we set up a committee to evaluate research proposals, created a process for doing so, and sent out a call. We were able to award four grants that year, three for $15,000 and one for $8,000, for PDM-related empirical studies.

Around 2003, the eminent child psychiatrist Stanley Greenspan became exasperated with what was happening in mental health treatment. He noticed, for example, that many parents who had consulted him in the previous decade for help with their psychologically troubled children seemed uninterested in understanding the meaning of their son's or daughter's behavior, or in how they might help their child with the problems they were witnessing. They wanted simple diagnoses, such as ADD, and easily administered medications for them. He was also weary of hearing that there is no "evidence basis" for the psychoanalytic therapies. Even though very few randomized controlled trials of psychodynamic treatments had been done by the early 2000s, he reasonably regarded the extensive empirical literature on personality, ego strength, defenses, attachment, development, neuroscience, general psychotherapy, and other areas as a strong evidence base for psychodynamic clinical work. Concluding that the social changes that were affecting his practice derived partly from the impact of official taxonomies, he spearheaded a new classification effort – this one directed at clinicians rather than researchers, record-keepers, and billing personnel.

Greenspan contacted the presidents of five major psychoanalytic organizations: the International Psychoanalytical Association, the American Psychoanalytic Association, the Division of Psychoanalysis of the American Psychological Association (Division 39, now the Society for Psychoanalysis and Psychoanalytic Psychology), the American Academy of Psychoanalysis, and the National Membership Committee on Psychoanalysis in Clinical Social Work (now the American Association for Psychoanalysis in Clinical Social Work). He solicited their support and asked them to nominate people for several task forces, including adult and child personality, mental functions, symptom syndromes, and outcome research. At the same time, he prevailed upon leading psychoanalytically oriented scientists (e.g., Sidney Blatt, Reiner Dahlbender, Peter Fonagy, Falk Leichsenring, Jonathan Shedler, Howard Shevrin, Joel Weinberger, Drew Westen, Daniel Widlocher), to provide articles summarizing their research legacy so that the proposed classification system would include incontestable empirical support.

I became involved in the original PDM project when Jaine Darwin, then President of Division 39, proposed me for its Personality task force. Eventually, I was asked to head that committee and to write up our section of what we began calling the "PDM." Once in that role, I was asked to be on the overall Steering Committee as well. As the contributions from task forces came in, Greenspan began to call on both me and Robert Wallerstein to copyedit the submissions. So while I was not part of the original conceptualization of the project, I got on the train at an early station and had a good overview of the immensity of the project.

I was impressed from the outset with the level of goodwill among participants. Despite Wallerstein's private warning that my committee comprised strongly opinionated individuals who would require my most exquisite diplomatic skills, I found that all members were eager to reach common ground. Interestingly, one of our rare disagreements concerned whether or not to characterize personality structure as on a continuum running from healthy through psychotic levels of organization. Jonathan Shedler and Drew Westen felt that including a psychotic "level of severity" would confuse readers who had become accustomed to thinking of psychotic phenomena in terms of discrete "disorder" categories rather than as a level of personality organization; Otto Kernberg, Eve Caligor, and I wanted to include a psychotic range of severity of personality disorder. In the absence of research showing that most psychoanalytic therapists endorsed the concept of a psychotic level of organization, we decided to write the continuum as going from healthy through neurotic and borderline levels to "the border with the psychotic conditions" (PDM Task Force, 2006, p. 21).

The original PDM had sections on (1) adults, (2) children and adolescents, and (3) infancy and earliest childhood, followed by the empirical articles Greenspan had solicited. Within the adult and child/adolescent sections, respectively, were subsections on personality structure (or, in the case of children, emerging structure), mental functions (9 capacities), and symptoms. In the symptoms part, Greenspan asked us to take the DSM categorical diagnoses *as is* and note the subjective experience of each disorder in terms of cognitive, affective, somatic, and interpersonal aspects. Finally, we included in each section a few fully formulated cases, often individuals who met criteria for the same DSM diagnosis but whose problems had discrepant meanings and different treatments of choice. The infancy section was an extensive discussion of problems of the earliest years that included many conditions that the DSM did not address at all.

In an effort to keep costs low for students, and because his organization, the Interdisciplinary Council on Development and Learning, had the means to produce the books in quantity, Greenspan chose self-publishing for printing and disseminating the manual. An unintended negative consequence of this decision was the loss of marketing services that would have been done by an established publisher. When Greenspan became ill and died within only months of the finished product, decisions about how many volumes to produce and how to distribute them fell on leaders of the ICDL, who had not been part of the PDM enterprise. Fortunately, Greenspan's widow, Nancy Greenspan, protected the PDM's interests, insisting, for example, that none of the profits from the volume became diverted from the intended fund for research to benefit clinicians.

Despite the downsides of the self-publishing decision and despite Greenspan's death soon after its publication, PDM-1 was quite successful. Greenspan had been able to herd all the psychoanalytic cats into getting a document finished in only two years – a remarkable accomplishment considering the tendency of analysts to bicker among themselves and resist speaking as one community. The manual was reviewed positively in several major professional publications and in the *New York Times*. In some countries, including most notably Italy and New Zealand, the PDM became well known, while in others, such as most countries in the Far East, it was mostly invisible. Overall, fora new and controversial endeavor, it sold well.

Greenspan had conceived the PDM as a preliminary document to be improved by critiques from both clinicians and researchers; upon publication, he invited comments from the mental health community. Most of the feedback was positive. We did, however, get one response that embarrassed us. Daniel Plotkin, a geriatric psychiatrist in Los Angeles, wrote us to ask why, in a putatively developmentally sensitive document with sections on infancy, childhood, and adulthood, there was no consideration of the elderly. The answer was that it had never occurred to us that we needed such a section! – a comical reality and a testimony to the power of denial, given that the modal age of members of the steering committee was in the seventies.

When Greenspan died, I thought the PDM would die as well. Most of the PDM-1 Steering Committee members were elderly, and those of us under age 70 did not want to devote the rest of our careers to the PDM, which had been entirely a labor of love, involving significant unpaid professional time. I did not anticipate the appearance of anyone who would take on the project of a revised PDM, and I was not willing to make the necessary sacrifices to do it myself. Then Vittorio Lingiardi, a clinician and a professor at Sapienza University in Rome, contacted me, emphasizing the need for a second edition, volunteering to lead the project, and urging me to co-edit it. Despite my misgivings, I eventually acceded to his plea. Greenspan's dream was not dead; the PDM-2 would be in the hands of one of the rare researchers who is also a seasoned clinician. The lion's share of the vision, organization, and oversight of the volume has fallen to Dr. Lingiardi (for an overview, See Lingiardi & McWilliams, 2018).

I have not regretted his talking me into that role. Overall, the project went smoothly notwithstanding some conflict on a couple of the task forces. Our first job was to obtain the support of all organizations that sponsored the original PDM, which turned out to be easy. Our second was to obtain support from some additional organizations, including the International Association for Relational Psychoanalysis and Psychotherapy, and the Italian Group for the Advancement of Psychoanalytic Diagnosis. This was also easy. Sponsors of PDM-2 include ten international organizations, including the original five.

Then we sought people to head task forces. Not so easy, but again, we found many energetic, highly qualified, and hard-working individuals willing to donate their time and effort most generously. Our chapter editors include Robert Bornstein, Franco Del Corno, Francesco Gazzillo, Robert Gordon, Norka Malberg, Johanna Malone, Linda Mayes, Nick Midgley, Emanuela Mundo, John O'Neil, Daniel Plotkin, Larry Rosenberg, Jonathan Shedler, Anna Maria Speranza, Mario Speranza, and Sherwood Waldron. Although PDM-1 involved scholars from enough geographical areas to justify our description of the manual as an international effort, PDM-2 includes a greater diversity of contributors, including experts from countries as different from Western Europe and North America as Turkey and Iran.

Then we approached Guilford Publications in the United States and Raffaello Cortina Publishers in Italy. Both were immediately interested in publishing PDM-2. Although it was complicated to handle the transfer of copyright from the ICDL, the good will and support of Nancy Greenspan made it possible. Jim Nageotte of Guilford supervised the manuscript with unflagging enthusiasm. The involvement of major publishing houses has meant that the PDM-2 has been well publicized and has not depended, as PDM-1 did, on word-of-mouth advertisement. This was perhaps the most consequential change from the first to the second edition. There were some other notable changes as well.

First, there are some additions. PDM-2 includes five rather than three developmental phases. We separated adolescence from childhood, on the commonsensical grounds that the psychology of a seven-year-old child is considerably different from that of a 17-year-old. We accepted Daniel Plotkin's recommendation for a section on the elderly and asked him and Franco Del Corno to oversee it. As a consequence, PDM-2 is the first major diagnostic system that explicates the special needs of the geriatric population. In the chapters on infancy, childhood, adolescence, adulthood, and old age, we considered homotypic as well as heterotypic developmental patterns. And on the basis of both research and clinical report, we added three capacities to the sections on mental functioning, for a total of 12, under the four rubrics of cognitive and affective processes, identity and relationships, defense mechanisms and coping, and self-awareness and self-direction.

Second, in response to feedback that the PDM-1 system of biopsychosocial diagnosis can be intimidating to learn for those unfamiliar with psychodynamic diagnosis and case formulation, we added a section on assessment of overall personality and mental functioning. In addition to comprehensive reviews of empirically sound instruments, PDM-2 includes the Psychodiagnostic Chart (PDC), a user-friendly tool for summarizing personality organization. Originally developed by Robert Bornstein and Robert Gordon for adults, the PDC has versions for children, adolescents, and the elderly. The cases in the second edition include forms on which the patient under consideration can be profiled via the PDC. Therapists can download these forms from the Guilford website.

Third, in the Personality section, consistent with Kernberg's structural personality diagnosis as well as with long-standing clinical observation, we included a psychotic level of personality organization. As I have noted, we did not include such a level on the continuum of personality functioning in PDM-1 because there was a difference of opinion among task force members and we lacked empirical studies supporting the concept. By the time we were developing PDM-2, however, research by Robert Gordon (2009) (e.g.), had demonstrated that most practitioners – not only psychoanalytic therapists but also those of other orientations – endorse and find clinically valuable the concept of a psychotic level of functioning.

Fourth, we included specific comparisons and contrasts among the ICD and DSM systems, relating relevant controversies to our decisions in PDM-2. These conversations are contextualized historically. They shed considerable light on what are otherwise confusing shifts and inconsistences in the use of professional terminology, and they illuminate many aspects of the social construction of psychopathology. The evolution of diagnostic nomenclature, with its cycles of sensitivity to some mental health issues and not to others, is an area of intellectual history that deserves more attention. Because clinicians had responded positively to the section in PDM-1 on the patient's subjective experience of DSM diagnoses, we expanded the comments on cognitive, affective, somatic, and interpersonal implications, contextualizing those issues similarly.

Finally, we made an omission and an integration. We eliminated the large section of articles by cutting-edge researchers at the end of the first edition of the PDM, preferring instead to incorporate citations to relevant research throughout the PDM-2. That decision allowed us to devote more pages to issues of diagnosis while continuing to honor the empirical legacy of our most clinically relevant scientists.

One other note of interest about a proposed change that we eventually did *not* make: We have had informal feedback from many directions, including therapists trained in humanistic, biological, and cognitive-behavioral approaches, that the PDM has been helpful to them. At the same time, in PDM-2, unlike the first edition, there is more attention to nonpsychoanalytic approaches, which the manual recommends for certain kinds of mental suffering. With a view to expanding the reach of the PDM classification system, we considered renaming the manual the "Psychological Diagnostic Manual," or perhaps the "Practitioner's Diagnostic Manual," thus explicitly welcoming its use by nonpsychoanalytic professionals. I was enthusiastic about this proposal, but Guilford Press was not. They argued that the PDM has become a "brand," and therefore should not be retitled. We deferred to their expertise.

Concluding comments

No diagnostic system can capture the complexity of anyone's psychology nor the uniqueness of an individual person. But therapists, especially less seasoned clinicians, need some overall "map" of relevant psychological territory, or else they risk feeling helpless in the face of infinite human variety. We need to be careful that the maps we are given describe the most important elements of the clinical terrain, and not just those that are useful to pharmaceutical corporations, administrators of health benefits, and a narrow group of researchers. We hope that in PDM-2, the clinical community will find a good-enough map of the territory of human strengths and weaknesses, health and suffering, that will be more useful to the coming generation of therapists and scholars than many of our official taxonomies of "disorders" have been.

References

Barlow, D. H. (2011). The development and evaluation of psychological treatments for panic disorder. In Gernsbacher, M., Pew, D., Hough, L., & Pomerantz, J. R. (Eds.), *Psychology and the real world: Essays illustrating fundamental contributions to society* (pp. 198–204). Worth Publishers.

Boswell, J. F., Kraus, D. R., Miller, S. D., & Lambert, M. J. (2014). Implementing routine outcome monitoring in clinical practice: Benefits, challenges, and solutions. *Psychotherapy Research*, *25*(1), 6–19. https://doi.org/10.1080/ 10503307.2013.817696

Campbell, L. F., Norcross, J. C., Vasquez, M. J. T., & Kaslow, N. (2013). Recognition of psychotherapy effectiveness: The APA resolution. *Psychotherapy*, *50*(1), 98–101. https://doi.org/10.1037/a0031817

Clegg, J. W. (2012). Teaching about mental health and illness through the history of the *DSM*. *History of Psychology*, *15*(4), 364–370. https://doi.org/10.1037/a0027249

Fonagy, P., Steele, H., Moran, G., Steele, M., & Higgit, A. (1991). The capacity for understanding mental states: The reflective self in parent and child and its significance for security of attachment. *Infant and Mental Health Journal*, *13*(3), 200–217. https://doi.org/10.1002/1097-0355(199123)12:3<201::AID-IMHJ2280120307>3.0.CO;2-7

Frances, A. (2013). *Saving normal: An insider's revolt against out-of-control psychiatric diagnosis, DSM-5, big pharma, and the medicalization of ordinary life*. HarperCollins.

Gabbard, G. O. (2005). Reflective function, mentalization, and borderline personality disorder. In Beitman, B. D. (Ed.), *Self-awareness deficits in psychiatric patients: Neurobiology, assessment, and treatment* (pp. 213–228). Norton.

Gordon, R. M. (2009). Reactions to the *Psychodynamic Diagnostic Manual (PDM)* by psychodynamic, CBT, and other non-psychodynamic psychologists. *Issues in Psychoanalytic Psychology*, *31*(1), 55–62. https://www.researchgate.net/profile/Robert-Gordon-10/publication/235683646_Reactions_to_the_Psychodynamic_Diagnostic_Manual_PDM_ by_Psychodynamic_CBT_and_Other_Non-_Psychodynamic_Psychologists/links/0fcfd512886138178b000000/Reactions-to-the-Psychodynamic-Diagnostic-Manual-PDM-by-Psychodynamic-CBT-and-Other-Non-Psychodynamic-Psychologists.pdf

Huppert, J. D., Franklin, M. E., Foa, E. B., & Davidson, J. R. (2002). Study refusal and exclusion from a randomized treatment study of generalized social phobia. *Journal of Anxiety Disorders*, *17*(6), 683–693. https://doi.org/10.1016/ S0887–6185(02)00238-4

Jurist, E. L., & Slade, A. (Eds.). (2008). *Mind to mind: Infant research, neuroscience, and psychoanalysis*. Other Press.

Kernberg, O. F. (1984). *Severe personality disorders: Psychotherapeutic strategies*. Yale University Press.

Klein, M. (1946). Notes on some schizoid mechanisms. *International Journal of Psycho-Analysis*, *27*, 99–110. https://pep-web.org/browse/document/IJP.027.0099A

Klerman, G. L. (1978). The evolution of a scientific nosology. In Shershow, J. C. (Ed.), *Schizophrenia: Science and practice* (pp. 99–121). Harvard University Press.

Lambert, M. J., Hansen, N. B., & Finch, A. E. (2001). Patient-focused research: Using patient outcome data to enhance treatment effects. *Journal of Consulting and Clinical Psychology*, *69*(2), 159–172. https://doi.org/10.1037/0022-006X.69.2.159

Lazar, S. G. (Ed.). (2010). *Psychotherapy is worth it: A comprehensive review of its cost-effectiveness*. American Psychiatric Publishing, Inc.

Lingiardi, V., & McWilliams, N. (2017). *Psychodynamic diagnostic manual*, 2nd ed. *(PDM-2)*. Guilford.

Lingiardi, V., & McWilliams, N. (2018). Introduction to the special issue on the *Psychodynamic Diagnostic Manual, 2nd Edition (PDM-2)*: The *PDM*: Yesterday, Today, Tomorrow. *Psychoanalytic Psychology*, *35*(3), 289–293. https://doi.org/ 10.1037/pap0000188

Morrison, K. H., Bradley, R., & Westen, D. (2003). The external validity of controlled clinical trials of psychotherapy for depression and anxiety: A naturalistic study. *Psychology and Psychotherapy: Theory, Research and Practice*, *76*(2), 109–132. https://doi.org/10.1348/147608303765951168

Müller, C., Kaufhold, J., Overbeck, G., & Grabhorn, R. (2006). The importance of reflective functioning to the diagnosis of psychic structure. *Psychology and Psychotherapy: Theory, Research and Practice*, *79*(4), 485–494. https://doi.org/10.1348/147608305X68048

Norcross, J. C., & Wampold, B. E. (2019). Relationships and responsiveness in the psychological treatment of trauma: The tragedy of the APA clinical practice guideline. *Psychotherapy*, *56*(3), 391–399. https://doi.org/10.1037/pst0000228

PDM Task Force. (2006). *Psychodynamic diagnostic manual (PDM)*. Alliance of Psychoanalytic Organizations.

Pilecki, B., Clegg, J., & McKay, D. (2011). The influence of corporate and political interests on models of illness in the evolution of the *DSM*. *European Psychiatry*, *26*(3), 194–200. https://doi.org/10.1016/j.eurpsy.2011.01.005

Rekers, G. A., & Lovaas, O. I. (1974). Behavioral treatment of deviant sex-role behaviors in a male child. *Journal of Applied Behavioral Analysis*, *7*(2), 173–190. https://doi.org/10.1901/jaba.1974.7-173

Sadler, J. Z. (2005). *Values and psychiatric diagnosis*. Oxford University Press.

Seligman, M. E. P. (1995). The effectiveness of psychotherapy: The Consumer Reports study. *American Psychologist*, *50*(12), 965–974. https://doi.org/10.1037/0003-066X.50.12.965

Spitzer, R. L. (1991). An outsider-insider's views about revising the DSMs. *Journal of Abnormal Psychiatry*, *100*(3), 294–296. https://doi.org/10.1037/h0046535

Stricker, G., & Trierwelier, S. J. (1995). The local clinical scientist: A bridge between science and practice. *American Psychologist*, *50*(12), 995–1002. https://doi.org/10.1037/0003-066X.50.12.995

Sullivan, H. S. (1973). *Clinical studies in psychiatry*. Norton.

Truijens, F., Zuhlke-van Hulzen, L., & Vanheule, S. (2019). To manualize, or not to manualize: Is that still the question? A systematic review of empirical evidence for manual superiority in psychological treatment. *Journal of Clinical Psychology*, *75*(3), 329–343. https://doi.org/10.1002/jclp.22712

Toward a science of the heart[1]

Romanticism and the revival of psychology

Kirk Schneider

> "When… we talk of "psychology as a natural science," we must not assume that that means a sort of psychology that stands at last on solid ground. It means just the reverse; it means a psychology particularly fragile, and into which the waters of metaphysical criticism leak at every joint, a psychology whose elementary assumptions and data must be reconsidered in wider connections and translated into other terms." (William James, 1892/1961, pp. 334, 335)

Throughout its history, psychology has been the locus of debate concerning the proper nature of the study of mental life. All have not agreed on how psychology ought to achieve scientific status or even whether psychology is best conceived and designed as a science at all. If some believe this debate has never been significant or if they believe it is now over, this is only because of the attempted hegemony of the logical positivist view, the well-established view that psychology is to be a science modeled on the natural sciences, and that its applications would follow just as successful technologies have risen from the development of the physical sciences.

There is a long, distinguished history of proposals to the contrary, starting with proposals of the founders of modern psychology. For instance Wundt (1900–1920), who is so well-known for establishing the first psychological laboratory in 1879, believed that laboratory research is quite limited in its relevance to psychological subject matter and spent a large part of his career developing his *völkerpsychologie* (cultural psychology), which was aimed at the study of higher, more complex organizations of psychological life. Giorgi (1970) has provided a detailed history of the ever-present protests that have criticized psychology. He showed that these various criticisms are of two basic types, namely that psychology lacks unity and that psychology is remote from its subject matter. If one considers that there are two fundamental criteria for truth that pervade both the sciences and the humanities—coherence (logical or empirical consistency) and correspondence (accurate reference to reality)—it is evident that these criticisms strike directly to the very heart of the truth value of psychological

DOI: 10.4324/9781003325512-13

knowledge. Giorgi (1970) convincingly argued that these problems are inevitable consequences of psychology's natural science approach and as such are unresolvable as long as psychology remains dominated by that approach.

It appears that times have changed in our discipline despite those who still cling to the identification of psychology with hypothetical-deductive-inductive methods. Perhaps the postmodern zeitgeist has brought about an awareness of the limits of an exclusively positivist discipline. The Kuhn–Popper debate during the 1960s and 1970s raised psychologists' consciousness of alternative metascientific approaches. Works with philosophical sophistication that addresses methodological issues and metascientific issues like those of Bernstein (1976, 1983) and Polkinghorne (1983, 1988, 1994) make it more and more difficult to deny the existence of a move toward alternative methods and of numerous legitimate ways to achieve psychological knowledge (Koch, 1993).

Despite these trends, however, there is another realignment taking place in psychology today. Just at the moment when psychology is opening up to a plurality of approaches, massive economic and political pressures are forcing a new reality—the reestablishment of a logical positivist hegemony. This realignment is dangerous in my view and threatens one of the most vital yet underappreciated metascientific alternatives in psychology—romanticism. Reflecting precisely those personalistic concerns that logical positivism seeks to supplant, romanticism warrants a sustained and serious reassessment in our discipline and a renewed appreciation for its virtues.

The origins and nature of romanticism

Romanticism is an artistic and intellectual movement that originated in the late 18th century. Although romanticism rebelled against formal (technical) reason, it was not, for the most part, an irrational movement (Jamison, 1993; Jones, 1969). To the contrary, romanticism attempted to enlarge rationality, to fortify it with affect and intuition, and to relate it to the most puzzling problems of life—love, freedom, and fear (Jones, 1969). Eighteenth-century writers such as Goethe, for example, rebelled against the sterile empiricism of their day; Goethe said in effect that awe is the highest dimension of humankind, in awe people experience the vast (May, 1991, p. 245). "The intensist light of reason," echoed Herman Melville, "cannot shed blazonings upon the deeper truths in man, as will sometimes proceed from his profoundest gloom" (1852/1964, p. 199).

To elaborate, romanticism rebelled against Enlightenment rationality. For the early romantics, Enlightenment rationality placed far too much emphasis on linear, causal knowledge. The search for causes, from the romantic standpoint, led to a search for superficial solutions—that which is readily apparent, measurable, and capable of isolation. For the romantic, however, the world was much too broad and interconnected to be "dissected" in such ways. According to the romantic, a return to the lived world and to childlike openness was needed. Correlatively, there needed to be a return to the tacit state of experience prior to intellectualization (See Polanyi, 1962). Although this tacit state was considered primitive by many Enlightenment onlookers, to thoughtful romantics it was neither primitive nor backward but deep, reverent, and comprehensive. Romanticism elucidated many layers of human experience from the individual to the collective and from the archetypal to the futuristic but always with an eye to what was basic or profound about a given standpoint. Although romanticism touched on religious themes, it did not champion any religion; it championed inquiry. The upshot is that romanticism emphasized three elements in its revolt against Enlightenment rationality: the interrelated wholeness of experience; access to such wholeness by means of tacit processes—affect, intuition, kinesthesia, and imagination; and qualitative or descriptive accounts of such processes (Barrett, 1958; Jones, 1969; Kirschner, 1996; McDermott, 1993; Tillich, 1952).[2]

The romantic conception of existence gave rise to a variety of theoretical and methodological positions in psychology. These positions drew on romanticism's ontology—holism, tacit awareness, and qualitative description. Among these positions are Dilthey's (1977) *Geisteswissenschaften* (human sciences), Husserl's (1962) phenomenology, Heidegger's (1962) philosophy of being, James's (1904/1987) radical empiricism, the personality and clinical formulations of many of the early humanistic, existential, and transpersonal psychologists (e.g., Jung, 1966; Maslow, 1971; May, 1958; Rogers, 1961), and psychodynamic formulations emphasizing relational factors (See Kirschner, 1987, 1996; Wertz, 1993). Romantic ontology is also apparent in narrative, cultural, and ethnographic spheres of psychological inquiry (Becker, 1973; Messer, Sass, & Woolfolk, 1988; Rank, 1996).

Romantic ways of knowing, as can be seen above, have a long and distinguished lineage in psychology. Despite this continuity, however, romanticism has played a relatively marginal role in American psychology. William James, for example, wrote extensively about the importance of emotions, intuition, and spirituality, but few works of his contemporaries resonated with these concerns (Meyers, 1986). Edmund Husserl formulated phenomenology at a time when traditional empiricism had already become the established methodology in psychology. Finally, the humanistic psychology of Rogers, Maslow, May, and others received favorable attention in the popular press and to a significant extent in the clinic, but it was received with disdain or indifference in academic circles (DeCarvalho, 1991).

The threats to romanticism

Today, psychology faces the extinction of the romantic perspective. Managed care, technocratic models for living, and funding cutbacks have profoundly impacted our discipline. Although there probably always will be a place for isolated romantic practices, these practices have fewer and fewer footholds in mainstream academia and virtually no influence on mainstream graduate training (Aanstoos, 1994; O'Hara, 1997). The responsibility for this situation, however, does not merely rest with romanticism's adversaries; it also, ironically, can be traced to romanticism's proponents. Long before managed care, for example, the holistic, flexible, and exploratory nature of romanticism led some clinicians to charge exorbitant treatment fees; it led others to engage in seemingly endless treatment regimens, producing little in the way of results; and it led still others to ignore the need to formally document or theorize about their work (Hillman & Ventura, 1993; Sedgwick, 1982). The result was that by the early 1960s, therapists, third-party payers, and even clients themselves began to turn away from romantically oriented practices (Garfield & Bergin, 1994). Concomitant with these developments, a growing number of clinicians began to formulate brief and focused therapy models (e.g., Bellak & Small, 1965; Sifneos, 1972). These models proved popular for the following reasons: They were cost-effective, increasingly well-researched, and helpful to many who could not otherwise afford treatment (Butcher, Stelmachers, & Maudal, 1983). Even when clients could pay, moreover, they did not, on average, remain in treatment for more than eight sessions (Butcher et al., 1983; Manning, Wells, & Benjamin, 1986). Although there is increasing controversy about the soundness of the above data—for example, the Consumer Reports (1995) study indicating that more clients than previously believed not only seek out but greatly benefit from long-term therapy (See also I. J. Miller, 1996a)—two points ring clear: First, a significant portion of clientele prefer brief and symptom-focused approaches; and second, romantically oriented therapy has to an extent courted its own fate.

The above conditions notwithstanding, however, the pendulum, in my view, has swung wildly to the opposite side—toward corporate control of costs, persistent undertreatment, and onerous formalization. The bases for this current state of affairs are many: the influence on mental-health delivery services of market forces; the emphasis of those forces on brief, standardized, and so-called cost-effective services; the aggressive bids by psychiatrists, psychologists, and master's-level clinicians to meet those market-driven needs; and the convergence of traditional research interests (e.g., randomized trials) with those of market-driven forces (e.g., managed care, for-profit HMOs, federal agencies) to evaluate mental health services (Barlow, 1996; Fensterheim & Raw, 1996). The evidence for these linkages derives from an increasingly vocal segment of the clinical community. At a recent symposium of distinguished psychotherapy researchers, for example, Hans Strupp cautioned that "the skillful, theoretically sophisticated therapist is being replaced by technicians with very limited training and expertise" (Garfield, 1997, p. 78). At the same meeting, Allen Bergin decried the "overemphasis on mechanistic/naturalistic conceptions of causality and therapeutic change processes" and called for increased attention to humanistic and phenomenological aspects of therapy as a countermeasure (Garfield, 1997, p. 83). Several recent surveys of psychologists corroborate Strupp and Bergin's concerns. For example, in a Colorado survey of 223 responding psychologists, 64% reported incidents of managed care companies discontinuing treatment when it was still indicated (Hipp, Atkinson, & Pelc, 1994). In a California survey of 173 responding psychologists, 55% reported incidents in which therapy had been denied on the basis of rigid criteria that failed to consider the specific case, and 57% reported that a client's progress had been damaged by managed care denials (Denkers & Clifford, 1994). Finally, in a national survey of 718 responding psychologists, 72% reported that their overall experience was that managed care negatively affected the quality of treatment (Tucker & Lubin, 1994). The fear of a market-driven, industrialized ethos in psychology has also inspired several notable protest movements: The National Coalition of Mental Health Professionals and Consumers, comprising 1,300 members (Wylie, 1995), and a Managed Care Task Force (Moldawski, 1997, p. 24) cosponsored by Divisions 42 (Independent Practice) and 29 (Psychotherapy) of the American Psychological Association are two examples.

As suggested previously, however, the prevailing ethos in psychology runs counter to these protests (Barlow, 1996; Goldfried & Wolfe, 1996). Spearheaded in part by concerns about funding for research and practice, there have been two prominent developments within the American Psychological Association, both of which rely heavily on standardization: The first is a template for establishing therapeutic guidelines (American Psychological Association, 1995), and the second is a recommendation by the clinical division of the American Psychological Association on the "training and dissemination of empirically validated psychological treatments" (Task Force on Promotion and Dissemination of Psychological Procedures, Division of Clinical Psychology of the American Psychological Association, 1995).

Some romantically oriented therapists and researchers who have established practices and reputations may not be especially fazed by the above developments; others are not so fortunate. Students, and hence the coming generation of romantically inclined professionals, are at a particular disadvantage. As increasing segments of the therapeutic population gravitate toward managed mental health care and as professional organizations—such as the American Psychological Association and the American Psychiatric Association—accede to these trends, the opportunities to learn about, let alone to practice, romantically oriented approaches are rapidly dwindling (Walls & Scholom, 1996).

Toward a romantic psychology

For the purposes of this chapter, I define romantic psychology in its broadest, dialectical sense. Drawing from the discussion by Sass (1988), I recognize two basic strains of psychological romanticism. The first strain derives from the literary and artistic legacy of 18th-century thinkers such as Lord Byron and Goethe and stresses individual depth and experience. This lineage was then extended and elaborated on by European and American thinkers, such as Schopenhauer, Kierkegaard, Emerson, and Thoreau, and subsequently by the phenomenological and existential philosophers, such as Husserl, Sartre, and Camus. The individualist lineage culminated, finally, in the humanistic and existential psychology movements of Europe and America.

The second strain of romanticism also derives from the 18th-century rebellion against 17th-century rationalism, but it emphasizes collective depth and experience. This heritage, which originated in the works of Schlegel, Herder, and Schiller in the 18th and 19th centuries and culminated in the philosophical and psychological works of Heidegger, Gadamer, Ricoeur, and others (e.g., Hillman, 1975; Jung, 1966), focused on the "need for tradition and social order" in self-expression, over and above subjective individualism (Sass, 1988, pp. 256–258).

The most recent manifestations of the romantic in psychology are seen in the orientations of existential-humanistic, hermeneutical, narrative, semiotic, cultural, relational, transpersonal, and ecological psychologies (Bevan & Kessel, 1994; Messer et al., 1988; O'Hara, 1994; Sass, 1988; Taylor, 1992; Walsh & Vaughan, 1993). Although each of these spheres of inquiry differentially accents the individual and the collective—as well as linguistic and prelinguistic modes of expression—they all converge with regard to one overarching concern: the human "lifeworld" or *lebenswelt* (Husserl, 1962; Valle & Halling, 1989). As suggested earlier, the lifeworld consists of three basic dimensions. The first dimension is the tacit state of experience prior to systematic reflection. This state is characterized by what Gendlin (1978) refers to as the "felt-sense" and comprises affect, intuition, kinesthesia, and imagination. The tacit state is further characterized by a sense of profundity, poignancy, and significance. It is the state in which we live. Second, the lifeworld is holistic, complex, and multitextured. Although distinct themes can be gleaned from the lifeworld, they are always contextualized by related themes in a continually evolving gestalt. One does not speak of linear causes from this standpoint, but of atmospheres, salient themes, and structures (Merleau-Ponty, 1962). Third, when the lifeworld becomes a theme of knowledge, it always includes the coconstitution of the investigator and participant. The investigator is a participant-knower and understands that he or she is part of the phenomenon that is being studied (Giorgi, 1970; Polkinghorne, 1988).

There is also a convergence among the above romantic strains regarding the need for qualitative–descriptive research methodologies to explicate the lifeworld. Although these methodologies, which include phenomenology, hermeneutics, grounded theory, ethnomethodology, field studies, and case studies, do not purport (at least in their modern forms) to formulate objectified laws about the lifeworld, they do endeavor to reflect the essential, situated meaning structures that emerge therein. The question for these romantic methodologies is what is the significance, impact, and meaning of psychological data for people's everyday lives? That is, what about the data really matters to people?

Experimental research, for example, may yield important data about symptom reduction and psychosocial adjustment following a particular therapy, but from the standpoint of the romantic there needs to be a much fuller inquiry. What role does such a transformation actually play in the day-to-day lives of those who are studied? To what degree are participants' fears, anxieties, and depressions addressed by such changes? How does this therapy relate to more personal, qualitative issues, such as participants' capacities to love and be loved, to use their imaginations, to innovate, or to live in a more culturally enriching environment? It is one thing to gauge therapeutic outcome by the norms and standards of paper and pencil tests. It is quite another, however, to gauge it by the broader textures and subtleties of real-life experience (Shedler, Mayman, & Manis, 1993). In an in-depth study of American social values, Bellah, Madsen, Sullivan, and Tipton (1985) reported that the kind of symptom reduction and adjustment described above has an increasingly low priority. What is important to a growing number of Americans, these researchers concluded, is a renewed sense of community, a revival of spiritual values, and a socially meaningful career path. Numerous other social critics, correspondingly, have pointed to the woeful inadequacy of both symptom reduction and adjustment as criteria for psychological health (Breggin, 1991; Laing, 1967; Maslow, 1971). When normality in America is associated with such conditions as spiritual and emotional emptiness (Cushman, 1990, 1995; Lerner, 1996), Type A personality (Moss & Dielman, 1986; Multiple Risk Factor Intervention Trial Group, 1979), and workaholism (Fassel, 1990; Schaef & Fassel, 1988), factors that have been demonstrated to erode physical and mental health (Bracke & Bugental, 1995; Lerner, 1996; Morin, 1995), there must be a redefinition of our assumptions as a culture. From my standpoint, psychology can and should be in the vanguard of such a redefinition. Rather than reflecting the expedient, short-term goals of mainstream culture, psychology can and should include the pursuit of long-term, holistic goals advocated by an emerging social consciousness (Elgin & LeDrew, 1997; Pauchant, 1995).

In short, romantic sensibilities can push mainstream psychology into considering the broader context of people's lived and intimate realities. It can ask systemic questions about health and dysfunction, love and work. The question naturally arises, but who will pay for the kind of long-term, qualitative outlook advocated by romantic psychology? Although this question is an important one, it should first be pointed out that psychology is not (nor should be) an exclusively market-driven enterprise. Although psychology—just as every other professional discipline—must consider the monetary impact of its services, this impact should not fundamentally compromise the field's knowledge base, which may or may not be compatible with economic interests (Albee, 1996). The second point is that there are emerging funding alternatives that are compatible with the position outlined in this chapter. Shore (1995), for example, has outlined a funding option called managed cooperation. Managed cooperation calls for insurance companies to fix their rate of reimbursement for therapeutic services at a level that is somewhat below a standard fee; it calls further for a regional board comprising consumers, clinicians, government representatives, and insurers to oversee this reimbursement process and recommend reasonable fee levels; and it envisions a copayment, negotiated between clients and therapists, on a sliding-scale basis. This copayment could range anywhere from $5 to $50 per session, depending on what is worked out. The upshot of this plan is that (a) the liability of insurers is limited but can be substantially stretched; (b) clients and clinicians "become more cost conscious"; (c) clients retain the "rights of choice, decision-making, and privacy"; and (d) "clinicians are guaranteed at least a minimum payment" for each service, and yet are still able to "set fees in accordance with their training, talent and [community] reputation" (Shore, 1995, p. 11).

Benefit packages such as the latter, it should be further pointed out, need not in principle require a *DSM-IV* diagnosis (*Diagnostic and Statistical Manual of Mental Disorders,* 4th ed., American Psychiatric Association, 1994). The Boston-based American Mental Health Alliance, for example, uses two basic reimbursement criteria: clinically determined treatment and progressive client copayments (Dan Kagan, personal communication, August 5, 1997). Still other funding programs that are compatible with romantic values include the medical savings account recently floated before Congress (I. J. Miller, 1996a) and single-payer mental health plans offering generous benefits.

To sum, I propose that the pendulum has swung too far in the direction of standardization and that the convergence between mainstream cultural forces and conventional psychology is detrimental to the long-term interests of society and psychology as a whole. My implication here is that mainstream psychology needs to reassess its dissociation from the romantic and its response to or reflection of cultural trends. Correspondingly, I hope to show how both mainstream psychology and society can benefit by acknowledging the romantic as well as how the romantic can gain by acknowledging conventional realities and that these respective positions can enhance and enrich one another. First, I consider the costs of psychology's present distancing from the romantic on two levels—the clinical and the methodological (particularly as it pertains to clinical practice). Next, I illustrate romantic psychology's benefits and complements to mainstream psychology. I propose that romanticism can be drawn on to reenergize our discipline. Finally, I consider the romantic position in light of certain postmodern alternatives to mainstream psychology. I show that although romanticism and postmodernism share much in common, their differences in certain cases should not be neglected.

The price of discarding the romantic

Although many sectors of psychology (e.g., research, biological, administrative) have been affected by managed mental health care, none has been as jarred as therapeutic practice (Barlow, 1996). In this field, there has been a growing emphasis on computer science, psychopharmacology, and short-term modalities to transform dysfunctional behavior (Norcross, Alford, & Demichele, 1992).

As noted previously, the American Psychological Association has authorized a template by which standards for evaluating psychotherapy guidelines are to be set, and the clinical division of the association has published its own recommendations to incorporate consideration of empirically validated treatments within clinical training. Although these officially sanctioned actions may on their face appear benign and even economically necessary, they portend an ill fate for the romantic dimension of psychology. This is because the template of the American Psychological Association, as well as the association's Clinical Division report, are biased in the direction of favoring some methodologies (e.g., randomized trials, causal modeling) over other methodologies (e.g., reflective practice, case studies) for evaluating therapies. Although these former methodologies may be endorsed by, say, cognitive-behavioral practitioners, they are not viewed as adequate for those who are concerned with more holistic processes and outcomes (Stern, 1994–1995; Wertz, 1995). There are two basic reasons for this conclusion. First, holistic therapies (such as those of the psychodynamic and existential-humanistic variety) tend to be long-term and flexibly or artistically delivered. Randomized trials, however, have been overwhelmingly applied to short-term, systematic frameworks (Seligman, 1996). Second, even if randomized trials could address flexible therapies, as has been suggested recently (Jacobson & Christensen, 1996), they would tend to address such therapies from within the confines of traditional empiricism, using the overt and measurable criteria of traditional empiricism. Yet these criteria, in the areas of say, diagnosis and outcome, are at odds with the broader and complex concerns of most flexible therapies (Bugental & Bracke, 1992; Goldfried & Wolfe, 1996). The upshot is that holistic therapies are likely to be increasingly debased in the years ahead, not merely by managed care, but by an exclusionary methodological vision.

The problem with basing psychotherapy research (or indeed psychotherapy) on the current nosology of mental disorders is that it restricts the range within which problems can be treated. Less and less do clients have therapeutic options, and more and more is the multidimensionality of suffering abrogated. Yet consider: Some therapy clients have multiple disorders that are related in larger patterns and require interventions that transcend standardized procedures (Bohart, Leitner, & O'Hara, in press). Some clients prefer therapy aimed less at symptom change and more at personal or spiritual growth (Consumer Reports, 1995). Other clients prefer therapy that addresses social and cultural issues (e.g., prejudice, value conflicts) that do not clearly conform to *DSM-IV* diagnoses or manualization (Faidley & Leitner, 1993). Still other clients prefer therapies because they work for them, regardless of expert opinion (I. J. Miller, 1996b). Finally, many clients prefer therapy that stresses personal and relational factors over prepackaged techniques (Krupnick, Sotsky, Simmens, Moher, Elkin, Watkins Pilkonisk, 1996; Lambert & Bergin, 1994). Such clients favor conditions for therapeutic change—honesty, respect, caring—over implemented procedures (Stein & Lambert, 1995).

To sum, the value of standardized procedures is that they can be delivered at relatively low cost in short time intervals. The drawback of these modalities is that they tend to address simple or highly circumscribed problems (I. J. Miller, 1996a). The romantic approaches, on the other hand, tend to require more time, effort, and expense than standardized approaches, but they also appear to be more effective than standardized approaches at addressing difficult or complex life issues (Howard, Lueger, Maling, & Martinovich, 1993; I. J. Miller, 1996a; Seligman, 1996). These are the issues with which many clients struggle today and with which more clients are likely to struggle in the future (Bugental & Bracke, 1992; Elgin & LeDrew, 1997).

The central question is, then, are we as a discipline willing to give up the rich veins of practice and inquiry described above? Are we willing to decisively sever our ties with artistic influences, eliminating them in principle from the education of our trainees? Do we see where the discipline is headed? I do not believe that enough of us do.

The benefits of the romantic to psychology

Many of the concrete benefits of the romantic can be understood when traced to America's founding psychologist and self-proclaimed romanticist, William James (Leary, 1992). Arguably James's finest statement (and a pioneering example of qualitative research) was his *The Varieties of Religious Experience* (1902/1936). Not only did this classic elucidate the nature and structure of spiritual transcendence, it also brought tangible scientific interest to a field that had hitherto been neglected and debased (Fadiman & Frager, 1976). Other major romantic psychological influences that have brought tangible benefits include those of Freud and Jung in the area of psychotherapy (Hillman, 1975; Kirschner, 1996), Luria (1979) in the domain of neuropsychology, and Giorgi (1970) in the realm of methodology.

Below is a brief sampling of the kind of qualitative–descriptive methodologies that have been elaborated in general terms by theorists such as Giorgi (1970) and Polkinghorne (1988). These studies show how careful accounts of the lifeworld can be structured so as to yield tangible psychosocial benefits.

Abraham Maslow's (1954) study of self-actualization is a case in point. Maslow began this study by drawing on feelings, hunches, and detailed field notes. He reflected deeply, for example, about his most influential teachers—Max Wertheimer and Ruth Benedict—and explicated that which made them stand out. Later, he immersed himself in the experiences of other historic and inspirational figures. Finally, he conducted in-depth interviews with such figures, consolidated his findings, and extrapolated his results to many different subdisciplines, such as clinical, personality, and organizational psychology (Maslow, 1971).

The concept of self-actualization and its associated "hierarchy of needs" plays a notable role in personology (Maddi, 1976), industrial organizational psychology (Masserik, 1994), and educational psychology (Richards & Combs, 1994). Thanks to the influence of Maslow and other existential-humanistic psychologists (e.g., Rogers), there have been significant increases in the trends toward worker participation in management, meaning-based jobs, and human relations training (Kramer, 1995; Masserik, 1994). There has also been an increased recognition of the roles played by empathy, emotions, and creativity within the educational setting (Goleman, 1995; Richards & Combs, 1994). Arguably, these factors are integral to the previously mentioned social responsibility movement in our culture and to a resurgent quest for meaning (Lerner, 1996; Pauchant, 1995).

In the clinical area, existential–humanistic therapists, such as Rogers, May, Perls, Laing, Bugental, and Gendlin, have proved equally prescient. By underscoring experiential and relational dimensions of therapy, these theorists anticipated that which the outcome literature reveals quantitatively—that factors such as warmth, genuineness, responsibility, mutuality, immediacy, affectivity, and kinesthesia account for significantly more change variability than do isolated techniques (Duncan & Moynihan, 1994; Lambert & Bergin, 1994).

The early introspections and case reports of James (1904/1987), Reich (1949), Goldstein (1963), Boss (1978), Maslow (1954), Lowen (1975), and others led directly to the development of the holistic health and medicine movement. Factors such as psychological hardiness and the physician–patient relationship and activities such as the caressing of infants, group therapy for cancer patients, and yoga and meditation to supplement physical healing have all been hailed as promising new dimensions in the medical community (Duggan, 1995; Kobasa, 1979; Sacks, 1990).

For a broader sampling of qualitative-descriptive studies that have benefited psychology, see Messer et al. (1988), Schneider (1993, 1998), Schneider and May (1995), Valle and Halling (1989), and Wertz (1994).

The complementary value of romanticism

One of the most critical questions facing psychology today is that of the relationship between romantic approaches and mainstream empirical approaches. To the extent that romantic contributions to the discipline are acknowledged at all by mainstream psychology, they are relegated to what philosophers of science (e.g., Giorgi, 1986) call the "context of discovery" in the scientific process. Phenomenological descriptions, personal experience and anecdote, linguistic analyses, cultural–historical reflections, and so on are thought to play a role in the earliest stage of scientific thought, that of the generation of theories or hypotheses. However useful they may be in particular instances of psychology, the work of scientific psychology proper is located, on the contrary, in the "context of verification" (Giorgi, 1986). This context involves transforming romantic might-be insights into testable propositions, operationally defining variables, designing an empirical test, and applying quantitative, inductive analyses to observations that alone could support a certification of the truth value or usefulness of these contributions.

There are serious difficulties inherent in this model of the relationship of romantic contributions to the body of psychology proper. First, because these contributions are viewed as being neither necessary nor sufficient, they are not identified as essential parts of the scientific process. Consequently, they are not encouraged in practice; they are often not used in the formation of theory and hypothesis; and most importantly, they are not developed or taught in light of such methodological norms as would be necessary for their rigorous, maximally sophisticated, and most fruitful enactment. The result is that psychological theories and hypotheses do not have to be, and often are not, grounded in and relevant to the real world of human existence (Giorgi, 1970; Polkinghorne, 1983).

A second problem has to do with insufficiencies in the context of justification as constituted within the mainstream positivist model of science. That is, even hypotheses that are strongly supported by empirical verification remain problematically related to the concrete lives of individual human beings. For example, the reader of an introductory psychology text, which presumably contains the best verified knowledge claims of the discipline, is hard pressed to know if and how the propositions are true of him or her or anyone else in particular life situations. If and how the above propositions apply to specific, complex life situations remain almost completely unexplored. Conclusions based on aggregate data may not even be applicable to particular individual participants in the research let alone to others or to individuals in different situations. Although at times the meaning of theories, hypotheses, experimental results, and so on is addressed, usually in discussion sections of research reports, there are no established methodological norms governing attributions of applicability and overall significance to the lifeworld. If psychology is to be a complete science and to provide truths that are applicable at the level of the actual lives of individual human beings, it must develop and regard as essential procedures guided by rigorous methodological norms that are appropriate to relating theoretical and empirical knowledge back to the lifeworld. This requires qualitative modes of knowledge distinct from those involved in hypothesis testing.

Is it possible to show how qualitative and quantitative research can interrelate with and benefit from one another? I believe so. Lukoff, Edwards, and Miller (in press), for example, have formulated a qualitative research design—the multiple case study—that may serve as a model for such complementarity. This design entails a formal set of guidelines that address the cornerstones of scientific investigation: discovery and verification, and validity and reliability. The first step in this methodology is to frame a research question based on hunches, speculations, or gaps in the relevant literature. The second step is to select participants who are relevant to the topic of study and to collect as much data as possible about them. To illustrate this procedure, I refer to an actual multiple case study conducted by Fox (1996; See also Fox & Serlin, 1996), concerning changes in high-risk youth as a result of a coping skills class. This study tracked four participants, ages 18–21, who participated in a one-year coping skills class over a three-year period. To guard against concerns about construct validity (e.g., does the study measure what it purports to measure?), the researcher is encouraged to select participants and collect data on the basis of converging lines of evidence. In Fox's study, participants were selected and data collected on the basis of observations by the investigator, interview data (i.e., from participants, teachers, parents), a rating scale administered by both the investigator and a school psychologist, and a variety of other archival data. Such data indicated that the participants were who Fox purported them to be—high-risk adolescents—and that their responses to the class were valid.

The third step in the procedure is to reduce the raw data about participants into a manageable form for both researcher and presentation. To guard against selection bias, the researcher (as was the case with Fox) uses independent judges to review both the raw data and data reduction. The fourth step entails data interpretation: "In this phase, new theory is developed... Validity depends on the quality of the arguments that link data to theory" (Lukoff et al., in press, p. 14). Fox (1996, pp. 267–269) concluded that after three years of gathering multiple sources of data, the coping-skills class resulted in "dramatic positive changes" in 14 distinct categories. The internal validity of this stage depends on the "extent to which alternative explanations of the phenomenon can be excluded" (Lukoff et al., in press, p. 14). "Hypotheses," Lukoff et al. continue, "are best supported if they are tested against a broad range of cases, and an active search is made for negative cases that might disprove a particular hypothesis" (p. 12). Using independent judges, relevant archival material, and interviews, Fox (1996) paid careful attention to both the limits and delimits of his design (pp. 165–169) as well as to alternative explanations of his results (pp. 269–276).

With regard to external validity—the extent to which data interpretations can be generalized to real-life settings—the multiple case design has some ideal qualities according to Lukoff et al. (in press). This is because, unlike experimental studies, which must be carried out in highly controlled laboratory settings, the case study is conducted directly in the naturalistic environment (e.g., in a school setting as in Fox's [1996] study). The downside of the case study, of course, is that it aims at depth of understanding more than breadth of verification. However, this limitation can be mitigated to some degree by working with as many participants as possible and by repeating the study. Bromley (1986) likened this process to the building up of case law in jurisprudence. Such a process, observed Bromley, "provides rules, generalizations and categories which gradually systematize the knowledge (facts and theories) gained from the intensive study of individual cases" (p. 2).

The upshot of this vignette is that despite notable limitations, the multiple case studies in particular and the qualitative framework generally have many virtues in the contexts of both discovery and verification (Bromley, 1986; Yin, 1989). Even an early skeptic such as D. T. Campbell has arrived at this position. In his introduction to Yin's (1989) book, he wrote: "More and more I have come to the conclusion that the core of the scientific method is not experimentation per se, but rather the strategy connoted by the phrase 'plausible rival hypotheses'" (p. 8). Accordingly, by using multiple sources of data, examining converging lines of evidence, and drawing convincing inferences from data, qualitative research can provide valid, reliable, and useful psychological knowledge. What then does the qualitative framework contribute to the quantitative paradigm? I suggest the following three elements: The generation of hypotheses, hunches, and speculations from which experimental data can be drawn (consider, for example, Fox's [1996] 14 categories of outcome as potential dependent variables); the investigation of naturally occurring phenomena, complex emotional experiences, and longitudinal perspectives that cannot readily be operationalized (e.g., raw case data); and the deepening of or elaboration on existing experimental findings.[3] (Compare, for example, Fox's ample findings regarding high-risk youths with those in the traditional literature [Fox, 1996; National Research Council, 1993].)

Experimental research, on the other hand, can complement qualitative investigations as follows: by limiting threats to validity and reliability, that is, by controlling confounding variables such as researcher and selection biases; by isolating causal relationships; and by broadening, at a greatly accelerated pace, the generalizability of findings (Jacobson & Christensen, 1996; Yin, 1989). In general, concluded Yin (1989), experimental research is optimal when the boundaries between phenomenon and context are clearly evident, whereas qualitative research is better suited to subtler and more complex phenomena and contexts.

For all their mutuality, however, there are areas—such as individually meaningful poetic, intuitive, and visionary states—where qualitative investigation resists experimental systematization altogether. These areas should be respected, in my view, as legitimate sources of psychological knowledge (See also James, 1904/1987, p. 1160). Although such states may not presently have the generalizability of traditional forms of evidence, this circumstance could change. (Consider Maslow's early hunches about self-actualization or Einstein's visions of relativity theory [Einstein, 1952, p. 43].)

Other romantically oriented research that supplements or is supplemented by experimental findings includes multiple case investigations, such as that by M. Miller (1996) on diet and psychological health; phenomenological studies, such as those by Stevick (1971) on the nature of anger, Colaizzi (1973) on the experience of learning, Wertz (1983) on the nature of perception, Churchill (1998) on the diagnostic experience, and Fischer (1985) on individualized assessment; and grounded theory inquiries, such as those by Rennie (1990) and Schneider (1984) on clients' perceptions of therapy.

The complementary potential of romanticism

The implications of a romantic complement to psychology are both provocative and far-ranging. I believe that the entire discipline of psychology could benefit by being grounded in a romantic context—the context of the lifeworld. The romantic is a ground in two senses: It is a ground for hypothesis generation and it is a ground for hypothesis verification. It both stimulates discovery and deepens and elaborates on empirical confirmations. Experimental research, in my view, operates somewhere between these romantic grounds of discovery and verification (as is true of quantitative research generally). Where appropriate, experimental research plays the vital role of specifying, clarifying, and broadly generalizing romantic insights; however, experimental research cannot entirely supplant those insights, and, on the contrary, in my view, needs to refer back to them. How is truth to be decided in such a framework? As in case-law jurisprudence, the answer would depend on (a) expert consensus, and (b) converging lines of evidence from both qualitative and quantitative data. (Consider, for example, the converging lines of support for relationship factors in psychotherapy.) Let us speculate now about a few more dimensions of a romantically grounded psychology.

In the field of psychotherapy, for example, research and practice could be conducted on a variety of levels, from the organic (physiological), environmental (behavioral), and cognitive, to the psychosexual (psychoanalytic), interpersonal (relational), and experiential (existential; Schneider & May, 1995). Each of these levels could be seen as ever-widening and ever-deepening spheres of liberation culminating, as implied, at the existential–experiential mode of change. Depending on clients' desires and capacities, change would occur flexibly within this model, with therapists offering a diversity of interventions. Research too would be conducted flexibly, contingent on questions asked and aims desired. For example, quantitative research and programmatic practice could be implemented for peculiarly organic, environmental, and cognitive spheres of concern (where functioning is quasimechanistic), whereas qualitative inquiry and holistic practice could be engaged for more intimate realms of concern, such as those of sexuality, interpersonal relationships, and kinesthesia. (See Schneider, in press, and Schneider & May, 1995, for an elaboration on this formulation.) The model might work something like this: Quantitative findings about, say, the reduction in negative self-statements in depression would be referred to qualitative studies about the meaning of such a phenomenon in clients' everyday lives. These data would then be fed back to the therapeutic context and used to determine treatment. This framework, of course, would require formidable time and resources. However, cost and time offsets in the forms of higher client satisfaction, improved life functioning, and improved psychosocial understanding may be the result (Bugental & Bracke, 1992; Howard et al., 1993; I. J. Miller, 1996a). On the practice side, time and cost may not be as daunting as they appear initially. Although some clients would choose longer term services, many others, because of their desires and capacities for change, would choose briefer versions (which is compatible with previously mentioned studies on this issue). For those who do choose longer engagements, cost-containing measures, such as managed cooperation, could be implemented.

The implications for training therapists in this context would also be far-ranging. Therapy would not necessarily or exclusively be taught in terms of the isolated norms of test data, the *DSM-IV,* or standardized manuals. Neither would it be taught only as a static enterprise in which the doctor is the sole authority. Although these latter standpoints would be recognized as useful in limited circumstances and therefore worthy of study, their role would be deemphasized. What would be emphasized is a broader and deeper approach to clients, one that values the immediate, affective, and kinesthetic experience of clients and not just theories about them (Schneider & May, 1995). Far from being a facile enterprise, the kind of training advocated here would require the utmost cultivation of personal and technical skills: skills devoted to understanding the whole person, his or her chief concerns, and his or her chief challenges in redressing those concerns (Bugental, 1987). In addition to formulating problem-oriented process notes or behaviorally anchored treatment plans, students would benefit from providing rich and sensitive qualitative descriptions of their clients. Students should attend to clients' whole behavioral and experiential repertoires and note their full affective, kinesthetic, and cognitive experience of those clients. Students should be schooled not merely in evaluating clients' progress toward treatment goals but in assessing the meaning of those treatment goals for clients' lives as a whole. In this way, students would have access to a full range of experiential data about their clients and would be in an optimal position to amalgamate that which is essential in the formulation of their treatment plan.

With regard to the clinical psychology curriculum, not only would qualitative–descriptive methodologies and approaches be taught alongside more mainstream approaches, but philosophical and literary studies would be added as well. There could be courses, for example, about art, music, narrative psychology, existential philosophy, and postmodernism alongside classes about diagnosis, psychophysiology, and social psychology. There could also be courses on meditative and contemplative approaches to psychotherapy, personal growth, and relational dynamics. The idea here would be to help to cultivate a sensitive and well-rounded human being as a ground for that human being's role as a therapist, researcher, or teacher. No less than Freud (1959) himself argued this point in his essay *On the Question of Lay Analysis*. Specifically, he contended that the best preparation for psychological studies is immersion in the study of art, culture, and the humanities in contrast to immersion in medicine and the natural sciences. Rollo May (1991) has also shown the therapeutic value of such literary dimensions in his discussion of Dante's *Divine Comedy* and Goethe's *Faust.*

Beyond the clinical arena, the romantic could complement many of the major subject areas of psychology—physiology and personality, social, and developmental psychology, and so on. As suggested earlier, the main criterion from the romantic standpoint would be what are the ways that this particular datum has meaning, impact, and significance in the life or lives of those affected, and how can we best explicate that meaning, impact, and significance? Such a reconception, of course, requires a shift in emphasis away from the laboratory and toward naturalistic settings and research.

The romantic dimension described above is not merely a prescientific heuristic for traditional empirical research but a needed and essential way of relating experimentally determined and quantitatively defined knowledge back to the lifeworld. This kind of research holds tremendous potential for informing us of the many qualitatively different problems that people bring to therapy, vocational settings, and interpersonal contexts, and the different ways in which people learn to transform these problems.

The upshot of these considerations is that psychological research and practice should begin and end with thoroughgoing and rigorous inquiry into the lifeworld. Such inquiries can (a) guide the development of relevant hypotheses, measures, and so on; (b) contribute valuable qualitative insights into the psychological processes involved in experimental situations; and (c) provide rigorous research in complex everyday situations. In addition, such inquiries must be regarded as scientific and legitimate in their own right, appropriate to the kind of questions they address, and not necessarily in need of supplementation. Theories, hypotheses, and quantitative research, however, are in themselves insufficient and require ways of knowing if and how they relate to the concrete lives of persons (Allport, 1961). In this context, romantic psychology provides a necessary supplement.

The postmodern challenge to romanticism

Traditional empiricism and clinical standardization are not the only challenges to psychology's romantic heritage; new and more subtle criticisms are emerging. The most prominent of these is postmodernist philosophy. Postmodernist philosophy has acquired an increasing visibility in American psychology (e.g., Cushman, 1990; Gergen, 1994; Sampson, 1993). This visibility is understandable; we live in postmodern times. By postmodern times, I mean our consciousness of the breakdown of premodern (e.g., religious) and modern (e.g., scientific) institutions, our relinquishment of absolute truths, and our recognition of socially constructed realities (O'Hara & Anderson, 1991). A distinction must be drawn, however, between acceptance of our postmodern predicament and advocacy or even celebration of that predicament. Although the romanticism I have described does not deny the postmodern context within which it operates, it does reject wholehearted endorsements of that context (See also Hoshmand & Martin, 1994). To the degree that advocates of postmodernity curb the conventional trend toward objectifying (and quantifying) psychological data, the romantic vision is in thorough agreement with postmodernism. Likewise, to the extent that supporters of postmodernity uphold the sanctity of unique and alternative psychosocial discourses, the romantic view is also compatible with postmodernism. However, to the degree that advocates of the postmodern make a shrine of those disparate discourses, approach them as self-sealing doctrines, and forget our collective (i.e., human) situation on this planet, these advocates cultivate a relativistic morass that directly counters the romantic sensibility (Grondin, 1995). For example, Sampson (1993) and Gergen (1994) directed psychology's attention to the unique identities of disparate groups in our society but failed to demand that same attention for (existential) conditions that inform and underlie those identities. The romantic orientation, on the other hand, goes beyond the unique viewpoint of the individual or culture in an attempt to understand their common challenges. Drawing on feeling and intuition, romanticism attunes to the life we share (our awareness of death, our journey through creation, our urges to love and be loved) as well as to our unique interests, conflicts, and concerns (Becker, 1973; Kirschner, 1987). My point here is that more of a balance is needed in the postmodern inquiry into identity (Smith, 1994). Not only is it important to investigate the cultural, linguistic, and political dimensions of the lifeworld, it is also necessary to explore the emotional and intuitive connotations of those dimensions (Merleau-Ponty, 1962; Polkinghorne, 1994). These connotations access people's felt impressions, bodily understandings, and existential awarenesses (Gendlin, 1978; May, 1981). They help us to empathize with one another and, in the long run, to learn from and coexist with one another. To quote Hoshmand and Martin (1994).

A surprisingly diverse set of philosophical opinions (including those of such prominent individuals as Wittgenstein, Gadamer, and Habermas...) hold that it may be possible to reflect critically on one's cultural heritage and experiences, to debate across cultures, and to seek transcendent understandings that might conceivably bridge diverse cultural practices in societies and in scientific communities. (p. 184).

Summary and conclusion: Whither the romantic?

When the 1994 president of the American Psychological Association, Frank Farley, suggested that we psychologists "stand very close to being a discipline concerned with superficial problems" and that spirituality, "deep feelings about soul and eternity... [and] a psychology of meaning in the broadest sense... placing the mystery of life in context, and most importantly, showing the road to generosity and love" will "become increasingly important" (cited in Martin, 1994, p. 12), he was sounding a romantic chord.

In this chapter, I have shown that, although marginal in its influence, romanticism has a long and distinguished lineage in psychology. I have also shown that today, romantic psychology faces a grave diminution of its influence. This development is based in part on the shortcomings of romanticism itself, but it is also in large part due to converging political, economic, and professional interests.

I have further proposed that there is a formidable price to be paid for the eroding of romanticism's influence in psychology. This price includes psychology's deepening neglect of its meaning and significance for the lifeworld; its further dissociation from the arts and humanities; and its widening reductionism.

As an antidote to this dire state of affairs, I hope that I have shown the many ways that romantic psychology not only benefits but also complements the evolving profession of psychology. Finally, I have suggested that romanticism and postmodernist philosophy have much in common as alternatives to mainstream psychological reductionism. However, I have also argued that strident advocates of postmodernism fail to see a middle ground of commonality in the midst of relativism, and they fail to find conviction in the face of doubt.

Is it beyond the present imagination to conceive of a romantic revival in psychology? Perhaps. At the very least, however, the romantic psychology that I have been discussing compels significantly more attention than it has heretofore garnered or is currently receiving. Although the kind of romantic revolution that I urge in this chapter (and that others have urged elsewhere) is far-reaching, and the resources necessary to meet it are formidable, psychologists, from my standpoint, would be remiss to overlook it. The real question is whether we as a profession are going to act in an expedient way—in conformity with fashionable trends—or in accord with our professional mandate? If no one stands up for principle (as opposed to fashion) in our field, there will surely be few capable of taking this stance in our stead. Even if one is a tough-minded empiricist, one must recognize our field's multidimensionality. One must recognize that psychology cannot simply stand for a monolithic curriculum or one-track science (Koch, 1993; Rychlak, 1993). It must open to the larger view of science embodied by a growing constituency, the view supported in many cases by clinicians but that relates to the field as a whole: that is, the view of psychology as a human inquiry, one tailored to people's lived realities. As the early romanticists taught, such a view may well help to salvage our planet as well as our discipline.

Notes

1 The phrase "science of the heart" was used recently by broadcast journalist and author Bill Moyers (Baccalaureate address, Brown University, May 25, 1997) to characterize the ancient Israelite conception of wisdom (or *hochma*). *Hochma*, according to Moyers, is very similar to this article's definition of romanticism: It combines intelligence, feeling, and perception

2 I acknowledge the complex and controversial nature of the so-called romantic movement in the arts and philosophy. The term has many connotations and many historical antecedents (Jones, 1969). However, I have distilled in this definition—a position that might be termed "romantic science" (Luria, 1979)—features that I believe to be relevant to psychology.

3 This point highlights one of the unique advantages of certain forms of qualitative research—the relationship that is cultivated between researcher and participant. Without this relationship, in my view, key disclosures are likely to be sacrificed.

References

Aanstoos, C. (1994). Mainstream psychology and the humanistic alternative. In F. J. Wertz (Ed.), *The humanistic movement: Recovering the person in psychology* (1–11). Lake Worth, FL: Gardner.

Albee, G. W. (1996). Revolutions and counterrevolutions in prevention. *American Psychologist, 51*, 1130–1133.

Allport, G. (1961). *Pattern and growth in personality.* New York: Holt, Rinehart, & Winston.

American Psychiatric Association. (1994). *Diagnostic and statistical manual of mental disorders* (4th ed.). Washington, DC: Author.

American Psychological Association. (1995). *Template for developing guidelines: Interventions for mental disorders and psychosocial aspects of physical disorders.* Washington, DC: Author.

Barlow, D. H. (1996). Health care policy, psychotherapy research, and the future of psychotherapy. *American Psychologist, 51*, 1050–1058.

Barrett, W. (1958). *Irrational man.* New York: Doubleday.

Becker, E. (1973). *The denial of death.* New York: Free Press.

Bellah, R. N., Madsen, R., Sullivan, W. M., & Tipton, S. M. (1985). *Habits of the heart.* Berkeley, CA: University of California Press.

Bellak, L., & Small, L. (1965). *Emergency psychotherapy and brief psychotherapy.* New York: Grune & Stratton.

Bernstein, R. (1976). *The restructuring of social and political theory.* New York: Harcourt Brace Jovanovich.

Bernstein, R. (1983). *Beyond objectivism and relativism.* Philadelphia: University of Pennsylvania Press.

Bevan, W., & Kessel, F. (1994). Plain truths and home cooking: Thoughts on the making and remaking of psychology. *American Psychologist, 49*, 505–509.

Bohart, A., O'Hara, M., & Leitner, L. (1998). Empirically violated treatments: Disenfranchisement of humanistic and other psychotherapies. *Psychotherapy research, 8*(2), 141–157

Boss, M. (1978). *Existential foundations of psychology and medicine.* (S. Conway & A. Cleary, Trans.). New York: Jason Aronson.

Bracke, P. E., & Bugental, J. F. T. (1995). Existential addiction: A model for treating Type A behavior and workaholism. In T. Pauchant (Ed.), *In search of meaning: Managing for the health of our organizations, our communities, and the natural world* (pp. 65–93). San Francisco: Jossey-Bass.

Breggin, P. (1991). *Toxic psychiatry.* New York: St. Martin's Press.

Bromley, D. (1986). *The case-study method in psychology and related disciplines.* New York: Wiley.

Bugental, J. F. T. (1987). *The art of the psychotherapist.* New York: Norton.

Bugental, J. F. T., & Bracke, P. E. (1992). The future of existential-humanistic psychotherapy. *Psychotherapy, 29*, 28–33.

Butcher, J. N., Stelmachers, Z. T., & Maudal, G. R. (1983). Crisis intervention and emergency psychotherapy. In I. B. Weiner (Ed.), *Clinical methods in psychology* (pp. 572–633). New York: Wiley.

Churchill, S. D. (1998). The intentionality of psychodiagnostic seeing: A phenomenological investigation of clinical impression formation. In R. S. Valle (Ed.),

Phenomenological inquiry: Existential and transpersonal dimensions (pp. 175–207). New York: Plenum.

Colaizzi, P. F. (1973). *Reflections and research in psychology*. Dubuque, IA: Kendall/Hunt.

Consumer Reports. (1995, November). Mental health: Does therapy help? *Consumer Reports*. pp. 734–739.

Cushman, P. (1990). Why the self is empty: Toward a historically situated psychology. *American Psychologist, 45*, 599–611.

Cushman, P. (1995). *Constructing the self, constructing America*. Reading, MA: Addison-Wesley.

DeCarvalho, R. (1991). *The founders of humanistic psychology*. New York: Praeger.

Denkers, G., & Clifford, R. (1994). *A survey of psychologists' experiences with managed care: Consumer issues*. San Mateo, CA: San Francisco Bay Area Psychologists Task Force on Managed Care.

Dilthey, W. (1977). *Descriptive psychology and historical understanding*. The Hague: Nijhoff. (Original work published 1894).

Duggan, R. M. (1995). Complementary medicine: Transforming influence or footnote to history? *Alternative Therapies in Health and Medicine, 1*(2), 28–33.

Duncan, B. L., & Moynihan, D. W. (1994). Applying outcome research: Intentional utilization of the client's frame of reference. *Psychotherapy, 31*, 294–301.

Einstein, A. (1952). Letter to Jacques Hadamard. In E. Ghiselin (Ed.), *The creative process* (pp. 43–44). New York: Mentor.

Elgin, D., & LeDrew, C. (1997, May). *Global consciousness change: Indicators of an emerging paradigm*. San Anselmo, CA: Millennium Project.

Fadiman, J., & Frager, R. (1976). *Personality and personal growth*. New York: Harper & Row.

Faidley, A. J., & Leitner, L. M. (1993). *Assessing experience in psychotherapy: Personal construct alternatives*. Greenwich, CT: Praeger.

Fassel, D. (1990). *Working ourselves to death*. San Francisco, CA: Harper.

Fensterheim, H., & Raw, S. D. (1996). Psychotherapy research is not psychotherapy practice. *Clinical Psychology: Science and Practice, 3*, 168–171.

Fischer, C. T. (1985). *Individualized psychological assessment*. Monterey, CA: Brooks/Cole.

Fox, G. K. (1996). *A multiple case study of a coping skills group for high risk, high school students*. Unpublished doctoral dissertation, Saybrook Institute, San Francisco, CA.

Fox, G. K., & Serlin, I. (1996). High-risk youth and the transition to adulthood. *Humanistic Psychologist, 24*(3), 349–363.

Freud, S. (1959). The question of lay analysis. In J. Strachey (Ed.), *The standard edition of the complete psychological works of Sigmund Freud* (*Vol. 20*, pp. 183–258). London: Hogarth Press. (Original work published 1926).

Garfield, S. L. (Ed.). (1997). The therapist as a neglected variable in psychotherapy research. *Clinical Psychology: Science and Practice, 4*, 40–89.

Garfield, S. L., & Bergin, A. E. (1994). Overview, trends, and future issues. In A. E. Bergin & S. L. Garfield (Eds.), *Handbook of psychotherapy and behavior change*, (4th ed., pp. 3–18). New York: Wiley.

Gendlin, E. (1978). *Focusing*. New York: Bantam.

Gergen, K. J. (1994). Exploring the postmodern: Perils or potentials? *American Psychologist, 49*, 412–416.

Giorgi, A. (1970). *Psychology as a human science*. New York: Harper & Row.

Giorgi, A. (1986). The "context of discovery/context of verification" distinction and descriptive human science. *Journal of Phenomenological Psychology, 17*, 151–166.

Goldfried, M. R., & Wolfe, B. E. (1996). Psychotherapy practice and research: Repairing a strained alliance. *American Psychologist, 51*, 1007–1016.

Goldstein, K. (1963). *The organism.* Boston: Beacon Press.

Goleman, D. (1995). *Emotional intelligence: Why it can matter more than IQ.* New York: Bantam.

Grondin, J. (1995). *Sources of hermeneutics.* Albany, NY: State University of New York Press.

Heidegger, M. (1962). *Being and time.* New York: Harper & Row.

Hillman, J. (1975). *Revisioning psychology.* New York: Harper & Row.

Hillman, J., & Ventura, M. (1993). *We've had 100 years of psychotherapy—and the world's getting worse.* New York: Harper/Collins.

Hipp, M. L., Atkinson, C., & Pelc, R. (1994). *Colorado Psychological Association legislative survey.* Denver, CO: Colorado Psychological Association.

Hoshmand, L. T., & Martin, J. (1994). Naturalizing the epistemology of psychological research. *Journal of Theoretical and Philosophical Psychology, 14*(2), 171–189.

Howard, K. I., Lueger, R. J., Maling, M. S., & Martinovich, Z. (1993). A phase model of psychotherapy outcome: Causal mediation of change. *Journal of Consulting and Clinical Psychology, 61*, 678–685.

Husserl, E. (1962). *Ideas: General introduction to pure phenomenology.* New York: Collier.

Jacobson, N. S., & Christensen, A. (1996). Studying the effectiveness of psychotherapy: How well can clinical trials do the job? *American Psychologist, 51*, 1031–1039.

James, W. (1936). *The varieties of religious experience.* New York: Modern Library. (Original work published 1902).

James, W. (1961). *Psychology: The briefer course.* New York: Harper Torch Books. (Original work published 1892).

James, W. (1987). A world of pure experience. In B. Kuklick (Ed.), *William James: Writings 1902–1910* (pp. 1159–1182). New York: Viking. (Original work published 1904).

Jamison, K. R. (1993). *Touched by fire: Manic–depressive illness and the artistic temperament.* New York: Free Press.

Jones, W. T. (1969). *Kant to Wittgenstein and Sartre: A history of Western philosophy.* New York: Harcourt, Brace, & World.

Jung, C. G. (1966). *Two essays on analytical psychology.* (R. F. C. Hull, Trans.). Princeton, NJ: Princeton University Press.

Kirschner, S. R. (1987). "Then what have I to do with thee?": On identity, fieldwork, and ethnographic knowledge. *Cultural Anthropology, 2*(2), 211–234.

Kirschner, S. R. (1996). *The religious and romantic origins of psychoanalysis: Individuation and integration in post-Freudian theory.* Cambridge, England: Cambridge University Press.

Kobasa, S. (1979). Stressful life events, personality, and health: An inquiry into hardiness. *Journal of Personality and Social Psychology, 37*, 1–11.

Koch, S. (1993). "Psychology" or "the psychological studies"? *American Psychologist, 48*, 902–904.

Kramer, R. (1995). Carl Rogers meets Otto Rank: The discovery of relationship. In T. C. Pauchant (Ed.), *In search of meaning: Managing for the health of our organizations, our communities and the natural world.* San Francisco: Jossey-Bass.

Krupnick, J. L., Sotsky, S. M., Simmens, S., Moher, J., Elkin, I., Watkins, J., & Pilkonisk, P. A. (1996). The role of the therapeutic alliance in psychotherapy and pharmacotherapy outcome. Findings in the National Institute of Mental Health Treatment of Depression Collaborative Research Project. *Journal of Consulting and Clinical Psychology*, *64*, 532–539.

Laing, R. D. (1967). *Politics of experience*. New York: Ballantine.

Lambert, M. J., & Bergin, A. E. (1994). The effectiveness of psychotherapy. In A. E. Bergin & S. L. Garfield (Eds.), *Handbook of psychotherapy and behavior change* (pp. 143–189). New York: Wiley.

Leary, D. E. (1992). William James and the art of human understanding. *American Psychologist*, *47*, 152–160.

Lerner, M. (1996). *The politics of meaning: Restoring hope and possibility in an age of cynicism*. Reading, PA: Addison-Wesley.

Lowen, A. (1975). *Bioenergetics*. New York: Penguin.

Lukoff, D., Edwards, D., & Miller, M. (1998). The case study as a scientific method for researching alternative therapies. *Alternative Therapies in Health and Medicine, 4*(2), 44–52.

Luria, A. R. (1979). *The making of mind* (M. Cole & S. Cole, Trans.). Cambridge, MA: Harvard University Press.

Maddi, S. (1976). *Personaliy theories: A comparative analysis*. Homewood, IL: Dorsey Press.

Manning, W. G., Wells, K. B., & Benjamin, B. (1986). *Use of outpatient mental health care: Trial of a prepaid group practice versus fee-for-service*. (R-3277-NIMH). Santa Monica, CA: Rand.

Martin, S. (1994, October). Farley sums up his '93–'94 presidential year. *APA Monitor*. p. 12.

Maslow, A. (1954). *Motivation and personality*. New York: Harper & Row.

Maslow, A. (1971). *The further reaches of human nature*. New York: Penguin.

Masserik, F. (1994). The humanistic core of industrial/organizational psychology. In F. Wertz (Ed.), *The humanistic movement: Recovering the person in psychology* (pp. 274–281). Lake Worth, FL: Gardner.

May, R. (1958). The origins and significance of the existential movement in psychology. In R. May, E. Angel, & H. Ellenberger (Eds.), *Existence: A new dimension in psychiatry and psychology* (pp. 3–36). New York: Basic Books.

May, R. (1981). *Freedom and destiny*. New York: Norton.

May, R. (1991). *The cry for myth*. New York: Norton.

McDermott, R. A. (1993). Transpersonal worldviews: Historical and philosophical reflections. In R. Walsh & F. Vaughan (Eds.), *Paths beyond ego: The transpersonal vision* (pp. 206–213). Los Angeles: Tarcher.

Melville, H. (1964). *Pierre: Or, the ambiguities*. New York: Signet Classics. (Original work published 1852).

Merleau-Ponty, M. (1962). *The phenomenology of perception*. London: Routledge & Kegan Paul.

Messer, S. B., Sass, L. A., & Woolfolk, R. L. (1988). *Hermeneutics and psychological theory: Interpretive perspectives on personality, psychotherapy, and psychopathology*. New Brunswick, NJ: Rutgers University Press.

Meyers, G. E. (1986). *William James: His life and thought*. New Haven, CT: Yale University Press.

Miller, I. J. (1996a). Managed care is harmful to outpatient mental health services: A call for accountability. *Professional Psychology: Research and Practice*, *27*, 349–363.

Miller, I. J. (1996b). Time-limited brief therapy has gone too far: The result is invisible rationing. *Professional Psychology: Research and Practice*, *27*, 567–576.

Miller, M. (1996). *Diet and psychological health: A multiple case study*. Unpublished doctoral dissertation, Saybrook Institute, San Francisco, CA.

Moldawski, S. (1997, July). Managed care and psychotherapy are incompatible. *APA Monitor.* p. 24.

View in article

Morin, E. (1995). Organizational effectiveness and the meaning of work. In T. Pauchant (Ed.), *In search of meaning* (pp. 29–64). San Francisco: Jossey-Bass.

Moss, G. E., & Dielman, J. (1986). Demographic correlates of SI assessments of Type A behavior. *Psychosomatic Medicine*, *48*, 564–574.

Multiple Risk Factor Intervention Trial Group. (1979). The MRFIT behavior pattern study 1: Study design, procedures, and reproducibility of behavior pattern judgment. *Journal of Chronic Disease*, *32*, 293–305.

National Research Council. (1993). *Panel on high-risk youth: Losing generations*. Washington, DC: National Academy Press.

Norcross, J. C., Alford, B. A., & Demichele, J. T. (1992). The future of psychotherapy: Delphi data and concluding observations. *Psychotherapy*, *29*, 150–158.

O'Hara, M. (1994). Relational humanism: Psychology for a pluralistic world. In F. J. Wertz (Ed.), *The humanistic movement: Recovering the person in psychology* (pp. 322–329). Lake Worth, FL: Gardner.

O'Hara, M. (1997). Emancipatory therapeutic practice in a turbulent transmodern era: A work of retrieval. *Journal of Humanistic Psychology*, *37* (3)7–33.

O'Hara, M., & Anderson, W. (1991, September). Welcome to the postmodern world. *Networker.* pp. 19–25.

Pauchant, T. C. (1995). *In search of meaning: Managing for the health of our organizations, our communities, and the natural world*. San Francisco: Jossey-Bass.

Polanyi, M. (1962). *Personal knowledge: Towards a post-critical philosophy*. Chicago: University of Chicago Press.

Polkinghorne, D. (1983). *Methodology for the human sciences: Systems of inquiry*. Albany, NY: State University of New York Press.

Polkinghorne, D. (1988). *Narrative knowing and the human sciences*. Albany, NY: State University of New York Press.

Polkinghorne, D. (1994). A path of understanding for psychology. *Journal of Theoretical and Philosophical Psychology*, *14*(2), 128–145.

Rank, O. (1996). *A psychology of difference: The American lectures*. Princeton, NJ: Princeton University Press.

Reich, W. (1949). *Character analysis*. New York: Orgone Institute Press.

Rennie, D. L. (1990). Toward a representation of the client's experience of the psychotherapy hour. In G. Lietaer, J. Rombauts, & R. Van Balen (Eds.), *Client-centered and experiential therapy in the nineties* (pp. 155–172). Leuven, Belgium: Leuven University Press.

Richards, A. C., & Combs, A. W. (1994). Education and the humanistic challenge. In F. Wertz (Ed.), *The humanistic movement: Recovering the person in psychology* (pp. 256–273). Lake Worth, FL: Gardner.

Rogers, C. (1961). *On becoming a person*. Boston, MA: Houghton Mifflin.

Rychlak, J. F. (1993). A suggested principle of complementarity for psychology: In theory, not method. *American Psychologist, 48*, 933–942.

Sacks, O. (1990). *Awakenings*. New York: HarperCollins.

Sampson, E. E. (1993). Identity politics: Challenges to psychology's understanding. *American Psychologist, 48*, 1219–1230.

Sass, L. (1988). Humanism, hermeneutics, and the concept of the subject. In S. B. Messer, L. A. Sass, & R. L. Woolfolk, (Eds.), *Hermeneutics and psychological theory: Interpretive perspectives on personality, psychotherapy, and psychopathology* (pp. 222–271). New Brunswick, NJ: Rutgers University Press.

Schaef, A. W., & Fassel, D. (1988). *The addictive organization*. San Francisco, CA: Harper.

Schneider, K. J. (1984). Clients' perceptions of the positive and negative characteristics of their counselors (Doctoral dissertation, Saybrook Institute, 1985) *Dissertation Abstracts International, 45*(10), 3345B.

Schneider, K. J. (1993). *Horror and the holy: Wisdom-teachings of the monster tale*. Chicago: Open Court.

Schneider, K. J. (1998). *The paradoxical self: Toward an understanding of our contradictory nature* (2nd ed.). Atlantic Highlands, NJ: Humanities Press.

Schneider, K. J. (in press). Existential processes. In L. Greenberg, G. Lietaer, & J. Watson (Eds.), *Experiential psychotherapy: Foundations and differential treatment approaches*. New York: Guilford.

Schneider, K. J., & May, R. (1995). *The psychology of existence: An integrative, clinical perspective*. New York: McGraw-Hill.

Sedgwick, P. (1982). *Psychopolitics*. New York: Harper & Row.

Seligman, M. E. P. (1996). Science as an ally of practice. *American Psychologist, 51*, 1072–1079.

Shedler, J., Mayman, M., & Manis, M. (1993). The illusion of mental health. *American Psychologist, 48*, 1117–1131.

Shore, K. (1995, November). *Moving America beyond managed care and managed competition*. Paper presented at the National Coalition for Mental Health Professionals and Consumers and the Georgia Mental Health Coalition on Managed Care, Atlanta, GA.

Sifneos, P. E. (1972). *Short-term psychotherapy and emotional crisis*. Cambridge, MA: Harvard University Press.

Smith, M. B. (1994). Selfhood at risk: Postmodern perils and the perils of the postmodern. *American Psychologist, 49*, 405–411.

Stein, D. M., & Lambert, M. J. (1995). Graduate training in psychotherapy: Are therapy outcomes enhanced? *Journal of Consulting and Clinical Psychology, 63*, 182–196.

Stern, E. M. (1994–1995, Winter). August 1994 APA council session. *Division 32 Newsletter*. pp. 3–4.

Stevick, E. L. (1971). An empirical investigation of the experience of anger. In A. Giorgi, W. F. Fischer, & R. von Eckartsberg (Eds.), *Duquesne studies in phenomenological psychology* (*Vol. 1*, pp. 132–148). Pittsburgh, PA: Duquesne University Press.

Task Force on Promotion and Dissemination of Psychological Procedures, Division of Clinical Psychology of the American Psychological Association. (1995). Training and dissemination of empirically-validated psychological treatments: Report and recommendations. *Clinical Psychologist, 48*, 3–23.

Taylor, E. (1992). William James and the humanistic tradition. *Journal of Humanistic Psychology, 31*(1), 56–74.

Tillich, P. (1952). *The courage to be.* New Haven, CT: Yale University Press.
Tucker, L., & Lubin, W. (1994). *National survey of psychologists.* Report from Division 39, American Psychological Association. Washington, DC: American Psychological Association.
Valle, R., & Halling, S. (1989). *Existential-phenomenological perspectives in psychology: Exploring the breadth of human experience.* New York: Plenum.
Walls, G. B., & Scholom, A. H. (1996, Winter). APA practice guidelines template jeopardizes clinical autonomy of practitioners. *APA Division 39 Newsletter, Psychologist/Psychoanalyst.* pp. 17–21.
Walsh, R., & Vaughan, F. (1993). *Paths beyond ego: The transpersonal vision.* Los Angeles: Tarcher.
Wertz, F. J. (1983). Revolution in psychology: Case study of the new look school of perceptual psychology. In A. Giorgi, A. Barton, & C. Maes (Eds.), *Duquesne studies in phenomenological psychology* (*Vol. 4*, pp. 222–243). Pittsburgh, PA: Duquesne University Press.
Wertz, F. J. (1993). The phenomenology of Sigmund Freud. *Journal of Phenomenological Psychology, 24*(2), 101–129.
Wertz, F. J. (1994). *The humanistic movement: Recovering the person in psychology.* Lake Worth, FL: Gardner Press.
Wertz, F. J. (1995). The scientific status of psychology. *Humanistic Psychologist, 23*(3), 285–304.
Wundt, W. (1900–1920). *Volkerpsychologie.* Ein untersuchung der entwicklungsgesetze von sprache, mythos, und sitte. (Vols. 1–10). Leipzig, Germany: Englemann.
Wylie, M. S. (1995). The new visionaries. *The Family Therapy Networker, 19*(5), 20–36.
Yin, R. K. (1989). *Case study research: Design and methods.* Beverly Hills, CA: Sage.

Writing this article has been an odyssey. My deepest thanks go to the many colleagues and friends who have supported me during my labors. In particular, I would like to thank Frederick J. Wertz, without whose encouragement, assistance, and impeccable scholarship this article may not have come to pass. I would also like to thank Jeffrey Bricker, Edward Mendelowitz, Ilene Serlin, Mark Stern, Maurice Friedman, Arthur Bohart, David Leary, Eugene Taylor, David Lukoff, Edward Sampson, Kurt Salzinger, Nicholas Cummings, Brewster Smith, Samuel Haramis, and Jurate Raulinaitis for their invaluable suggestions.This article is indebted to the spirit, teaching, and life of Rollo May.

Section III

Implications and future actions

11

Going beneath the surface

What people want from therapy

Santiago Delboy and Linda L. Michaels

Background

Mental healthcare and ways to deal with emotional suffering are top of mind for many in our country. The traumas of the COVID-19 pandemic have heightened suffering for many, and racial and social inequities – long-standing and harrowing – have contributed to outrage and anguish. Stigma seems to be declining, especially among the younger generations, as celebrities and professional athletes are increasingly speaking out about their own mental health journeys. All of this is driving increased interest in and demand for mental healthcare, and, understandably, people have questions about what the best care is for them and how to find it. At the same time, general knowledge about therapy seems to be low, and misconceptions about depth therapy, in particular, as seen in ongoing stereotypes, seem prevalent. Thus, many do not have ready answers for their questions, and they are unsure about how to identify the type of care they need, how to find it, and how to assess whether it's of high quality. This void has, for the most part, been filled by the advertising and marketing messages from for-profit tech companies, insurance companies, and Silicon Valley investors looking to disrupt and dominate another industry. These entities have products to sell and profits to make, and see an opportunity among vulnerable people faced with a fragmented collection of independent clinicians. Even as our media channels are inundated with advertising from these tech companies, we wonder if these messages align with what people want and need. Do people resonate with their quick-fix appeals? Are people equipped with the information and education to assess their needs and identify what might help them best? What do people really want from therapy?

In the context of these questions, we believe that the public should know more about mental health care in general, and more about therapies of depth, insight, and relationship in particular. They might even find these therapies highly appealing, as they offer desirable benefits – they are highly effective and long-lasting. There is a robust, high-quality evidence base (Shedler, 2010; Gerber et al., 2011) showing that depth therapies are highly effective treatments (Steinert et al., 2017; Abbass, 2006; De Maat et al., 2009; Bateman & Fonagy,

DOI: 10.4324/9781003325512-15

2008; Leichsenring et al. 2013; Leichsenring & Rabung, 2008, 2011; Driessen et al., 2013). The treatments have been tested in many ways, including randomized control trials with thousands of patients, and found to be highly effective for a variety of conditions and populations, and especially for complex cases such as personality disorders, chronic depression and anxiety, and comorbidities (Lazar, 2018). Studies also show that many people need to receive a certain amount of therapy in order to show improvement; for example, one study showed that the average client needs 50–75 sessions, and the large Consumer Reports study suggested two years of weekly sessions (Lambert, Hansen & Finch, 2001; Morrison, Bradley & Westen, 2003; Seligman, 1995). Importantly, the effect sizes, or improvements due to these treatments – high at the end of many studies – continue to increase over time (Abbass, 2004; Lazar, 2018). This is in stark contrast to the finding that relapse rates of short-term therapy are unacceptably high, with the majority of patients receiving "evidence-based" treatment seeking additional treatment within 6–12 months for the same condition (Westen, Novotny & Thompson-Brenner, 2004). Although the benefits of depth therapies – effective, tested therapies that last for the long term – are likely what many people want, we do not see them reflected in the public narrative about therapy and we are concerned that these therapies have been missing, if not pushed out, from the public conversation by a variety of forces.

Along with limited awareness and understanding about therapy among the general public, we can identify multiple, powerful, vested, and monied interests promoting specific therapy brands, cultivating customers, and communicating to the public for years. It is not uncommon to see articles in the popular press touting "evidence-based treatments" or, more specifically, "cognitive behavioral therapy" (CBT). For example, NBC News published "What is cognitive behavioral therapy and how does it work" (DiGiulio, 2019), which presented CBT as the "gold standard" treatment for an enormous range of emotional and physical symptoms. While it is understandable that the popular press is not fully apprised of the entire evidence base of research in the field, we were surprised and dismayed to see that same article re-posted uncritically by the American Psychological Association on its LinkedIn account. Unfortunately, articles such as these are misleading for the public, which has little access to the evidence for the effectiveness of various treatments, and even less access to the skills to evaluate it. (For a review of the misleading claims of so-called "evidence-based" therapy, See Shedler, 2015). A layperson is probably not the typical reader of the Journal of the American Medical Association and thus would not have read JAMA's article asking "Is Cognitive Behavioral Therapy the Gold Standard for Psychotherapy?" (Leichsenring & Steinert, 2017) and learned that the answer was clearly "No."

In addition to the popular press, many individuals look to their insurance companies for mental health information and treatment options. For-profit insurance companies, beholden to quarterly financial results, are heavily incented to prefer those services that minimize cost – namely, medications or short-term, time-limited psychotherapy – and have seemingly worked diligently to restrict coverage for and access to quality mental healthcare. One strategy is to limit the number of therapists in their provider networks, which they may do by restricting therapists' reimbursement to below-market rates, or by having "ghost networks," meaning many of the therapists listed as in-network either have full practices, have retired, or are dead (Holstein & Paul, 2017). Another strategy is more hidden, yet more troubling. The 2019 class-action victory in a lengthy lawsuit filed against United Behavioral Health (Wit v UBH) reveals how deeply financial incentives infected, and indeed directed, UBH's coverage decisions. UBH was found to have systematically applied treatment coverage criteria developed by United's finance team, over the objections of United's own clinicians. UBH relied on these internal criteria to deny mental health treatment coverage, which, according to the lawsuit, resulted in individuals' suffering, relapsing, and dying. The Judge also found that UBH's criteria fell short of meeting generally accepted standards of care. Importantly, the Standards of Care outlined in the Judge's ruling have become the backbone of new legislation for parity and medical necessity guidelines for mental health care in multiple states.

In addition, individuals who are suffering will likely have seen some of the many direct-to-consumer ads for psychiatric medications. These ads, for which the industry spends $4.5–5.5 billion per year, make medications seem more appealing, more effective, and less risky (Ventola, 2011). From these ads, the public is unlikely to learn that the efficacy of medication has been overstated by approximately one-third (Carroll, 2018). Most recently, the next wave of direct-to-consumer advertising arrives from a different industry entering the mental health field technology. Silicon Valley investors and technopreneurs are aggressively developing products – mobile apps, websites, artificial intelligence – and aggressively advertising them online, on the radio, on the side of many a city bus. Despite scarce evidence that such products work, they are attracting staggering levels of investment. In 2020, digital behavioral health funding increased substantially over 2019, with $2.4 billion in funding across 67 deals (Wang & Zweig, 2021) and, in the first quarter of 2021, investments in new digital health deals were at a high of $6.7 billion, with mental health investments once again topping the list (Oss, 2021). These investments respond to the size of the opportunity: Talkspace estimates the "total global addressable market" for its services at $480 billion (Talkspace, 2021a). Employers and insurance companies are attracted to these services, often based on programmable algorithms, and see a quick way to cut costs. As of March of 2021, for example, Talkspace, which recently went public for $1.4B, reported contracts with 10 health plan clients and 91 enterprise clients, claiming that the number of people eligible to receive services through these partnerships exceeds 55 million (Talkspace, 2021a).

Some of these technology companies are positioning themselves as offering therapy or comprehensive mental healthcare, yet in fact, they do not. For example, some companies market asynchronous texting services as "therapy," even though there is no synchronous therapist-client communication let alone opportunities to share real-time conversation or exploration of issues, or emotional reactions that can be some of the most powerful aspects of one's experience in therapy. Others promote the ease of "seamlessly switching therapists, at no extra cost," (Talkspace, 2021b) which provides a way to avoid engaging with difficult emotions or conflict with one's therapist, and thus eliminates the opportunity to leverage some of the most important functions of the therapist-patient relationship. Other companies sell online self-help services, such as mindfulness or breathing exercises, or coaching services. The public likely does not know that anyone can call themselves a coach, and there is no graduate degree or state license for coaching. These deprofessionalized services offer an even further incentive for profit-maximizing corporations. It seems as though reach and efficiency and profitability have superseded questions of quality, let alone depth, insight, and relationship.

Many of our professional organizations and academics seem unlikely to stand up for therapies of depth, insight, and relationship; on the contrary, they seem to be limiting their focus to short-term, manualized treatments. Academics can complete research studies more quickly when they are studying a 10-session treatment protocol vs a two-year therapy process, and thus publish more prolifically. The American Psychological Association Division 12 maintains a list of empirically supported treatments and 90% of the treatments on its list are CBT, despite criticisms, from psychologists themselves, of this list and the problematic usage and definition of "evidence" and the corruption of the evidence-based practice model, (Wachtel, 2010; Tolin et al, 2015). In fact, despite the strong and robust evidence base for depth therapy highlighted earlier, evidence-based treatments have come to be synonymous with "short-term, technique-oriented, diagnosis-specific, symptom-reducing, protocol-following interventions… based on one type of evidence – the 'gold standard' of scientific investigations – randomized controlled trials," (Gnaulati, 2018, p. 2). These trends make it less likely that the therapists of tomorrow will be exposed to therapies of depth, insight, and relationship.

Thus, whether from insurers, pharmaceutical manufacturers, technology firms, and even our own mental health professions, almost every resource and message available to the public is steering them toward short-term, algorithm-based, depersonalized, quick-fix solutions, whether in the form of a medication or a time-limited, manualized treatment. Risks and costs are understated, while efficacies are overstated. These dynamics are reinforced by a cultural zeitgeist that values "quick-fixes" over reflection and long-term solutions. Thus, therapies of depth, insight, and relationship find themselves squeezed out of the public conversation around how to help those who are suffering. Specifically, many don't see psychoanalytic therapy as a credible source, and it is often perceived as antiquated, ineffective, never-ending, too expensive, and mainly for the privileged. There have been intentional efforts to discredit psychoanalytic and other depth treatment in multiple realms, for example by suggesting there is no "evidence" supporting it and further research is not indicated (Marcus et al., 2014; Mayo-Wilson et al., 2014; Steinert et al., 2017). To be sure, some of the problems have been generated by the psychoanalytic community itself, as fragmented as it is and disconnected from the mainstream population as it can be.

One way to conceptualize the challenges faced by therapies of depth, insight, and relationship is to think of them as a branding problem. This means centering the associations, emotions, mental models, and expectations about depth therapies – the way these therapies have come to "live" in people's minds and hearts – as a core part of the issue. Using this perspective highlights the need to first listen to the public, the users and potential users of therapy, in order to find ways to engage with them that are meaningful, relevant, impactful, and on their terms. Our ultimate goal is not to help therapists or professional organizations profit from this understanding, but to support people's informed decisions and right to choose from a wider range of therapeutic alternatives, and to bring therapies of depth, insight, and relationship back to their consideration set. With this in mind, our original research focuses on understanding people's values and preferences for therapy and therapists – a component of evidenced-based practice often ignored but critical for the success of mental health treatment. The corporate world has a long history of using and refining methodologies to do similar research, asking people questions directly in order to understand their needs, attitudes, preferences, and associations. While our objectives are very different from those traditionally pursued by for-profit corporations, these tools and methodologies are nonetheless useful for our goals. In general, nonprofits can benefit from leveraging frameworks and techniques from the for-profit world (e.g., Delboy et al., 2010; Kylander & Stone, 2012).

This effort is significantly different from other types of research in the mental health field, focusing on either clinical outcomes or on clinicians' perceptions. Our project was led by the authors, both of whom had significant education and experience in the marketing and marketing research fields prior to becoming clinicians. Except for access to the sample for our survey, the entire project, including contributions from project leaders and the rest of the research team, was conducted on a pro-bono basis. Working with limited financial resources limited the breadth of what we were able to cover in our research, but did not compromise its quality or adherence to marketing research best practices. Moreover, while the authors identify as advocates of therapies of depth, insight, and relationship, multiple measures were taken to minimize any bias in the research design, the questions we asked, and the people we talked to.

Methodology

A basic market research design when studying a new issue, topic, or population, typically considers two sequential stages. First, a qualitative phase using an unstructured discussion or observation guide, in order to explore the topic in more depth, develops an initial understanding and set of hypotheses and provides input on key topics to investigate and language to use in the second stage. The second stage consists of quantitative research, typically conducted using a structured questionnaire presented to a representative sample of the population of interest. Our overall objective was to understand the general public's needs, attitudes, and associations regarding mental health and psychotherapy and develop a way in which we could meaningfully communicate the value of therapies of depth, insight, and relationship.

Qualitative research

For our qualitative phase, we conducted a total of 46 in-depth interviews in three iterative waves, between September of 2018 and May of 2019. Our specific objectives were to explore themes associated with mental health issues, treatment modalities, psychotherapy effectiveness, associations to types of therapy, and assessment of a concept describing therapies of depth, insight, and relationship.

We developed an interview guide with specific themes and questions, while allowing flexibility to deepen exploration as needed. The interview guide was written based on the key issues we wanted to address and refined in each wave based on preliminary findings. The interviews, lasting between 30 and 90 minutes, were conducted in person or over the phone by members of the research team. During the third wave, we received additional support from graduate Marketing Communications students from a university in the Chicago area.

The interviewees were recruited from the personal networks of members of the research team and of the Psychotherapy Action Network, excluding clinicians, clinical students, or their close relatives, as their views and opinions might not represent those of the general public. The majority of interviewees are residents of the Chicago area and has different levels of experience with therapy. While we attempted to have a balanced representation of different demographics, the sample for qualitative research does not aim to be statistically representative of the general population.

Quantitative research

The quantitative phase of our project included an online survey, completed by a final U.S. representative sample of 1,535 respondents (margin of error is ± 2.53% for the total results, with a 95% confidence level) during early March of 2020. The sample is representative of the population in terms of age, gender, ethnicity, geographic region, and household income. It is important to note that fieldwork for our survey took place before lockdowns due to the COVID-19 pandemic were commonplace, and before remote mental health services became prevalent. The specific objectives of this phase were to quantify attitudes and behaviors associated with mental health, treatment options, and psychotherapy in particular. We also measured people's associations to two specific treatment modalities, psychoanalysis, and CBT. During the quantitative phase, the research team consisted of the research leads and two graduate students from a dual program in Business Administration and Market Research.

Online survey research is the most widely used quantitative method in market research. By one account, 89% of market research professionals globally use it regularly (Statista, 2021). In the United States, where 93% of adults say they use the internet (Pew Research Center, 2021), this method has the potential to reach the majority of the total population, making it the standard approach for commercial survey research. Other data collection methods used in quantitative research (e.g., phone or in-person surveys) might help in reaching highly specific low-incidence groups, which is not a requirement for our project, and are also prohibitively expensive for our endeavor.

The instrument utilized in this phase was a structured questionnaire, created by the research team, based on the main themes captured in the qualitative phase. The questions took different forms (e.g., Likert scales, multiple choice) depending on what they were capturing (e.g., attitudes, associations, awareness, behaviors). The questionnaire was programmed for online distribution using a survey software that allows for complex questionnaire flow and skip logic, and implementation of best research practices (e.g., response and statement randomization). The online survey took respondents about 15–20 minutes to complete.

A critical step in conducting survey research is to clearly define the population under study. While our goal was to understand and "listen to" the general population, we wanted to gather responses from people with at least some awareness of the issues we would be asking about in the survey. Thus, the research population was defined as those who reported being aware of therapy or counseling. This became our main screening criteria, as it defined who qualified to take the survey and who did not, and was captured using a multiple-choice question in the first section of the survey, also known as "screener." Everyone contacted to participate in the survey answered the screener and was then either allowed to proceed to the main questionnaire, if they met the screening criteria, or terminated, ending the survey for them at that point. A number of respondents were eliminated if they failed standard market research quality control checks (e.g., "speeding" through the survey, selecting "decoy" response alternatives, and reporting employment in the sector of interest). In total, we contacted approximately 3,000 people and 61% of them met our screening criteria. After applying the other filters and quality control checks, our final sample consisted of 1,535 complete and valid surveys. The screener also included key demographic questions (age, gender, race/ethnicity, state of residence, and household income range), asked to everyone we contacted, regardless of whether or not they qualified to complete the survey. This information was required from everyone for data weighting purposes (see below).

Following common practice in online survey research, the sample was recruited from an online panel. An "online panel" is, at its core, an extensive list of people who have agreed to provide some personal information and be contacted periodically to participate in market research. Panels are actively maintained and managed by dedicated Online Panel Providers (OPP). OPPs ensure diversity in the composition of their panel, actively ensure data quality, offer incentives to their panelists, and keep their panelist's information updated. The OPP does *not* provide its panelists' personal information to organizations doing market research. Instead, our research team shared with the OPP a link to the online survey we programmed, so that the OPP could email its panelists directly, inviting them to participate in the survey. The OPP followed market research best practices to minimize sampling bias when distributing the link.

In addition to working with a professionally managed OPP, we took steps to make sure that the final sample adequately represented our research population on five key demographics: age, gender, race/ethnicity, household income, and geographic region[1]. One of the most widely used techniques to ensure that survey data is statistically representative is data weighting (Mercer, Lau & Kennedy, 2018). This method allows different groups to be fairly and adequately represented in the data analysis, leading to more representative and accurate results. In addition, weighting survey data can also address issues of coverage created by systematic differences between groups with different levels of internet access (Dever, Rafferty & Valliant, 2008). In order to conduct this process, we collaborated (pro-bono) with a Marketing Analytics Expert.

The process involves identifying "weighting targets" and creating "weighting factors" for each respondent, based on their demographics, so that their responses will be subject to a statistical correction once aggregated. The data weighting method we used is called Iterative Proportional Fitting (IPF). IPF takes the marginal population distributions and, through an iterative statistical process, calculates individual weighting factors for each survey respondent. When those weighting factors are applied (i.e., when the sample is "weighted"), the aggregate results will be distributed to reflect the desired weighting targets. Thanks to the sampling precautions taken during the data collection process, all weighting factors in our sample fell under a reasonable range, thus avoiding any significant distortion in the data.

Because the demographic distribution of our research population (as defined by our screening criteria) was unknown, we followed a two-step IPF process, starting with U.S. Census demographic data as a weighting target for the *total number of screeners* we collected. On the weighted data for all screeners, the team calculated the distribution of each of the five demographic variables of interest, among those respondents who *qualified* for the survey (i.e., those who met the screening criteria). These distributions became the *weighting targets* for the final sample of 1,535 respondents. As a result, the aggregate data the team analyzed and presented is representative of the research population across the five target demographics.

One important item to note is the difference between the demographic distribution of the overall U.S. population and that of our research population. As observed in Exhibit A, the distribution in both populations is very similar in terms of gender, income, and geographic region. However, there are differences when it comes to age and race/ethnicity. Those who qualified for our survey (e.g., people aware of therapy) are more likely to be white (vs the overall U.S. population) and skew older (vs the overall U.S. population). Because of the two-step weighting approach we followed, we can determine that these differences are *not* due to sample bias, but a result of relatively higher therapy awareness among people identifying as white and those who are older.

Exhibit A

Demographic distribution comparison between U.S. Census and our final sample

Demographic Distribution

	U.S. Census (%)	*People Who Qualified to the Survey (%)*
Gender		
Male	49	46
Female	51	54
Ethnicity		
White (non-Hispanic)	62	74
Black or African-American	13	7
Hispanic or Latino (any race)	19	13
Asian or Asian American	6	5
Other	1	1
Age		
18–24	14	7
25–34	21	13
35–44	19	16
45–55	19	22
55–70	28	41
Annual HH Income		
Under $25,000	19	18
$25,000–49,999	21	23
$50,000–74,999	17	19
$75,000–99,999	13	11
$100,000–149,999	15	15
$150,000 or more	16	13
Region		
Northeast	17	16
Midwest	21	24
South	38	37
West	24	23

Notes:

- Left column is publicly available U.S. Census data, used as weighting targets during the first step of the data weighting process.
- Right column is the estimated distribution of those who qualified to the survey (i.e., people aware of therapy), used as weighting targets during the second step of the data weighting process.

Research findings

In this section, we provide an overview of the findings and insights from our research. We focus on the results from our quantitative survey, while providing direct quotes from the qualitative interviews in order to provide the reader with additional perspectives in people's own words.

Attitudes and perceptions about therapy

A high-level finding from our survey is that people, despite their reported awareness of therapy, do not appear to have strong opinions about mental health or mental health treatment. In the 56 statements evaluated, most people selected one of the two middle points of the six-point agreement scale we used. Only eight statements had a Top-2 Box higher than 50% and only nine of them had a Bottom-2 Box[2] higher than 50%.

When asking people what they want from psychotherapy (multiple choices could be selected), the top two answers received the same level of support (about 70%): "learning skills and coping strategies," a focus of most manualized treatment modalities, and "better understanding yourself and the root of your issues," a focus of therapies of depth, insight, and relationship. These are closely followed by "sharing your feelings and thoughts without being judged or shamed" (66%) and "feeling heard and understood by someone who cares about you" (60%), both of which suggest the value placed on aspects of the therapeutic relationship. A similar percentage stresses the role therapy can play in becoming empowered to make their own choices in life. Interestingly, only 37% of people believe that the main goal of therapy is to help people change their behavior. These last two findings might suggest a distinction made between therapy as *helping people feel empowered to change* in contrast to therapy *aimed at behavioral change*, which would suggest the value people place on change coming from within. Indeed, one of our qualitative participants stated that "[therapy] *is empowering because you hopefully get to discover the root of the issue.*" Another participant stated, "*people think something is wrong with them and an outside force will fix it, but real changes come with an inward focus.*"

We were pleasantly surprised to discover that about two-thirds of the population recognize that therapy takes time, acknowledging that "emotional and psychological problems inherently take time to understand and resolve." A similar proportion believes that going to therapy is an investment that is worth making. Only a relatively small proportion of respondents, one in ten, does *not* appear to see value in focusing on understanding problems (as opposed to finding practical solutions) or on examining past issues and childhood experiences (as opposed to present-day problems). Our qualitative interviewees added more depth to these responses, stating that "[therapy] *is a liberating way for you to expose yourself to yourself*" and that it presents "*an opportunity to examine your thought process with guidance.*" In addition, only a few respondents in our survey

(10%) expressed stigmatized views, such as the belief that going to therapy implies the presence of significant psychological issues, or that seeing a therapist is like "paying to have a friend." However, a higher percentage (36%) perceives therapy as a way to "fix" something that is not working.

People's views on the therapeutic experience seem to be weaker than opinions about other topics, as suggested by the lower Top-2 Box scores. For example, the statement with the highest percentage of agreement only reached 32%, representing people's views on the usefulness of talking about the relationship between therapist and patient. The majority of people do not seem to see the value of exploring those dynamics. Moreover, in our qualitative interviews, we tested several different descriptions of transference (without the technical terminology) and most people had a negative reaction to this concept, occasionally leading to drops in mood during the interview itself. One qualitative participant said it clearly: "*I don't have a problem with the therapist, I have problems in other relationships!*" At the same time, the majority of people seem to recognize and value, even if implicitly, the interpersonal aspects of the therapeutic relationship. This is suggested by the very low percentages of people who believe that the therapist's personality does not matter much (8%), or that are skeptical about the therapist's genuine feelings of care (7%).

The remaining attitudinal statements we evaluated in our survey provide insights into a number of categories, summarized below:

- **Origin of mental health issues.** About half of people consider patterns and relationships as an important source of mental health issues and a reason to seek therapy. Less than 20% of people think that "mental health problems" mainly stem from other sources (e.g., chemical imbalances, irrational thoughts).
- **Comfort with feelings and vulnerability.** About a third of people feel able to handle their feelings on their own, and about the same percentage feels comfortable opening up to others.
- **Structure of therapy sessions.** We found that most people are not necessarily looking for structured or concrete sessions. Around 20% of people would prefer a therapist who sets the agenda for each session, who gives homework, or who gives advice. This is a significant proportion of the population but does not seem to represent the opinion of the majority.
- **Racial and cultural identity.** Only 15% of people stated that they would strongly prefer a therapist of their same racial or cultural background. These proportions are somewhat higher among those who identify as Black/African American (25%) and Hispanic/Latino (22%) but do not reach the high percentages that we would have anticipated.
- **Appeal of "evidence-based."** "Evidence-based" claims make about 40% of people more trusting of a therapy modality. Interviews in our qualitative interviews reflected these mixed views. While some valued the understanding that "*evidence-based means that research supports it*" and keeps therapy

from being *"touchy-feely or poking around in the dark,"* others highlighted the importance of the *"therapist's intuition and skill"* and *"the therapist having used practices with others and having real-world experience."*

- **Remote vs In-person therapy.** A little over 10% of people believe it makes no difference if therapy happens in person or not, which would suggest that people place value on in-person sessions. After the expansion of teletherapy due to the COVID-19 pandemic, attitudes in this area have most likely shifted since the time the survey was conducted.
- **Medications.** Medications are generally accepted, viewed positively, and seen as providing helpful and important benefits. Participants in our qualitative interviews stressed the importance of medications as an adjunct to therapy, as they can *"provide some relief,"* but they *"don't fix the root cause; meds enable you to do talk therapy."*

As an alternative way to measure people's preferences for different types of therapy, we asked respondents in our survey to choose one of two options presented to them: "therapy that takes longer but addresses the root cause of your symptoms, so that it can offer lasting results" or "therapy that takes fewer session and helps you manage your symptoms, but doesn't necessarily address the root cause of the problem." In hindsight, we recognize the wording of the two options in this forced choice was not equitable. However, we were surprised by the magnitude of relative support for the type of therapy that addresses "the root causes" of symptoms: 91% of respondents selected that option, while only 9% selected the shorter therapy that focused on symptom management.

Behavioral intentions and experience with mental health treatment

When people were asked to select which actions they might take if they were feeling "frustrated, sad, anxious, or not in control of their thoughts and emotions," the top two responses reflect contrasting preferences: About 58% stated that they would talk to friends and family, and a similar percentage said that they would keep themselves active and busy as a coping mechanism. About half of the respondents also indicated that they would try to remain optimistic and think positively. These top three responses were the leading responses across all demographics investigated in our survey. A bit under half of the respondents (48%) said that they would consider speaking with a therapist. It is worth noting that this percentage is higher among older respondents (e.g., 54% for those between 55 and 70 years old, versus 36% for those 18–24) and for white respondents (51%, versus 42% for non-white respondents). Motivation for considering therapy was described by one of our qualitative interviewees, who stated *"it's such a shame that there's a stigma, that needing help is a sign of weakness and personal failure."*

All other possible coping behaviors in our hypothetical scenario received lower percentages. For example, 39% of people would consider praying or seeking spiritual guidance and 32% stated that they would practice yoga, meditation, or mindfulness. A third of our respondents (32%) stated that they would keep it to themselves and get through their problems on their own. While this is a significant percentage of the population, it would suggest that other "independent" coping strategies (e.g., staying active, remaining optimistic) do *not* necessarily imply that people would choose to go through difficulties in isolation. Additionally, only 23% would consider taking medication to regulate their thoughts and emotions, and a similar percentage would search for ideas on social media. Only one in ten respondents stated that they would consider using a mental health app to feel better; this percentage has likely increased after mental health apps gained more prominence during the COVID-19 pandemic. Importantly, only 15% of people would explicitly take an avoidant approach to mental and emotional difficulties, stating that they would avoid thinking about it until the problem went away.

As mentioned above, a little under half of our respondents stated that they would consider speaking with a therapist in the scenario we described. When asking those who did *not* select that option why they would not consider talking to a therapist, the most common answer (41%) was the belief that therapy is too expensive. This suggests an important access barrier to seeking therapy, one that might be both realistic and also significantly based on perceptions. The next group of reasons why people would not consider seeking therapy includes the belief that they can handle problems on their own, the presence of family and friends they can rely on, and the discomfort of talking to a stranger about their problems. These responses were selected by, on average, 25% of the respondents. Only a minority of people expressed concerns associated with their perception of therapy, including the belief that therapy is too time-consuming (14%), that it is for people suffering from "major" mental health disorders (11%), or that therapy doesn't really work (6%). Finally, only 9% acknowledged that they believe that talking to a professional is a sign of weakness.

We asked people what steps they would take and what criteria they would follow if they were hypothetically considering starting therapy. As a result, their responses reflect behavioral *intentions* rather than people's actual behavior or unconscious decision-making factors. Most people (59%) said they would ask their physician for recommendations, highlighting the gate-keeping role that physicians play in recommending treatment, and perhaps specific types of therapy. A bit over half of people (53%) would also look for the mental health providers covered by their insurance, which is consistent with the concerns about the cost of therapy reported above. These two steps were the top two responses across all demographics. In contrast, only a third of respondents would ask their family or friends for referrals, and a quarter of respondents would use an online search engine like Google. Notably, younger people are significantly more likely to engage in these two behaviors.

When asked for the criteria people would follow when choosing a therapist, the factor mentioned by most (65%) is whether the therapist is in-network with the patient's insurance. This, again, is consistent with the concerns about the potential cost of therapy, and possibly a lack of awareness of other variables in selecting a therapist or type of therapy. The second most mentioned factor (52%) is the location of the therapist's office; we believe that, with the increased prevalence of teletherapy due to the COVID-19 pandemic, the importance assigned to this factor may have shifted. Interestingly, the third decision factor, selected by half of the population, is "the therapist's personality." We consider this as an acknowledgment of the importance of interpersonal factors in the therapeutic relationship. As one qualitative interviewee stated, therapy's effectiveness "*depends on if the therapist fits your personality even if he's a good therapist.*" The fourth decision driver (47%) is the recommendation by the person's physician, which is consistent with the gatekeeper role previously mentioned. Importantly, the physician's recommendation seems to be more important for older people, while younger people would likely assess a wider range of consideration factors.

In a second cluster of decision criteria, selected by 35–39% of people, we find aspects related to the experience levels of the therapist, specifically "experience working with people like me" (we found no significant differences across demographics) and the therapist's expertise in the specific issues the person would want to work on. A third cluster of factors, selected by 25–28% of people, includes "word of mouth" aspects (recommendations from friends and family and online reviews), as well as the number of years the therapist has been in practice. It is worth noting that, besides the therapist's personality, the perceived relevance of their clinical experience, and their years of practice, all other characteristics of the therapist appear to be much less important when selecting a therapist. For example, the therapist's theoretical orientation is a decision factor for only 15%. Even lower percentages are associated with the therapist's degree type (12%), the school they attended (6%), or their publications (5%).

We also wanted to know what people had actually done to deal with mental health, emotional, or psychological difficulties. We found that about half of our sample (47%) had direct experience with therapy or counseling, almost 90% of them as an adult; 25% of those with direct experience were current patients (we did not ask for the type of therapy people received). Two-thirds of our total sample had "indirect" experience, as defined by having close friends or family members who had ever received therapy or counseling. One-third of our sample had direct experience with psychiatric medications, and about 28% reported having used mindfulness/meditation or self-help books, the former being more significant among younger respondents. Other modalities (e.g., in-patient treatment, self-help groups) were selected by around one in ten participants. Only 5% stated having direct experience with therapy apps, although we believe this percentage may have increased as a result of the COVID-19 pandemic. Finally, almost a third of the population (31%) reported not having direct experience with any of the presented alternatives.

We also investigated people's willingness to consider mental health apps. 36% of people said they would consider apps for meditation and mindfulness practice (e.g., Calm, Headspace), 31% were open to apps that connect them to an actual therapist (e.g., BetterHelp, Talkspace), and only 18% said they would be open to journaling or AI-based apps (e.g., Woebot, Moodnote). A total of 43% said they would *not* consider using any of these types of apps, implying that almost three-fifths of people (57%) would consider them. These percentages may have shifted since our fieldwork, as teletherapy and mental health apps gained prominence due to the COVID-19 pandemic and advertising campaigns. The data showed clear variation based on the age of the respondents. Whereas 82% of people aged 18–24 and 75% of those 25–34 said they would consider using apps, 54% of people 45–54 and only 44% of those 55–70 years old said the same.

Most valuable aspects of therapy

We wanted to understand what people considered as the most valuable aspects of therapy. For current or former therapy patients, we asked this question in the context of their personal experience. For those with no direct experience, we asked it in the context of a hypothetical scenario. As expected, people who had been to therapy selected more choices, probably as a result of a broader appreciation and experience of the therapeutic process. For example, "talking to someone who is not judgmental" and "feeling understood and heard by another person" were two of the most valuable aspects of therapy as reported by those with direct experience (62% and 57%, respectively), but they were not as dominant among those without such experience (48% and 39%, respectively). "Becoming more self-aware" and "talking to someone with an objective perspective" are two other elements more valued by those with direct experience with therapy than by those without (54% vs 42% and 52% vs 40% respectively). As we can observe, the interpersonal experience of an empathic therapist is, understandably, considered in higher regard by those who have actually gone through therapy. Our qualitative interviews also suggest that a safe environment with an empathic, nonjudgmental therapist is seen as a key ingredient of therapy. As one of our qualitative interviewees stated, therapy is "*a place of constancy, safety,* [where] *I can be whoever I am and say whatever I want to say, without judgment or shame, with one person who will take what I say and guide me further in a more wholesome way.*"

It is important to note that, among those with direct therapy experience, learning new coping skills to manage thoughts and emotions is considered one of the most valuable aspects of therapy by a significant number of people (59%). About half of those with no direct experience (51%) also consider this would be valuable. In the group with no direct experience, that aspect of therapy is considered as valuable as getting to the root of their problems (51%). This speaks to the importance of "getting to the root" in the value people perceive in therapy. Near half of those with direct experience (46%) also consider getting to the root as one of the most valuable aspects of therapy.

Concept testing

We wanted to understand what people thought and felt about therapies of depth, insight, and relationship. In order to do this, we developed a description (a "concept") that we presented to our participants to gauge their reactions. We did not name the therapy we were describing, since there is no public-facing "name" that would encompass our description. This technique, called Concept Testing, is widely used in market research in order to get feedback from the public about a product idea, as part of the product development process. During our survey, we used a description first tested and refined successively during our qualitative interviews. The concept we used in the survey is presented in Exhibit B.

Exhibit B

Therapy description used in concept testing during online survey

This therapy can be useful for symptoms like depression, anxiety, or unhappiness, or for more serious mental health conditions. Its main focus is on understanding and dealing with the underlying causes of those issues. People gain self-awareness and self-understanding, which can lead to new ways of seeing and handling problems in life.

During therapy sessions, people are encouraged to talk openly about whatever is on their mind, at their own pace and on their own terms. The therapist listens in a curious and nonjudgmental way, asking questions and providing their perspective, but does not follow a pre-defined agenda or focus on teaching "skills." There is no predetermined duration for this kind of therapy; it may take as long as the person continues to see benefits.

People will likely talk about their past, including their childhood, and how it may still influence their present-day life. There may also be an emphasis on understanding past and present relationships, experiences, and patterns. This therapy believes that our thoughts and feelings might have important meaning. Thoughts and feelings are considered neither "negative" nor "irrational," and making sense of them is a big part of what helps people feel better.

With this therapy, many people experience not only a reduction of their symptoms, but can live a richer and freer life. They may continue to improve even after they stop going to therapy, because this therapy addresses underlying patterns that affect many areas of their life. People can recognize and stop old patterns, look at their past in different ways, change how they feel about themselves and others, and open up new possibilities for living going forward.

Note: This description was included as a part of the online survey in our quantitative research. Prior iterations of the description were used during the qualitative interviews.

The overall feedback to this description of a therapy of depth, insight, and relationship during our qualitative interviews was positive. Some of the positive comments centered on its individualized nature, the appreciation to go deeper to identify underlying issues, its long-lasting impact, and the non-judgmental stance toward the patient and their feelings. Some of the concerns we heard involved the unknown and potentially lengthy duration of treatment and lack of clear direction. Some people reacted against what they perceived as a minimization of the impact of their symptoms and their wish for symptom relief. As one interviewee put it: *"My symptoms **are** my worries, troubles, and problems. If you're telling me there are underlying issues, it makes my problems seem not legitimate."* Significantly, almost all our interviewees seemed confused or turned off by the notion that understanding and exploring the therapeutic relationship could be a part of this type of therapy (an aspect included during our qualitative phase). Following this homogeneous consensus, we decided to remove that part of the description in the final version we tested quantitatively.

In our online survey, after people had an opportunity to read the concept, we asked for their reactions along three dimensions, with consistent results across multiple demographics:

1 *Differentiation*: We found that most people (51%) found that this form of therapy was slightly different or not at all different from their current perception of therapy. This suggests that the way people think about therapy is consistent with a description of therapy that values depth, insight, and relationship.
2 *Interest*: 37% said they would be extremely or very interested in learning more about this type of therapy (a similar percent said they would be just interested). While the expressed interest does not reach a majority, it makes sense that not many people would want to learn about a form of therapy in the abstract.
3 *Willingness to consider*: An overwhelming 58% stated that they would definitely or probably consider this form of therapy (30% said they may or may not, and only 12% said they would probably or definitely not seek it).

When asking people for the most important benefits perceived in the concept, most of the items were selected by around half of our sample as one of the "most important" benefits; not a single or a few of them stood out. This might be a result of the complexity of the description we presented and an expression of how this form of therapy can be appreciated from different angles. The benefits selected the most (by around 53% of people) include recognizing and stopping old patterns, focusing on the underlying causes of psychological and emotional problems, and increasing self-awareness and self-understanding. Toward the bottom of the list, with around 40%, we found benefits that may not have been phrased in layperson language, or that might have sounded too abstract, including how this therapy can "open up new possibilities for living" or "help people live a richer and freer life." Interestingly, the benefit *least* selected (33%), which would suggest it may not be considered a benefit altogether, is the possibility to continue in therapy for as long as the person wants. Finally, only 4% stated that they don't see any benefits in this kind of therapy.

When asking for the most important concerns people had about our therapy description, the results were also widespread, although people seemed to have fewer concerns than benefits. The clear top two concerns involved worries about cost (39%), given that there is no predetermined duration, and the possibility that it might take a very long time to see any effects (34%). Again, stating the long-term nature of this kind of therapy might be a source of concern rather than being perceived as a benefit. The third most mentioned concern (24%) involved the possibility that, without a predetermined structure, people could "talk about things that don't matter." All other possible concerns were selected by less than 20% of our sample. Moreover, 24% of people stated that they did not have any concerns with this type of therapy. Interestingly, very few people (less than 10%) expressed concerns that, by focusing on underlying causes or "talking the past," this therapy would not focus enough on or help solve current problems. This would reinforce the notion that, while "current problems" are important, people recognize the value of understanding their underlying and historical causes.

Awareness of types of therapy

During the qualitative phase, we asked about people's awareness of specific types of therapy. It became clear that the two modalities with greater overall awareness were psychoanalysis and CBT. This finding was confirmed during our quantitative survey. Two-thirds of the population stated being aware of "Psychoanalysis/Psychoanalytic Therapy" (66%) and a similar proportion (64%) of CBT. Self-reported awareness does not, understandably, imply that people have a complete or accurate understanding of what these therapies are about. Awareness levels only indicate how much exposure these "brands" of therapy have had among the general public. In third place, "Mindfulness-based Therapy" was selected by 42% of people, and 30% stated being aware of "Humanistic Therapy (e.g., client-centered, existential)." All other types of therapy included in the survey received 16% awareness or less. Notably, "Psychodynamic Therapy" was among the brands we included and awareness was only 16%. While the term psychodynamic is common among professionals, it does not appear to have much recognition among the general public. Awareness of other types of branded therapies, ranging between 10% and 16%, included EMDR, ACT, DBT, and IFS (acronyms and full names were provided in the survey).

Comparing psychoanalysis and CBT

Since psychoanalysis and CBT were the only two modalities with significant levels of awareness, we measured the associations, in people's perception, between each modality and a number of attributes. Overall, psychoanalysis is mostly associated with self-understanding, getting to the "root cause" of problems, being able to help people from all demographics, and being an individualized yet expensive treatment option. CBT, on the other hand, is mostly associated with changing behaviors, being able to help people from all demographics, helping people gain control over their lives, and being a relevant, effective, and updated form of therapy for current psychological problems.

However, when compared side by side, psychoanalysis appears to be perceived less favorably than CBT by the general public along most dimensions. We observed this in both phases of our research, with both our qualitative interviewees and our quantitative survey respondents. The following sections summarize the findings in four areas. All the percentages shown are Top-2 Box scores, i.e., the percentage of people who indicated they "Agree" or "Strongly Agree" that a specific attribute represents each of the two modalities. The percentages measure the strength of the association of each attribute with each therapy modality.

1 How psychoanalysis and CBT help Psychoanalysis is more strongly associated than CBT (56% vs 45%) with the idea that it helps people "get to the root cause of their problems." Albeit by a smaller margin (58% vs 54%), psychoanalysis also trumps CBT in the perception that it "helps people know and understand themselves better." These two aspects, as noted previously, are important aspects that people value in therapy. As we heard in our qualitative interviews, psychoanalysis is "*for exploring yourself in more depth.*" On the other hand, CBT is more strongly associated than psychoanalysis with helping people "think and feel in different ways" (56% vs 49%) and helping people "get more control over their lives" (60% vs 48%). Finally, people overwhelmingly associate CBT (64% vs 42% for psychoanalysis) with the help it provides to "change behaviors." As one qualitative interviewee told us, CBT "*is about changing how you think or behave, about breaking the cycle of negative mental and recurring patterns.*"
2 What the therapy process is like The attributes more strongly associated with psychoanalysis are not necessarily favorable ones. More people believe that psychoanalysis, compared to CBT (40% vs 30%), "requires a long time to see any changes or results." One of our qualitative interviewees stated that psychoanalysis took "*years and years,*" while another stated that CBT "*doesn't take as long as other therapies.*" In addition, psychoanalysis is more strongly perceived (35% vs 26%) as being "more emotionally demanding and stressful than other forms of therapy." Both modalities were tied in two attributes where we would have expected that psychoanalysis, given

the way it thinks of itself, would have had an advantage. First, about 41% believe, equally for psychoanalysis and for CBT, that whether either modality works or not, "depends on the relationship between patient and therapist." Second, about 55% see both modalities as "individualized and tailored to each patient and situation." Finally, CBT is more strongly associated by a significant margin (57% vs 40%) with being focused on "offering tangible solutions or guidance."Importantly, during the qualitative interviews, several people shared perceptions about psychoanalysis being conducted by therapists who are "*cold*" and "*unempathic*" and particularly passive. One interviewee stated that a psychoanalytic therapist is "*not a good listener* [and] *wouldn't validate what I'm saying*", and another one stated that "*the doctor lets you talk and takes notes, but therapy is more helpful if doctor and patient are talking together.*" These perceptions are relevant to consider since, as discussed above, the experience of an empathic therapist is one of the most valued aspects in therapy. Thus, for some people, psychoanalysis may not even be included in their consideration set of therapies, as they view psychoanalysts as cold, unempathic and not meeting their general conceptions of a trusted therapist. Some of our respondents acknowledged that these perceptions are associated with long-standing stereotypes or "*cliches*" seen in popular media. Some interviewees also shared negative perceptions of CBT (e.g., as being "*mechanical*", "*one-size-fits-all,*" or "*what insurance companies like* [because it is] *short term*"), but these comments were less prevalent than the negative associations to psychoanalysis.

3 Who psychoanalysis and CBT are for Psychoanalysis is significantly more strongly associated (44% vs 33% for CBT) with helping "people with serious mental health issues or personality disorders." In contrast, CBT has a stronger association and a similar advantage (55% vs 44%) with being "for people with everyday problems like anxiety, depression, unhappiness, and relationship issues." This apparent split in people's associations was also observed in our qualitative interviews and might represent a challenge for psychoanalysis to be considered a viable mainstream therapeutic option. In addition, more than half of people consider that both psychoanalysis and CBT can be "helpful for everyone, regardless of age, gender, race, orientation, etc.," although CBT holds an advantage in this perception as well (62% vs 56%). Finally, when asked if they would consider each modality if they were looking for a therapist for themselves, more people stated that they would consider CBT than psychoanalysis (48% vs 39%). While this is an important metric that conveys which modality people feel would be a better "match," based on their own perceptions, it is also important to remember that, based on a separate question in our survey, the therapist's theoretical orientation is not a significant decision factor when choosing a therapist.

4 General perceptions of psychoanalysis and CBT The only attribute with which psychoanalysis has a strong association is the perception of being

expensive (55% vs 46% for CBT). Three attributes were related to the modalities' effectiveness, and CBT has an advantage in all of them based on people's perceptions. CBT is more strongly perceived as "one of the most effective forms of therapy" (51% vs 37% for psychoanalysis), as providing "long-lasting results" (50% vs 41%), and as having "extensive research showing that it works" (53% vs 48%). These attributes were echoed in some of our qualitative interviews, with one person stating that it is "*proven that* [CBT] *works with very challenging problems, not just easy ones*", while another expressing that "*even though it's a fundamental theory in psychology, I don't know if* [Psychoanalysis] *produces good results in a therapeutic sense.*" CBT is also more strongly associated with being a "very popular form of therapy," (53% vs 44%) and "relevant and updated to treat psychological problems in today's day and age" (60% vs 47%). These results are consistent with comments during our qualitative interviews about psychoanalysis being "*outdated*" and, as one interviewee told us, the perception that "*CBT is talk therapy.*"

Discussion and recommendations

The breadth of our research provides the most extensive dataset on people's opinions, needs, and attitudes about psychotherapy that we are aware of. Here we will synthesize and discuss the most salient themes, which apply to multiple demographic segments. We did not find systematic differences for any particular demographic group throughout the sample, suggesting that the overall findings apply to the whole research population. This was surprising, given the differences, such as varying utilization rates, among different racial and economic groups. It may be a reflection in the lay public of a lack of clear information or detailed familiarity with the therapy process or different therapies. Perhaps defining "awareness of therapy" as a screening criterion served as an "equalizing" function that smoothed demographic differences. It may also point toward aspects of our shared humanity.

First, people told us that they want to work with an empathic, nonjudgmental therapist, and they want to learn how to make important changes in their lives and open up new choices for themselves. While many types of therapy claim to offer these elements and benefits, people seem to want specific benefits that only depth therapies offer. Specifically, we learned that, when it comes to figuring out how to alleviate their suffering, what many people want is to get to the root of their problems, to understand themselves deeply, and to address the issues underlying their symptoms. An important segment of the public knows and understands that it will require time and effort, and they do not want to settle for symptom relief or quick fixes. We learned that many people intuitively know that there is more beneath the surface, believe that therapy is a process that takes time, and are willing to make and take that time.

These hopes for therapy are clearly distinct from the packaged solutions and messaging that currently predominate in the marketplace, and counter to the common narrative that's dominant in many of the public conversations about therapy – that it should be quick, easy, in the palm of your hand, at any moment of the day, and perhaps even with an interchangeable therapist. For example, despite the promises of "therapy anywhere/anytime" that large corporations, most of them relatively new in the mental health space, are selling, and even despite a cultural zeitgeist defined by quick fixes, there are people who want to make an investment in themselves, and are willing to spend their time and resources on this most valued investment – their self, their mind, their future. When it comes to specific types of therapy, namely CBT and psychoanalysis, our research confirmed the perception gaps we anticipated between these two most recognized forms of therapy, and also identified new ones. While analyzing the origins and development of these gaps in people's minds is beyond the scope of our project, we believe that it may result from a two-pronged process. On one hand, the ways in which CBT, with the support of multiple stakeholders, has become closely aligned to the entire category of "psychotherapy," has resulted in people associating CBT with a number of benefits which technically stem from other therapies. On the other hand, psychoanalysis may have contributed in various ways to its own disconnection from the public discourse.

In addition to understanding the general public, our project aimed at addressing a practical issue. Our central goal is to identify how to engage with the general public in order to communicate the value of therapies of depth, insight, and relationship in ways that are meaningful and impactful. In order to do so, we need to define a clear value proposition and design our communications based on the attitudes, needs, and preferences of the general public, rather than those of clinicians and professional organizations. We have developed a framework, grounded in our research, that includes four key elements that should be present in any efforts to communicate with the general public about depth therapy. They represent the most important dimensions, based on people's perceptions and attitudes, that communicate the value of therapies of depth, insight, and relationship.

1 **Basic must-have: "Feel Heard"** At a basic level, "feeling heard" is an expectation people have from *any* form of therapy. As such, it must be considered in any attempt to engage with the general public. The core message of this dimension is that therapy is a place where people will be heard and understood without judgment. Based on our research, two-thirds of people believe that the most valuable aspect of therapy is sharing thoughts and feelings without feeling judged. About 60% think that "feeling heard and understood" is one of the most important benefits of therapists in general. In addition, the majority of people consider that talking to someone who is not judgmental and feeling understood are the main benefits of therapy.

In qualitative interviews, these themes also came up consistently as a core part of therapy.

2 **Key rational benefit: "Change and Choice"** "Rational" benefits, also known as "functional" benefits, refer to what someone would "get" out of participating in therapy. Based on our research, we believe that the core message to convey is that therapy can help people change old patterns of behavior, thoughts, feelings, and relationships, so that they can then make different choices in their life. In fact, about 60% of people believe that the most important part of therapy is becoming empowered to make your own choices in life. Similarly, the majority of respondents believe that a key reason to seek out therapy is to change repeating patterns. Consistently, the majority also considered "stopping old patterns" as one of the main benefits in the therapy concept we tested. In qualitative interviews, people emphasized the value of therapy as a way to identify changes they would like to make, change repeating patterns, find new ways to feel and behave, pursue personal growth, and feel empowered to make choices.

3 **Key emotional benefit: "Worth It"** It has been long recognized in the marketing and branding literature (e.g., Gobe, 2001) that rational benefits are not enough; people's choices are to a large extent motivated by an emotional connection leading to the experience of emotional benefits. The core emotional benefit we recommend focusing on is encompassed in the concept of worth: therapy is worth the effort, the time, and the investment, because *you* are worth getting to know and grow. The emotional benefit embedded in this message is two-fold: it speaks to the value of doing something valuable and worthwhile for oneself, and to the experience of being seen as a worthwhile human being. These benefits are supported by the finding that two-thirds of people believe that emotional and psychological problems inherently take time to understand and resolve, and that going to therapy is an investment in oneself that is worth making. People also value and understand the importance of self-awareness and self-understanding. Moreover, in qualitative interviews, people with experience in therapy considered it a powerful process that takes time and offers the possibility to understand oneself better and feel liberated.

4 **Most differentiating factor: "Get to The Root"** In order to stand out relative to other forms of therapy, therapies of depth, insight, and relationship need to highlight how they are different and unique. Based on our research, a key way to convey this difference is through the message that therapy is a way to increase self-awareness and to "get to the root of the problem." Over two-thirds of our sample believe that the main goal of therapy is to better understand yourself and the root of your issues. The majority considered this aspect of the concept we tested (its focus on underlying causes) as one of the most important perceived benefits, and about half of people considered "getting to the root of the problem" the

most valuable aspect of therapy. In addition, 91% said they would prefer therapy that addresses root causes of symptoms, rather than only providing ways to manage symptoms (even if the latter would require fewer sessions). Finally, in our qualitative interviews, people see increasing self-awareness and "getting to the root" as empowering and helpful to make sense of inner experiences and to find new ways of dealing with relationships and life.

It is important to note that, while our research provides strong support for communication strategies that incorporate these four elements, they will not necessarily be equally appealing for every member of the general public. A fundamental marketing principle is that no product, service, brand, or experience will be equally appealing to all people. Similarly, no type of therapy can be everything to everyone, and we should not attempt to be so. Therapies of depth, insight, and relationship – just like any of their alternatives – will be appealing only to a subset of the general public. The four elements we recommend are the pillars of a research-based strategy to communicate and engage with that segment of the population. Importantly, our research suggests that this segment is not defined by specific demographics, but rather by their attitudes toward mental health and therapy itself.

Along these lines, our research also suggests a number of public-facing messages *not* to convey to the general public, as they elicited negative reactions in our research and might be confusing, irrelevant, or off-putting to the public. When communicating directly to the public, one should not:

- Downplay the value of "learning" skills and strategies to "manage" thoughts and feelings (i.e., symptoms).
- Disparage claims to "evidence" (e.g., EBT) as merely a marketing ploy.
- Dismiss people's questions or desires for structure, guidance, or assistance.
- Discourage or downplay a focus on symptoms and symptom relief.
- Denigrate medications and their use.
- Dismiss concerns about the expense or duration of treatment.
- Focus on the dynamics of the therapeutic relationship (e.g., transference, enactments), even if we use them as part of our clinical approach.
- Focus on the duration of treatment one way or the other – whether on long duration of depth therapy or in suggesting that short-term treatments might not be as effective.

Even if not well-publicized, it's clear that the evidence base for depth therapies is strong, valid, and substantive. It's indisputable that these therapies are highly effective, and they receive the support of many clinicians. What we know now, thanks to our research, is not only that these therapies work, but that they resonate with a large number of people who value them and want the benefits that only they can offer. We need to start talking about therapy and mental health care in new and different ways. If we don't, we run the risk of either alienating a big part of the public, who would not find their needs and preferences represented in contemporary narratives about therapy, or of keeping them from understanding the full range of benefits that therapy can offer. If we do – and our research points the way – we would be returning to the full definition and true spirit of "evidence-based practice," which encompasses research, therapist wisdom and clinical experience, *and* patient preferences and values (American Psychological Association, 2021). While our research does not assume the preferences of any individual, specific patient, it provides data and insights to inform that third component of EBP. There is a significant portion of the general public whose "preferences and values" resonate with those of therapies of depth, insight, and relationship. Engaging with the public using the insights from our project would help ensure that those who suffer can have the opportunity to think of therapy as providing the care and experience that resonates with their attitudes, needs, preferences, and values.

In order to bring therapies of depth, insight, and relationship back to the table, however, listening to the general public is only the first step. In order to effectively *engage* with the general public, organizations and clinicians advocating for these types of therapy need to work together. Engagement and communication need to be consistent, ongoing, and systematically managed efforts. One-off activities (e.g., a press release, a viral internet video, an isolated advertising campaign) will not work. Educating and engaging the public is a process that needs to be sustained. Like all relationships, it needs to be built, tended to, and nurtured over time. It is critical that supporting organizations are aligned around the messaging recommended by our research, so that public communications and messages are consistent with one another, and take action to engage their members and other constituents in this endeavor.

Because the expertise and capabilities required for communicating with the public effectively fall outside of the scope of most clinically-oriented professional organizations, it is critical that external experts, providers and agencies (e.g., social media, digital marketing, advertising) are enlisted to become part of our efforts. Finally, but equally important, is the need for financial resources to support ongoing initiatives and capabilities. While we can use tools and frameworks that are commonplace in the corporate world, non-profits do not have access to the financial resources that large businesses can use. While appropriate funding will be a challenge for any initiative that attempts to engage the general public, basing our communication on what we learned from our research, where we listened directly to the general public, will make any investments more efficient.

Future directions

While it is our hope that our research will offer the foundation to build a meaningful and productive relationship with the public through an effective and relevant communications strategy, we also know that there are other audiences involved in the mental health landscape. Future research efforts with therapists, academics, graduate students, referral sources or gatekeepers, and policymakers will be critical. The challenges experienced by therapies of depth, insight, and relationship are multi-faceted, and so must be their solution. Additionally, the impacts of COVID-19 and telehealth have not been sufficiently addressed in our research, due to timing. There could also be an opportunity to research specific sub-segments of the general population, to understand their needs, values, and associations in more depth. Our research, being the first of its kind, focused on understanding the public broadly. We did not find many systematic significant differences in our results, whether by different demographic groups or experience with therapy. Nevertheless, additional research aimed at understanding specific segments of the population would be a welcome addition to this body of work. Large corporations are already doing this kind of research (e.g., Facebook, 2019/2021). While we don't have their financial resources, we cannot afford to leave the understanding of the general public to them alone.

Our research findings and recommendations contain the ingredients for building a relationship with the public in which there is renewed trust, respect, and consideration of therapies of depth, insight, and relationship, leading to the revitalization of these therapies in the mind of the public. If therapists and professional organizations can carry out our recommendations, we are confident we can achieve our goals of providing the public with important information and education, enhancing access to mental health treatments that work, and elevating depth therapies as an effective, relevant, and valued treatment option.

Notes

1 Gender and race/ethnicity were direct questions. Respondents reported their exact age, which was grouped in predefined ranges by the survey program. Household income (before taxes) was asked by presenting income ranges. Respondents provided their state of residence, grouped into regions following a predefined algorithm.

2 Top-2 Box is the percentage of people who selected "Strongly agree" or "Agree" with a specific attitudinal statement. Bottom-2 Box is the percentage of people who selected "Strongly disagree" or "Disagree."

References

Abbass, A. A., Hancock, J. T., Henderson, J., & Kisely, S. (2006). Short-term psychodynamic psychotherapies for common mental disor- ders. *Cochrane Database of Systematic Reviews,* Issue 4, Article No. CD004687. doi:10.1002/14651858.CD004687.pub3

American Psychological Association. (2021). *APA Guidelines on Evidence-Based Psychological Practice in Health Care.* American Psychological Association, retrieved on October, 2021: https://www.apa.org/about/policy/psychological-practice-health-care.pdf

Bateman, A. & Fonagy, P. (2008). 8-year follow-up of patients treated for borderline personality disorder: Mentalization-based treatment versus treatment as usual. *American Journal of Psychiatry, 165,* 631–638. doi:10.1176/appi.ajp.2007.07040636

Carroll, A. (2018). Do Antidepressants work? *New York Times,* retrieved on October, 2021: https://www.nytimes.com/2018/03/12/upshot/do-antidepressants-work.html

De Maat, S., De Jonghe, F., Schoevers, R.A. & J.J.M. Dekker. (2009). The effectiveness of long-term psychoanalytic therapy: A systematic review of empirical studies. *Harvard Review of Psychiatry*, 17(1), 1–23.

Delboy, S., Gibb, C., Law, J., Sichel, B. & L. Taliento. (2010). *Activists, Pundits, and Quiet Followers: Engaging the public in social issues.* McKinsey & Company, retrieved on September, 2021: https://www.mckinsey.com/industries/public-and-social-sector/our-insights/needs-based-segmentation-helping-nonprofits-take-outreach-to-the-next-level

Dever, J.A., Rafferty, A. & R. Valliant. (2008). Internet surveys: Can statistical adjustments eliminate coverage bias? *Survey Research Methods*, 2(2), 47–62.

DiGiulio, S. (2019). *What is cognitive behavioral therapy and how does it work?* NBC News, retrieved on October, 2021: https://www.nbcnews.com/better/lifestyle/what-cognitive-behavioral-therapy-how-does-it-work-ncna975811

Driessen, E., Henricus, L.V., Don, F.J., Peen, J., Kool, S., Westra, D., Hendriksen, M., Schoevers, R.A., Cuijpers, P, Twisk, J.W.R. & J.J.M. Dekker. (2013). The efficacy of cognitive-behavioral therapy and psychodynamic therapy in the outpatient treatment of major depression: A randomized clinical trial. *The American Journal of Psychiatry*, 170(9), 1041–1050.

Facebook. (2019/2021). Instagram Teen Mental Health Deep Dive. Facebook, retrieved on October, 2021: https://about.fb.com/wp-content/uploads/2021/09/Instagram-Teen-Annotated-Research-Deck-2.pdf

Gerber, A., Kocsis, J., Milrod, B., Roose, S., Barber, J., Thase, M., Perkins, P. & A. Leon. (2011). A Quality-Based Review of Randomized Controlled Trials of Psychodynamic Psychotherapy. *The American Journal of Psychiatry*, 168(1), 19–28.

Gnaulati, E. (2018). Overlooked ethical problems associated with the research and practice of evidence-based treatments. *Journal of Humanistic Psychology*, 1–16. doi: *10.1177/0022167818800219*

Gobe, M. (2001). *Emotional Branding: The New Paradigm for Connecting Brands to People.* Allworth Press; New York, NY.

Holstein R. & D.P. Paul 3rd. (2017) Access to Behavioral Health Care Services in New Jersey. *Hosp Top.* 95(3), 51–56.

Kylander, N. & C. Stone. (2012). *The Role of Brand in the Nonprofit Sector.* Stanford Social Innovation Review, retrieved on September, 2021: https://ssir.org/articles/entry/the_role_of_brand_in_the_nonprofit_sector

Lambert, M., Hansen, N., & A. Finch. (2001). Patient-focused research: using patient outcome data to enhance treatment effects. *Journal of Consulting and Clinical Psychology*, 69(2), 159–172.

Lazar, S. G. (2018). The place for psychodynamic therapy and obstacles to its provision. *Psychiatric Clinics of North America*, 41(2), 193–205. https://doi.org/10.1016/j.psc.2018.01.004

Leichsenring F., Abbass A., Luyten P., Hilsenroth M., Rabung S. (2013). The emerging evidence for long-term psychodynamic therapy. *Psychodynamic Psychiatry*, 41(3), 361–84. doi: 10.1521/pdps.2013.41.3.361.

Leichsenring F. & Rabung S. (2008). Effectiveness of long-term psychodynamic psychotherapy: a meta-analysis. *Journal of the American Medical Association*, 300(13), 1551–65. doi: 10.1001/jama.300.13.1551.

Leichsenring, F. & Rabung, S. (2011). Long-term psychodynamic psychotherapy in complex mental disorders: update of a meta-analysis. *The British Journal of Psychiatry*, 199, 15–22.

Leichsenring F. & Steinert, C. (2017). Is cognitive behavioral therapy the gold standard for psychotherapy? The need for plurality in treatment and research. *Journal of the American Medical Association*, 318(14), 1323–1324.

Marcus D.K., O'Connell D., Norris A.L., Norris, A. & A. Sawaqdeh. (2014). Is the Dodo bird endangered in the 21st century? A meta-analysis of treatment comparison studies. *Clinical Psychology Rev*iew, 34(7), 519–530.

Mayo-Wilson, E., Dias, S., Mavranezouli, I., Kew, K., Clark,D., Ades, A. & S. Pilling. (2014). Psychological and pharmacological interventions for social anxiety disorder in adults: A systematic review and network meta-analysis. *The Lancet Psychiatry*, 1(5), 368–376.

Mercer, A., Lau, A. & C. Kennedy (2018). *For weighting online opt-in samples, what matters most?* Pew Research Center, retrieved on September, 2021: https://www.pewresearch.org/methods/2018/01/26/for-weighting-online-opt-in-samples-what-matters-most/

Morrison, K., Bradley, R., & D. Westen. (2003). The external validity of controlled clinical trials of psychotherapy for depression and anxiety: A naturalistic study. *Psychology and Psychotherapy: Theory, Research and Practice*, 76, 109–132.

Oss, M. (2021). *How virtual behavioral health organizations fit in the healthcare ecosystem.* Open Minds Daily, 4/13/21 and 4/19/21, retrieved on September 2021: https://openminds.com/market-intelligence/executive-briefings/how-virtual-behavioral-health-organizations-fit-in-the-health-care-ecosystem

Pew Research Center. (2021). *Internet/Broadband Fact Sheet.* Pew Research Center, retrieved on September, 2021: https://www.pewresearch.org/internet/fact-sheet/internet-broadband/

Seligman, M.E.P. (1995). The effectiveness of psychotherapy: The Consumer Reports study. *American Psychologist*, 2, 965–974.

Shedler J. (2010). The efficacy of psychodynamic psychotherapy. *American Psychologist*, 65(2): 98–109. https://doi.org/10.1037/a0018378

Shedler J. (2015). Where is the evidence for "evidence-based" therapy? *Journal of Psychological Therapies in Primary Care*, 4(May), 47–59. https://jonathanshedler.com/wp-content/uploads/2015/07/Shedler-2015-Where-is-the-evidence-for-evidence-based-therapy-R.pdf

Statista Research Department. (2021). *Most used quantitative methods in the market research industry worldwide 2020*. Statista, retrieved on September, 2021: https://www.statista.com/statistics/875970/market-research-industry-use-of-traditional-quantitative-methods/

Steinert, C., Munder, T., Rabung, S., Hoyer, J., & F. Leichsenring. (2017). Psychodynamic *therapy*: As efficacious as other empirically supported treatments? A meta-analysis testing equivalence of outcomes. *American Journal of Psychiatry*, 174(10), 943–953.

Talkspace. (2021a). SEC Filing, Form S-1. Retrieved October 2021: https://investors.talkspace.com/node/7031/

Talkspace. (2021b). Retrieved October 2021: https://www.talkspace.com/#how

Tolin, D.F., McKay, D., Forman, E., Klonskly, E.D. & B.D. Thombs. (2015). Empirically Supported Treatment: Recommendations for a New Model. *Clinical Psychology: Science and Practice*, 22(4), 317–338.

Ventola C.L. (2011). Direct-to-Consumer Pharmaceutical Advertising: Therapeutic or Toxic? *P & T: A peer-reviewed journal for formulary management*, 36(10), 669–684.

Wachtel, P.L. (2010). Beyond "ESTs:" Problematic assumptions in the pursuit of evidence-based practice. *Psychoanalytic Psychology*, 27, 251–272.

Wang, E., & M. Zweig. (2021). *A defining moment for digital behavioral health: Four market trends*. Rock Health. Retrieved October 2021: https://rockhealth.com/insights/a-defining-moment-for-digital-behavioral-health-four-market-trends/

Westen D., Novotny C., & H. Thompson-Brenner. (2004). The empirical status of empirically supported psychotherapies: Assumptions, findings, and reporting in controlled clinical trials. *Psychological Bulletin*, 130(4), 631–663.

Mirror and window

What each reveals

Todd Essig

This chapter began with a dream from the early 90s, one I had near the end of my analysis. The dream both symbolized termination and foreshadowed much of my subsequent "zeitgeist-y" professional life:

> I'm in a room that's part office and part foyer with a mirror and a window through which one could see a green-grassed public space bustling with activity. My attention is drawn to both. With physics-defying dream-logic I end up attending to both simultaneously: mirror and window.

Flash forward to the mid-aughts when, after more than a decade starting and running The Psychoanalytic Connection (psychoanalysis.net), I'm offered a chance to write a regular column for a news start-up called *True/Slant.* First there and then at *Forbes,* after they bought *True/Slant,* I've been trying to take lessons learned in the introspective mirror of psychoanalysis and apply them to the issues of the day from out there in the *agora* (Essig, 2020a; Stein, 2020). This chapter reverses that direction. It shares with a professional audience curated excerpts and summaries of articles from *Forbes* I wrote for the general public. The selections, made from over 300 articles, were based on the potential relevance to what I see as a vital, central challenge of the 20s: how to help psychotherapies of depth, insight, and relationship thrive and make it to the 30s, hopefully to a future where the view out the window includes clinical psychoanalysis.

The War for the Future of Psychotherapy[1]

Written in December 2019 following PsiAN's first conference, this piece contextualizes some dark trends threatening psychotherapy's future but does so from the perspective of encouraging activism rather than pessimism. For those of us who provide such care, the darkness of these trends is obvious. But this is not so in the wider culture where so many find it so difficult to access helpful care. There, a feeling of "who cares that the therapists are fighting" is strong. But if psychotherapies of depth, insight, and relationship are to have a future

DOI: 10.4324/9781003325512-16

then the threats to practice need to be seen as a problem shared by all, not just a guild issue. So, this is how the piece starts:

> Maybe you heard. There's a war brewing. At stake is the future of psychotherapy. Will manuals, algorithms, and automatons prevail? Or will we be able to preserve the centrality of unique and responsive human relationships? The fight will determine the kinds of care available to people with problems in living. And you better pay attention. This fight concerns you; after all, who doesn't have such problems at some point in life, or care about someone who does?

The combatants in this war were clear, at least to me. One side defined the very essence of psychotherapy in human terms, as an I-Thou relationship (Buber, 1970; Stern, 2017). Everything emerges from that. The other side wants to eliminate human factors as much as possible. They define psychotherapy as deploying an algorithm for a previously specified problem where success or failure is independent of the delivery system used. People are indistinguishable one from another—and maybe not necessary at all:

> I see two factions coalescing into an algorithmic alliance. The first is those technology entrepreneurs building, marketing, and envisioning products to replace rather than extend and enrich therapeutic relationships ... Unfortunately, some are chasing profit not by trying to improve quality of care or access to that care. They are trying to disrupt and dehumanize the very definition of what psychotherapy is; who needs a therapist to be a person when you can have a cute chatbot trained to provide cognitive behavioral therapy (CBT). Often framed as a creative solution to the very real problems of access, solving those problems is not really their agenda. They are entrepreneurs, not altruistic policy-makers or healthcare providers trying to fix our badly broken mental healthcare delivery system. Quantity of profit, not quality of care is the goal. At the extreme you have those trying to fulfill the dream of artificial intimacy where a program provides a fully automated simulation of empathy and care, chatbots like yesterday's ELIZA or today's Woebot.

There are also threats from the converse of that extreme, as Linda Michaels recently noted (2021). Some technology companies, like the marketing behemoth Talkspace, operate by turning clinicians into simulations of a chatbot. They create platforms and procedures that push people to function in as chatbot-like a way as is possible. They do this by, for example, providing and requiring scripts for specific situations, programming required response times, and monitoring retention rates to keep users on their platform. What a clear example of our culture taking a wrong turn. They are using marketing power to push us to expect more from technology and less from each other, what Turkle has called our "robotic moment." (Turkle, 2016; Turkle, Essig, & Russell, 2017).

> The second faction in the algorithmic alliance is inside the profession; those reducing and then limiting psychotherapy to a set of procedures encoded in instruction manuals, i.e., to an algorithm. The group supporting instruction-manual therapies includes psychotherapy researchers designing treatment procedures based on how easily they can be studied under controlled circumstances. Rather than taking seriously the unique features of specifically psychological treatments, this research is built on a serious case of medicine-envy: if the drug companies do it then so too should we! The goal is not to help but be testable with a randomized controlled trial (RCT). Providing actual help to actual people under real word conditions is at best secondary. And, as other research shows, when tested in real world conditions these treatments often fail. The evidence for so called "evidence-based treatments" does not travel well into the real world of real people with problems in living. Its like a drug company testing a medication in a lab for a short period of time on paid volunteers in perfect health other than a pure form of the specific diagnosis being studied and then marketing that drug without seeing how well it works, or doesn't, for people living in the real world.

The article then described other members of the algorithmic warrior class: media, insurance companies, and the American Psychological Association (APA).

> Consider media support. Instruction-manual based CBT (cognitive behavior therapy) is frequently called the 'gold-standard' in various media reports. But this exalted status is as commonly invoked as it is undeserved ... [see] ... a pair of recent books (Dalal, 2018; Gnaulati, 2018), and a special issue of the prestigious journal *Psychotherapy*. (Courtois & Brown, 2019).

Insurance companies are also an important member of an algorithmic alliance. Instruction-manual therapies are a bean counters dream! They routinely twist, and as found in the class action suit Wit v. UBH, distort research to limit reimbursement to specific acute symptoms. This lets them ignore underlying causes and chronic conditions. Imagine you go to your doctor with a high fever caused by a fulminating bacterial infection. If you were treated by the rules of managed mental healthcare, you would merely be given an aspirin to reduce the acute symptom of fever rather than a more expensive antibiotic to address the underlying cause. Pretty crazy, I know. But, that's what's happening. By saying time-limited instruction-manual treatments are the generally accepted standard of care insurance companies get around complying with parity legislation that mandate mental illnesses and injuries be treated on par with physical ones. But the more algorithmic and the less human the treatment, the more profit.

> Professional organizations, like the APA (American Psychological Association) are another powerful member of the algorithmic alliance leading us to a future of dehumanized care and automated psychotherapy. In a mis-guided effort to have a seat at the table with insurance companies and policy-makers they are giving their imprimatur of respectability to instruction-manual treatments solely based on the number of RCTs done.

In fact, as the article continues, "the APA crafted 'clinical practice guidelines' for treating PTSD and depression based on research guidelines used for the evaluation of medications." Unfortunately, as Jonathan Shedler presented at the PsiAN 2019 conference,

> (a)bout 2/3 of PTSD patients treated according to the algorithmic clinical guidelines publicized by the APA will still have PTSD at the conclusion of treatment. Depression is slightly worse. He noted that 70% of those treated according to those algorithmic practice guidelines either didn't improve or quickly relapsed.
>
> What this means is that if you have PTSD or are depressed, the chances are pretty good that you will not (that's a NOT) be helped by a clinician who follows APA practice guidelines. And the only way to understand this is to realize that even well-intentioned professional psychologists can become entrapped by the seductions algorithms afford. Instead of embracing our messy, fleshy all too human complexity, the APA has apparently thrown in with the alliance that views people as reliably programmable respondents to properly sequenced instructions: Who cares that the treatments don't help most people! They are reliable and well-studied!

Finally, with a warning and a plea for both-and thinking that grew in importance during the pandemic, there is a way all of us may be unwitting collaborators with the algorithmic warriors:

> We just may be complicit by the way we're sleepwalking towards a future of artificial intimacy. What I see as a dystopian future of fully dehumanized and automated psychotherapy will not come about solely because the algorithms and devices reach a level of sophistication so far only imagined in science fiction. It will happen because we step-by-sleepwalking-step reach a point of numbly accepting relationships with and through machines as routinely good-enough replacements for actually being together. To be clear, the antidote to this is not to turn our backs on technology. We should expect more and more from the tools we make. But we also have to start expecting more and more from each other, and ourselves. The answer is

> not less technology. The answer is more humanity; messy, fleshy, conflicted, complicated, horrendous, and wonderful other people. Only by learning to cherish each other more will we find ourselves in an anti-dystopian future.
>
> *Sleepwalking Towards Artificial Intimacy: How Psychotherapy Is Failing the Future*[2]

Psychotherapy's unintentional participation in building a future of artificial intimacy (what I have called "the other AI" to contrast with the typical meaning of AI as artificial intelligence) was a topic in a June 2018 article I co-wrote with Sherry Turkle and Gillian Isaacs Russell. We took on the "dream that technologies like artificial intelligence and robotics will soon be able to simulate the emotional experience and consequences of physically being with another person." We started with a robotic-moment (Turkle, 2011, 2016; Turkle, Essig, & Russell, 2017) observation that "there will only be widespread acceptance of artificial intimacy if we are willing to reduce what we expect from relationships to what technology can provide. And that's what we seem to be doing: sleepwalking toward this future by undermining what we expect from close relationships."

We asked "(h)ow did we get to a place where the idea of artificial intimacy seems so appealing, where our expectations for each other have so deteriorated?" Our answer was incrementally, by small steps. Obviously, things like texting rather than talking and then asking Siri or Alexa for a joke all play a part. But we also noted how "psychotherapy, a profession that would seem most committed to the power of person-to-person talk, has been part of this cultural shift toward settling for what machines can provide." Before the tectonic shifts in professional practice made necessary by the Covid-19 pandemic, there was already

> 'a taste for 'remote treatment.' For decades, remote treatment, beginning with talking to patients on the phone, has been a useful tool in psychotherapy when someone is ill, traveling for business, or on vacation. Sometimes patients can't find a therapist locally. And for ongoing treatments it has been the 'better than nothing' solution when a patient relocates. But gradually, Skype and Facetime have turned remote treatment into what many therapists consider the new normal: good-enough routine practice.

Of course, during the pandemic, at the delta-variant time of this writing, and the still to emerge post-Covid world, teletherapies have become part of routine practice. How could it responsibly be otherwise? But all is not lost. What inoculates psychotherapy against sleepwalking toward a future of artificial intimacy is awareness of difference, making the inevitable losses of relating through screens and speakers central to the practice of psychotherapies of depth, insight, and relationship (Russell and Essig, 2019; Essig & Russell, 2021). Practicing as though a technologically-mediated simulation of in-person practice is functionally equivalent to in-person practice rather than a *sui generis* form of treatment in its own right, one that can be helpful in its own terms, both does cultural harm and attenuates the potential clinical value of the treatment being offered. Acting as though screen relations are the same as in-person intimacies does not serve our patients well and takes us step-by-step closer to a world of artificial intimacy.

We closed with a plea:

> It is not inevitable that we will move toward the acceptance of artificial intimacy whether we are talking about care-bots, friendship-bots or therapy-bots. There is still time to demand more. After all, empathy, authenticity and embodied relationships most define us as human. These capabilities create human children who can most fully interact with their parents and peers and who can most richly reflect on their lives. They are bedrock for the experiences most central for a well-lived life. When we settle for images on screens or algorithms programmed to generate moments of pretend-understanding, we risk losing each other and we risk losing ourselves.

Direct to consumers

What to do if your therapy app didn't help your depression[3]

The attention economy in the post-social media world is vicious and harsh. Offering something well-written and useful does not necessarily attract readers at a level commensurate with the quality of the offering. To compensate, people writing for online distribution deploy many strategies in the competition for eyeballs, for example, and one of my favorites, commenting on a study that is itself gathering media attention. I used this piggybacking strategy in this post that also tried to get attention by talking directly to people who might be needing mental healthcare. It began:

> If you've tried a therapy app to deal with depression and it hasn't worked, relax. It's likely them, not you. Don't be discouraged. Help and healing are possible. I hope you'll continue with your efforts to build a better life—just maybe not with a therapy app.
>
> An app that cures depression sure sounds like a good idea. Help for everyone all the time. What could be better. There are lots of them fighting for as big a slice as possible of the 300 billion dollar mental health market, oftentimes making claims light years ahead of the available evidence. With all that marketing there's no reason not to give something a try. But if you're depressed and you reached out to an app for help only to drop it for one reason or another, take note that new research shows you are close to the majority of users. A recent meta-analysis (that is a study of the available studies) of

> clinical trials of smartphone apps for depressive symptoms showed drop-out rates approaching 50%. That's a lot of people who do not fully engage with a so-called treatment that was designed specifically to help them.

Part of therapy app appeal is the claim they are innovations, i.e., new and better! I wanted to discredit this notion because these apps are typically not at all innovations in providing mental healthcare. Even if they use a new technology or are a new application of an existing technology to helping people with depression, they almost always make things worse. To make this argument, I talked about research from Clayton Christensen, author of *The Innovator's Dilemma* (2013), who died the week before I wrote this piece in January 2020. His work makes clear that these apps are not in any way genuine innovations, despite all the marketing, because they don't, in his language, "get the job done" of being significantly better at making people less depressed. Using a new tool does not make the practice innovative if the results are not any better. Many if not most therapy apps, no matter how whiz-bangy the programming, are what the economists Daron Acemoglu and Pascual Restrepo termed "so-so technologies" (Roose, 2021, p. 56). The piece continues:

> In fact, a therapy app just might be today's version of a long discredited 'just get over it' or 'pull yourself up by the bootstraps' approach to depression. After all, when someone is depressed, they don't engage their life as fully as they need/want to. An app that requires engagement to do the job of helping people get back to a place where they can engage with things is, to be blunt, kind of (a) silly idea. Success requires that its hoped for result is present at the beginning.
>
> But I must admit that when it comes to depression I'm no stranger to silly ideas like this. I remember years ago when the anti-depressant, perhaps serotonin-boosting, effects of exercise were first becoming known. Since exercise, like technology, is one of my favorite things I thought, "whoa, cool." So I gently but enthusiastically recommended to a depressed patient that he take advantage of these new findings and start a 3 times per week exercise program. He raised his slumped head from his chest, fixed my gaze with sad eyes and said "if I could do that I wouldn't need to." Similarly, therapy apps for depression just might be something that works for people who don't need the help. And perhaps those who do need help engaging drop out, hence the large drop-out numbers.
>
> But the problem may even go beyond that. Exercise wouldn't make you more depressed, not if you do it right. But turning away from a human relationship when you need one and towards an algorithm playing out on a screen just may. It just may reinforce loneliness and alienation ... When someone is alienated, lonely and lacking in vitality, feeling perhaps helpless and hopeless, turning to a screen just may be the last place one should look. The problem with therapy apps with near 50% drop-out rates may not be

that the developers need to build better apps. The problem may be the simple fact that they are apps.

What To Expect From Psychotherapy On Screen: A Consumer's Guide[4]

How To Make Remote Psychotherapy Work Better For You: A Consumer's Guide[5]

Thirteen months before the pandemic exploded in March 2020 making it necessary for almost all psychotherapists to become emergency telehealth providers, as well as making us fellow victims of the global pandemic, I wrote a two-part "consumer's guide" for those seeking, considering, or receiving psychotherapy via technologically-mediated screen relations. The substance of the second, "*How To Make …*" was later refined into remote session guidelines published elsewhere (Russell & Essig, 2019; Essig & Russell, 2020).

I started "*What To Expect …*" by noting "(i)f you're thinking about meeting with a psychotherapist remotely on screen, there's something you should know: it's not the same as meeting in person." I then noted something the pandemic has made obvious.

> Remote treatment is getting lots of attention. It was one of the American Psychological Association's top 10 trends for 2018 … But the enthusiasm is well in excess of the evidence. And some, like me, are deeply worried that remote treatment is failing the future by helping push us towards a culture of artificial intimacy. In any event, it seems pretty clear that the time is ripe for consumers of these services to learn more about what they might be getting themselves into.

I continue with the theme of there being significant differences between meeting in-person and meeting on screen. Unfortunately, there is a tendency in the wider culture, one often embraced by psychotherapists of depth, insight, and relationship, to move from observations of difference into a polarized stance of being either for or against technology or a particular use of technology like teletherapy, or video games. It's a clash between excessive enthusiasm on the one hand and resistance on the other resulting in a stagnant stalement where a nuanced both-and appreciation of both promise and peril becomes hard to find. I have not been immune to participating in that, on both sides at various points. At times I've used fiery language both to urge technology-use and to ignite awareness of perils, especially when confronting excessive, unfounded, and uncritical enthusiasms. Sometimes I unfortunately made it harder to see the "both-and," seeing both the promise of care at a distance and the significant perils of ignoring difference and inevitable loss. Here was my attempt at balance in this consumer's guide to expectations:

> I want to be very clear that therapy delivered remotely can sometimes be helpful. There is too much good research and too many good stories to even consider saying otherwise. Being on screen together really will at times feel

like you can reach out and touch someone. But not always. Other times you'll feel the limits, the losses of isolation and distance that even the best technologies can't erase. The bottom line is that sometimes remote treatment can indeed be a better-than-nothing compromise worth the unavoidable costs. And sometimes not.

In my clinical practice I do provide care remotely, just not routinely and always with difference in mind. That way my patients and I can help minimize the inevitable losses.

And that risk-benefit way of thinking organized my response to the emergency conversion to telehealth made necessary by the pandemic (Essig, 2020b; Russell & Essig, 2020). There was no choice but to make it work.

My pandemic response

Want to see your therapist in-person mid-pandemic? Think again[6]

This was written in June, 2020 (and for reasons later explained, this was my last piece for *Forbes*) while serving as co-chair of the APsaA Covid-19 Advisory Team and co-teaching workshops about how to make teletherapy work during the pandemic (Essig & Russell, 2021; Russell & Essig, 2020). At the time of this writing, 14 months later and in the midst of the delta-variant surge, it remains as apt as it was a mere four months into the pandemic.

Resuming some version of normal life is incredibly appealing, especially for psychotherapy. Like I wrote about for the American Psychological Association (APA) (Essig, Russell & McWilliams, 2020), what takes place on screens, while workable, is fundamentally different and more difficult than when people are together. But mid-pandemic in-person psychotherapy may not be such a good solution for the limitations of screens and speakers, and it's not at all a return to normal life. In fact, and it's not obvious, the balance of risks and rewards argues against returning to the office however much one may want to. For almost everyone, video- or audio-based telehealth will remain a better choice than meeting in-person behind masks, screens, face shields, disinfectants, physical distance, ventilation, symptom monitoring, contact tracing, and the like.

However good it may feel, there's always danger when wishing something were true gets in the way of rationally balancing of risks and rewards. This is especially true for wishing mid-pandemic in-person work were a return to normal. There is a specific and imminent danger that regulators and insurance companies will ignore the harsh realities of the Covid-19 pandemic by prematurely terminating emergency waivers for telehealth. You may be forced to do something you do not want to do,

> either pay out-of-pocket or work in-person when you do not feel it safe or worthwhile to do so. We have to find the courage to engage the harsh realities of the pandemic however desperately one might wish things to be otherwise, and despite how some political leaders despicably try to pretend otherwise.

With this, hopefully balanced, start I continue by describing the decreased rewards and increased risks of mid-pandemic in-person work. First the diminished rewards:

> Let's start with the reward side of the equation. Mid-pandemic in-person psychotherapy won't be the same. The main problem is that necessary procedures for viral safety inevitably undermine fundamental experiences of psychological safety so necessary for effective psychotherapy. Like two people tethered together to keep each other safe while scaling a cliff, the experience of mid-pandemic in-person psychotherapy will be replete with dangers requiring constant vigilance and inter-dependence.
>
> Psychotherapy is built on a promise; you bring your suffering to this private place and I will work with you to keep you safe and help you heal. That promise is changed by necessary viral precautions. First, the possibility of contact tracing weakens the promise of confidentiality. I promise to keep this private changes to a promise to keep it private unless someone gets sick and I need to contact the local health department.
>
> Even more powerful is the fact that a mid-pandemic in-person psychotherapy promise has to include all the ways we will protect each other from very real dangers, hardly the experience of psychological safety. There will even be a promise to pretend we are safe together even when we are doing so many things to remind us we are each the source of a potentially life-altering infection.

Next were the increased risks that go along with diminished reward. After reviewing the then current understanding of infection risks from a typical psychotherapy practice, I considered psychological risks:

> The possibility of psychological risks in mid-pandemic in-person psychotherapy also needs to be considered. Will someone stop needed treatment because they feel the office is too dangerous, or maybe the trip to and from the office is a problem? Will some see the risks being taken and use that to trash the gains from three months of emergency telehealth? Will the anxiety of change increase substance abuse? We know that many mental health issues have physical co-morbidities that make people significantly more vulnerable to being ravaged by Covid-19. Will they stop needed treatment if emergency telehealth waivers are eliminated? And to name just one more from a list of possible risks, there's the additional stress and tension among

> the most emotionally vulnerable who will have to decide whether or not to continue risky care.

I closed, both this piece and my time at *Forbes*, with a warning still applicable today.

> No one should feel regulatory or insurance reimbursement pressure to take on these additional risks to provide or access psychotherapeutic care. Reason dictates that emergency waivers on telehealth restrictions should continue as long as the pandemic rages. While the virus makes the future even more uncertain than it usually is, the reduced clinical rewards and increased risks do make one thing clear: the only reason an insurance company would end emergency telehealth waivers would be a cynical attempt to reduce utilization by making psychotherapeutic care virally risky and less useful so that fewer people would access the care they need.
>
> Let's hope that doesn't happen.

What's next

The world has changed, several times, since I had the window/mirror dream that enriched decisions to spend my professional life looking both inward and out. Starting in the early 90s what I saw out the window was that the need to get connected and become fluent in using the Internet was the cutting-edge intersection of technology, mind, society, and psychotherapy. This was when AOL disks rained down like manna from heaven and when I became an enthusiastic techno-evangelist with The Psychoanalytic Connection, helping hundreds of colleagues get online and even more have experiences, sometimes their first experience, of online psychoanalytic scholarship and learning. But that cutting edge soon dulled. By the early aughts social media and mobile emerged as a new cutting edge. This was the so called Web 2.0 revolution. Being online started to mean creating content, not just being connected so one could access content others created. People started walking around with always on connection devices. We were always in touch with everyone all the time, amply able to document our now curated online lives. Mobile devices became ubiquitous with content creation king. In response, I turned my attention away from enthusiastically promoting the value, actually the necessity of getting connected and wrote, and then wrote some more. I became a content creator. With experience online increasing, my initial techno-enthusiasms wavered. They were then further undermined by all the accumulating scholarship asking urgent and fundamental questions about what using communications technologies was doing to us, especially our relationships with both self and other (Carr, 2011, 2015; Jackson, 2007; Powers, 2010; Turkle, 2016).

Which brings us to today. Now, in the midst of a pandemic fog that makes it difficult to see anything but it, there is, I think, another professionally relevant profound shift taking place, and I am not referring to the adaptations, surprises, and disappointments from everyone having become emergency telehealth providers. What I am seeing is a world so saturated with "content" that creating or finding meaning is becoming harder and harder. It seems that everyone has a blog or a podcast. Instagram and Twitter feeds feud for attention with TikTok. And what the social media vortex reveals is that the best, or at least the most popular, really do lack all conviction while the worst are full of passionate intensity.[7] Forget about the center not holding. Our culture no longer has any center. Instead, there are multiple, non-overlapping centers in which content is consumed in ever-deepening and narrowing silos of personal taste and tribal loyalty. Our culture is now defined by confirmation bias run amok; so much so that the more one writes, the less one is read.

Looking ahead one sees a new cutting-edge emerging. Just as connection gave way to mobile content that become tribalized, tribalized mobile content is now ceding its cutting-edge status to AI, deep learning models, and big data. More and more, these systems are and will be organizing what we will read, watch, and listen to; what we do; how to live; and even who we will become (Iansiti & Lakhani, 2020; Metz, 2021; Pasquale, 2020; Roose, 2021: Susskind & Susskind, 2016). Machine learning even promises a ladder for climbing out of our media silos. Whether and how psychoanalysis and all psychotherapies of depth, insight, and relationship will confront and relate to this world being remade by AI is the question occupying my mind right now. But I have no idea what, or even if, a specific professional praxis will emerge from this new cutting edge, like what happened with connection and then content. But I do know that the time for writing at a place like *Forbes* is over. And I am confident that in the next phase of my zeitgeist-y professional life I'll be trying to both look in the mirror and out the window.

Notes

1 Available at https://www.forbes.com/sites/toddessig/2019/12/27/the-war-for-the-future-of-psychotherapy/.
2 Available at https://www.forbes.com/sites/toddessig/2018/06/07/sleepwalking-towards-artificial-intimacy-how-psychotherapy-is-failing-the-future/.
3 Available at https://www.forbes.com/sites/toddessig/2020/01/31/what-to-do-if-your-therapy-app-didnt-help-your-depression/.
4 Available at https://www.forbes.com/sites/toddessig/2019/02/26/what-to-expect-from-psychotherapy-on-screen-a-consumers-guide/.
5 Available at https://www.forbes.com/sites/toddessig/2019/02/26/how-to-make-remote-psychotherapy-work-better-for-you-a-consumers-guide/.
6 https://www.forbes.com/sites/toddessig/2020/06/27/want-to-see-your-therapist-in-person-mid-pandemic-think-again/.
7 Lines borrowed from W. B. Yeats' poem "The Second Coming."

References

Buber, M. (1970). *I and thou* (W. Kaufmann, Trans.). New York, NY: Charles Scribner & Sons. (Original work published 1923).

Carr, N. (2011). *The shallows: What the internet is doing to our brains*. New York, NY: W. W. Norton.

Carr, N. (2015). *The glass cage: How our computers are changing us*. New York, NY: W. W. Norton.

Christensen, C. M. (2013). *The innovator's dilemma: when new technologies cause great firms to fail*. Boston, MA: Harvard Business Review Press.

Courtois, C. A., & Brown, L. S. (Eds.). (2019). Special Issue: APA Clinical Practice Guideline for PTSD: Coordinated Special Issue with Psychotherapy and Practice Innovations. *Psychotherapy*, 56(3).

Dalal, F. (2018). *CBT: The cognitive behavioural tsunami: Managerialism, politics and the corruptions of science*. New York, NY: Routledge.

Essig, T. (2020a). "Training Done? Write!" A Response to Alexander Stein. *Psychoanalytic Perspectives*, 17(2), 173–182.

Essig, T. (2020b). Emergency Conversion to Tele-treatment: Making it work [Video]. YouTube. https://www.youtube.com/watch?v=hZW1LBrtveo

Essig, T., & Russell, G. I. (2020). Remote Session Guidelines for Periods of Restricted Travel. Retrieved 8/2/21 from https://apsa.org/sites/default/files/Guide3-24.pdf.

Essig, T., & Russell, G. I. (2021). A Report from the Field: Providing Psychoanalytic Care during the Pandemic. *Psychoanalytic Perspectives*, 18(2), 157–177.

Essig, T., Russell, G. I., & McWilliams, N. (2020). Providing psychodynamic care during COVID-19: How to deepen the treatment with telehealth during the pandemic. American Psychological Association. Retrieved 8/2/21 https://www.apaservices.org/practice/news/psychodynamic-care-covid-19

Gnaulati, E. (2018). *Saving talk therapy: How health insurers, big pharma, and slanted science are ruining good mental health care*. Boston, MA: Beacon Press.

Iansiti, M., & Lakhani, K. R. (2020). *Competing in the age of AI: strategy and leadership when algorithms and networks run the world*. Boston, MA: Harvard Business Press.

Jackson, M. (2008). *Distracted: The erosion of attention and the coming dark age*. Amherst, NY:: Prometheus Books.

Metz, C. (2021). *Genius Makers: The Mavericks Who Brought AI to Google, Facebook, and the World*. New York, NY: Random House.

Michaels, L. (2021). After being sued by Talkspace, I never thought I'd be agreeing with them. Or am I? Retrieved 8/11/21 from https://medium.com/@psian/stranger-things-after-being-sued-by-talkspace-i-never-thought-id-be-agreeing-with-them-ee2f79e45980

Pasquale, F. (2020). *New Laws of Robotics: Defending Human Expertise in the Age of AI*. Cambridge, MA: Belknap Press: An Imprint of Harvard University Press.

Powers, W. (2010). *Hamlet's blackberry*. New York, NY: HarperCollins.

Roose, K. (2021). *Futureproof: 9 rules for humans in the age of automation*. New York, NY: Random House.

Russell, G. I., & Essig, T. (2019). Bodies and screen relations: Moving treatment from wishful thinking to informed decision-making. In Govner, A. & Mills, J. (eds.) *Innovations in Psychoanalysis* (pp. 228–249). Routledge.

Russell, G. I., & Essig, T. (2020). Remote Therapy Webinar: Presented by Gillian Isaacs Russell and Todd Essig, 11/07/2020, British Psychotherapy Foundation [Video]. YouTube. https://www.youtube.com/watch?v=HfebHoYLES4

Stein, A. (2020). Psychoanalysis in the Public Sphere: A Call for Taking Analytic Thinking, Writing and Action into the Broader World. *Psychoanalytic Perspectives,* 17(2), 141–160.

Stern, D. B. (2017). Interpersonal Psychoanalysis: History and Current Status. *Contemporary Psychoanalysis*, 53:1, 69–94, doi: 10.1080/00107530.2016.1274870.

Susskind, R., & Susskind, D. (2016). *The future of the professions: How technology will transform the work of human experts.* Oxford, UK: Oxford University Press.

Turkle, S. (2011). *Alone together: Why we expect more from technology and less from each other.* New York, NY: Basic Books.

Turkle, S. (2016). *Reclaiming conversation: The power of talk in a digital age.* New York, NY: Penguin.

Turkle, S., Essig, T., & Russell, G. I. (2017). Afterword: Reclaiming psychoanalysis: Sherry Turkle in conversation with the editors. Psychoanalytic Perspectives, 14(2), 237–248.

13

Psychoanalytic applications in a diverse society

Pratyusha Tummala-Narra

In his paper, "Wild Psychoanalysis," Freud (1910) cautioned against the loose interpretation of psychoanalytic theory and technique, as he offered a glimpse into a broader usage of psychoanalytic ideas by those not formally trained as psychoanalysts. Inherent in his critique was a cautionary statement about the analyst's interpretation of psychoanalytic ideas, and an emphasis on self-discovery by the client without the analyst's imposition. The notion of loose interpretation of psychoanalytic ideas is complicated. On one hand, psychoanalysis itself has been interpreted differently in some important ways within different schools of thought, such as ego psychology, the British school of object relations, and relational psychoanalysis. If psychoanalysis were not subject to interpretation and modification, then these schools of thought would not have as much to offer as they do today. On the other hand, broader interpretations of psychoanalytic principles may still be experienced as precarious, particularly in the way that psychoanalytic ideas may be applied to understandings of diversity within clinical and non-clinical contexts (e.g. community-based interventions). In some cases, the integration of concepts from other perspectives, such as multicultural and community psychologies, in practice and consultation may be viewed as diluting psychoanalysis.

In a way, this dilemma concerning the looseness of interpretation raises questions about who decides what psychoanalysis should look like in theory and practice. I believe that this dilemma is especially relevant to contemporary times, as we have experienced unprecedented changes in demography in the U.S. and elsewhere, and globalization characterized by rapid exchange of ideas through the media and internet. This dilemma is also current in that psychoanalysis continues to face challenges to its scientific legitimacy or at least the public awareness of this legitimacy, despite evidence for the effectiveness of psychoanalytic psychotherapy (Shedler, 2010). Additionally, questions about the elite status of psychoanalysis and its relevance to helping clients remain largely controversial.

This chapter addresses some important ways in which psychoanalysis can be interpreted through broader and more inclusive lens as a way of moving toward a more complete understanding of racial and cultural diversity across

DOI: 10.4324/9781003325512-17

clinical and community applications. This type of reshaping departs from the ways that psychoanalysis and other Euro-American theories have historically been applied to racially and culturally diverse communities, either through neglect of issues of diversity or through oversimplified modifications of existing psychoanalytic ideas. An example of the latter is the application of the concept of Oedipus Complex to non-Western cultures that lacks a consideration of indigenous narratives of family dynamics (Tang & Smith, 1996). This has essentially been a colonizing approach (Altman, 2010), rather than an approach that considers multiple subjectivities and indigenous narrative. From the perspective of a 1.5-generation Indian American (born in India and immigrated to the U.S. as a child) female psychologist, this chapter considers a psychoanalytic perspective that interfaces with multicultural psychology and community psychology frameworks, with the aim of addressing the complexity of racial and ethnic diversity within individual- and community-level interventions and of considering how practice across settings (e.g. psychotherapy, community work) informs how social context can be addressed in psychoanalytic theory.

Contemporary psychoanalytic perspectives hold the potential for privileging individuals' and communities' subjective experiences over theoretical principles that have been defined under a cultural lens that either diverges from or devalues individuals and communities that vary in significant ways from mainstream cultural context. This approach is not counter in fact to the way that Freud and his contemporaries engaged in extending the practice of psychoanalysis to individuals and communities who were marginalized along social class lines. Such efforts culminated in the establishment of free clinics in Vienna and other parts of Europe, where psychoanalysis was made accessible to students, laborers, factory workers, farmers, domestic servants, and several others who were unable to pay for their treatment (Danto, 2005). As Elizabeth Ann Danto (2005) recognized in her notable book, "Freud's Free Clinics," many early psychoanalysts, such as Erik Erikson, Melanie Klein, Anna Freud, and Eric Fromm, although known today for their theoretical revisions of Freud's theories, saw themselves as "brokers of social change" (p. 4) who challenged political conventions of their time.

Psychoanalysis indeed has revolutionary roots, not to mention a history of persecution and exile. The history of exile that is part of the psychoanalytic movement in England and the U.S. has marked a retreat from these efforts centered on social justice. It is only recently that psychoanalysts have written about exile and its impact on the psychoanalytic movement outside of Europe (Danto, 2005). Just as this part of psychoanalytic history has been disavowed for decades, contemporary times demand that we reexamine history and social context and revisit the notion of social change when we conduct practice. In the following sections, I will review recent developments in psychoanalytic theory concerning diversity, applications of psychoanalytic theory in community intervention, and then describe two vignettes, one from psychoanalytic psychotherapy and one from a community intervention. This will be followed by a discussion of the applicability of psychoanalytic ideas across settings, and of how psychoanalytic theory can be informed by practice and consultation with racially and culturally diverse individuals and communities.

Psychoanalytic theory and attending to diversity

Over the past 15 years, psychoanalysts, particularly those using the lens of object relations theory and relational psychoanalysis, have written about internal representations of gender, race, culture, sexual orientation, and social class. For example, scholars have described the importance of the therapist confronting his or her own feelings of the racial other in order to address cross-racial and similar-racial interactions effectively (Altman, 2010; Bonovitz, 2005; Leary, 2006, 2012; Yi, 1998). Emotional insight in psychotherapy, within their perspectives, lies in the conceptualization of therapeutic interaction as co-constructed by the therapist and client, and the ability to tolerate ambivalence, anxiety, sadness, guilt, and shame as negotiated within the therapeutic dyad. These perspectives emphasize attachment, separation, and related mourning as essential components of the individual's growth process, where the client and the therapist are changed by virtue of relating to one another (Mitchell, 1988; Stolorow, 1988).

Psychoanalysts have also explored intrapsychic and interpersonal changes in the context of immigration. Akhtar (1999, 2011) has described the many challenges of the mourning process for immigrants, including regression into earlier stages of development, culture shock and discontinuity of identity, disorganization, and a third separation-individuation process. Various aspects of immigrant adjustment and identity, such as bilingualism, pre- and post-migration character, challenges with acculturation, and the role of fantasy about country of origin and adoptive country, have been described in the psychoanalytic literature (Ainslie, 2009; Akhtar, 2011; Eng & Han, 2000; Foster, 2003; Tummala-Narra, 2009a). Additionally, in recent years, issues of spirituality (Aron, 2004; Roland, 2005; Tummala-Narra, 2009b), sexual orientation/identity, and gender identity (Drescher, 2007; Suchet, 2011) have been recognized as central to individual development. Indeed, there have been considerable advances in the psychoanalytic understanding of diversity within the context of the therapeutic relationship.

Psychoanalytic ideas on diversity have been further developed by scholars who would consider themselves as psychodynamic, feminist thinkers. Scholars who integrate perspectives from psychoanalysis and multicultural psychology have approached psychoanalytic concepts such as culturally and racially based transference in the therapeutic relationship with an emphasis on the role of power, privilege, and social hierarchies in interpersonal and intrapsychic experience (Comas Diaz, 2006; Greene, 2007; Tummala-Narra, 2007). These developments in psychoanalytic perspectives and diversity are largely influenced by multicultural and feminist frameworks which have been instrumental in raising awareness of the unique experiences of gender, racial and cultural groups, and related structural power dynamics inherent to mainstream society. The influence of multicultural psychology in particular is evident in research, practice, and training guidelines that emphasize psychologists' awareness, knowledge, and skills in effectively working with individuals from diverse sociocultural backgrounds (Sue, 2001; Vasquez, 2007).

Psychoanalysis has the potential to provide depth and meaning to various aspects of diversity (e.g. race, culture, social class, sexual orientation, dis/ability) within the profession of psychology. Indeed, psychoanalytic literature has increasingly recognized the need to attend to social context in the therapeutic dyad. For example, Flores (2007) noted the importance of "a mode of psychoanalytic listening" (p. 255) that involves the psychic and social aspects of the therapeutic dyad. The decontextualization of individual experience in psychotherapy has been thought to be as a dissociative process that interferes with therapeutic work (Bodnar, 2004). Smith (2006) noted that psychoanalysts work with the specifics of clients' intrapsychic lives, and as such the analyst should consider the specifics of experiences with diversity and how they shape the psyche. He further cautioned that we have to be in a position to recognize the specifics in order to "analyze what is manifest or infer what is unconscious" (p. 9). The alternative to this, of course, is to disavow relevant aspects of our clients' and our own identities, and render these dimensions of the psyche invisible. Unfortunately, this has been the case for a good part of psychoanalytic history, as evidenced in Freud's ambivalence toward and rejection of cultural specifics, reducing cultural dimensions to neurotic adaptation (Akhtar & Tummala-Narra, 2005; Altman, 2010).

Psychoanalytic theory and community intervention

Psychoanalytic concepts have been increasingly applied in community-based interventions over the past decade. Some theorists have integrated concepts such as transference, enactments, defense mechanisms, and working through to understand their experiences of working with clients in community interventions (Borg, 2004; Darwin & Reich, 2006; Miller, 2008; Twemlow & Parens, 2006). Borg (2004) described a project with a low-income community in Los Angeles in the aftermath of the riots following the Rodney King verdict in 1992. In this account, he noted the shared emphasis on collaboration in community empowerment theory and interpersonal psychoanalysis and emphasized the importance of addressing tensions related to conflicting points of view within this collaborative approach. Borg coined "community character," which "reflects unconscious internalization" of patterns of behavior and unspoken rules that help the community cope with anxiety (p. 151). In the case of the riots in Los Angeles, he conceptualized the relational patterns of community residents as characterized by racial, ethnic and gender stereotyping, and hostility toward outsiders, reflecting both actual relationships with significant others and the broader social context (Borg, 2004). Relatedly, King and Shelley (2008) drew connections between community psychology and psychoanalysis, highlighting Adler's valuing of social context and community feeling as essential to the individual's adjustment to communal life.

Twemlow and Parens (2006) further described the overlap between psychoanalysis and community psychology, including the use of a developmental perspective, respecting and privileging all sides of conflict in the working through process, the importance of holding and containing, appreciation of subjectivity, and assessing for a sufficient level of anxiety to motivate change. They suggested that psychoanalytic knowledge is critical for community-based work and advocated for an actively supportive community psychoanalytic method with less emphasis on interpretation. This approach (Twemlow & Parens, 2006; Volkan, 2001) involves several features: establishing a point of similarity between participants allowing for tolerance of differences and negative emotions, collaboration, developing personal relationships such that the process becomes humanized, establishing mutual respect for differences that can trigger racial, religious, gender, and ethnic stereotypes, developing a common language for better communication, accepting that the process requires ongoing maintenance, understanding that collaborative nonblaming promotes change, and the adoption of a neutral position of the facilitator who encourages mutual problem-solving. Such an approach may pose challenges to the psychoanalytic practitioner's sense of identity, as it requires an integration of multiple theoretical perspectives in a non-clinical context.

Several psychoanalytic practitioners have written about how their experiences of working in community settings, many of which suffered considerable trauma, raised questions about their psychoanalytic identity. For example, Miller (2008) described his experience working with a New York City firehouse in the aftermath of severe loss at the World Trade Center on September 11, 2001. In his account, Miller recognized his role as requiring flexibility to best suit the needs of the community. In one example, noted potentially conflicting roles, as he questioned whether his identification with the traumatized members of the community interfered with his sense of neutrality. In a different account, Granatir (2004) described how his personal experience as a Jew and minority helped him identify with and relate to boys and girls in a school-based program in Washington, D.C. He noted how his training as an analyst prepared him to listen with openness, curiosity, and acceptance of differences across people. In each of these examples, psychoanalytic practitioners point to the ways in which their personal and professional identities expanded through their efforts with integrating psychoanalytic perspectives beyond the clinical setting.

Liang, Tummala-Narra, and West (2011) reviewed several psychoanalytic concepts, such as intersubjectivity, transference, enactments, and the role of affect, as highly relevant to community-based interventions. They encourage all practitioners and consultants involved in community-based work to actively integrate a psychodynamic understanding of interpersonal aspects of interventions, including racial and cultural conflicts, with a collaborative approach that fosters empowerment and meaningful change. In this perspective, psychoanalytic theory approaches the study of power and social injustice with complexity and multidimensionality, such that community collaborators (e.g. consultants and community members) can more effectively address individual, group, and environmental stress.

Interestingly, although recent psychoanalytic applications in community interventions have raised interest in how best to conceptualize group dynamics in the community setting from a psychoanalytic perspective, few scholars have addressed how community-based work may better inform an understanding of social context within psychoanalysis more broadly (Twemlow & Parens, 2006; Twemlow et al., 2011). In the following sections, I describe two case vignettes that include components of my work in a psychoanalytically oriented psychotherapy and a community-based intervention, both focusing on racial and cultural dynamics. These vignettes are presented with the purpose of 1) illustrating potential applications of psychoanalytic concepts and an integration of multicultural and community psychologies in addressing racial and cultural dynamics in two distinct settings, and 2) considering the implications of therapeutic practice and community consultation with racial and ethnic minority clients for psychoanalytic theory and identity.

Case example: psychoanalytic psychotherapy with "Reena"

Reena is a 30-year-old Hindu, Indian American woman, born and raised in the Northeastern part of the U.S. She works full time, and sought psychotherapy to cope with her increasing anxiety at work. She was referred to see me by her primary care physician. She had never previously worked with a psychotherapist. I worked with Reena in weekly psychotherapy for approximately three years.

Reena's parents immigrated to the U.S. from a northern region of India in the late 1970s, during a time of mounting violence between Hindus and Muslims in the region. Her parents spoke little English and worked in a family business when they first arrived to the U.S. Reena has a younger sister with whom she feels close. She described her childhood as feeling "hectic," with her parents working most of the time, and her relatives (aunts, uncles at varying times) taking care of her and her sister. She stated that this experience was mixed in that she felt safe when her parents were there, and most of the time with her relatives. However, she did recall that between ages 5 and 8, she periodically witnessed her maternal uncle physically abuse his wife, during times when they were babysitting her and her sister. She did not tell her parents about these incidents, as she did not want to upset them, and felt as though there wasn't another alternative. In one session, she told me that she felt scared during these times, especially for her aunt.

Reena spoke in Hindi primarily at home, and in English outside of the home. She and her sister would often translate for their parents outside the home. She recalled this experience as generally a good one in that she felt that she was contributing to her family, and that her parents appreciated her help. The family's visits to India were infrequent, due to limited financial resources. Reena was encouraged to excel academically and took on this role as a shared dream with her parents. She completed her graduate education and feels that she has fulfilled her wishes as well as that of her parents. Reena reported having a closer relationship with her mother than her father, and that she felt sorry for her mother who carried the burden of working outside the home and taking care of children at home. She stated, "It's like she never had a break until we left home." At the time that, I met Reena, she had been living far away from her parents' home, and maintained frequent contact with them by phone and email.

Reena's school experiences were characterized by considerable anxiety. She recalled having few friends in her school and mostly interacted with friends in her neighborhood. Most of the children in her school (elementary through high school) were from middle-class White European American backgrounds. Reena recalled being teased because of her Hindu background, her brown skin color, and for wearing her hair in a braid and a bindi (dot) on her forehead when she was in elementary school. As she entered middle school, she told her parents that she no longer wanted to wear the bindi. Difference at school, more generally, was considered to be bad. Reena recalled an experience in high school where a Sikh boy was teased to a point when his parents moved to a different school district. She remembered feeling afraid of being seen as different, and at the same time angry about what had happened to this boy. Reena began to hide her Indian identity when she was around her non-Indian friends in high school and found partial success in doing this. She felt that she was more included by others, and yet, felt that her Indian and American worlds were disconnected. In college, she began dating men whom she never introduced to her parents. In fact, she worked hard to keep these relationships a secret from them.

In her late 20s, Reena began to feel pressured by her parents to marry an Indian American man. When I met her, Reena had been dating a White American man who was of Italian and French heritage for about one year, and she felt increasingly anxious about her intimacy with him. This fear was in part related to her memories of her abusive uncle, and in part to her concerns about racial and cultural differences. She worried about the difference in their cultural background and further separating from speaking in Hindi. However, she felt somewhat more comfortable with his working-class background as it resembled her own social class background growing up. At the same time, she was upset about what she experienced as racist attitudes of his parents. In one incident, when she went out for dinner with his family, his father made derogatory statements about African Americans. Reena was taken aback and wondered about how he felt about her racial background, and her brown skin color. While she felt as though she loved her boyfriend, she remained cautious about their relationship. She found herself increasingly worried at her workplace as well, having thoughts about others viewing her as inferior in some way. Her concerns at her workplace were especially salient when some co-workers commented on how "exotic" she looked, which she experienced as derogatory.

In psychotherapy, Reena and I worked on better understanding her anxiety both within and outside of the therapeutic relationship. She asked me on two different occasions if I felt that her contact with her parents was too frequent. She spoke with them twice a week by phone and emailed them twice a week. I asked her if she enjoyed talking with her parents. She said "Yes, it's important to me that I talk with them." When we talked about her questioning herself, she expressed that most of her friends who are not Indian told her that she was too dependent on her parents. I believe that it was important for her to hear that it is fine to talk with her parents as much as she wanted, and to be able to speak in Hindi with them. Early in our work, we began to challenge some of these assumptions that were based on Western, European-American ideas about parent-child relationships about which she felt ambivalent.

As our work progressed, Reena expressed concern that I wouldn't approve of her relationship with a non-Indian man, especially one that comes from a "racist family." In one session, she stated, "You're probably thinking about why I'm with this guy. I don't know that I really understand." When I asked her to say more about what she was imagining about my response, she said, "I don't know if you would think this is ok, I mean to be with someone not Indian. You are probably married to someone Indian. I've wondered about this. Then, I wonder what it will be like to tell my parents, when I don't even know if I want to be with him." I responded, "What would it be like for you if I was married to an Indian man?" She stated, "Well, it would be good, I guess. You would be doing all the right things, you know being a professional and marrying the right type of person, bring a good Indian woman." We went on to explore the "right type of Indian woman" and her feelings of difference from me. Difference was also apparent in the contrast between Reena's light brown skin tone and my darker brown skin tone. Through our discussions of our skin color differences, Reena understood her fantasy of me being married to an Indian man as reflecting her association between darker skin color and a stronger Indian identification. These discussions about skin color provoked anxiety for both of us, as we had each brought to our interaction complicated histories with race and skin color as Indian American women. For example, Reena felt unsure about what her relationship with her boyfriend and his family would mean for her own racial identity development, specifically that her racial minority status and her experiences with discrimination would be invisible to them. Memories of my own experiences with racial and skin color discrimination outside of the Indian American community and within the Indian American community, respectively, were elicited while working with Reena. As I identify with a bicultural Indian American orientation and as a person of color in the U.S., I recognized that I shared some of Reena's experiences, and at the same time wanted to help her become more aware of the conscious and unconscious meanings accompanying her experiences with race and ethnicity. Attending to our differences in skin color facilitated an exploration of authenticity as Indian-origin women and a sense of belonging within and outside of the Indian American community (Tummala-Narra, 2007).

We further struggled with difference and similarity as Reena later revealed that she felt as though I could understand her Indian American and Hindu backgrounds, but perhaps not her working-class background. Reena imagined that our shared cultural experience was disrupted by the possibility that I am married to an Indian man. I was also aware of the absence of the Hindi language in our work, another point of separation for us. Some of my countertransferential reactions included feeling rejected by her, as I felt that she had not seen my experiences with social class. I immigrated to the U.S. as a child and experienced shifts across social class throughout my life. Somehow, in our interactions, Reena had not recognized this part of my life, and it disappointed me. Perhaps, I too felt distant from her and my own past in these moments. Like Reena, I had struggled with separation from my parents and acculturating to the Western cultural context. At the same time, I recognized that we were both experiencing ambivalence about our relatively privileged positions, with cultural identifications, and separation from parents. My experience was invisible to her, as hers was invisible to her parents, her peers in school, her boyfriend, and his family. Our work evoked questions about the position of the therapist or analyst whose multiple identities are both seen and unseen by the client.

In the course of our work together, we increasingly talked about her experience of hiding aspects of her life from important people in her life (e.g. parents, boyfriend), and the experience of talking about these "hidden parts" with me. This discussion of her social context and identity, particularly with respect to culture, race, gender, and social class, helped to create a space in which Reena could more fully explore her racial and cultural identities, an essential component of her conflicts with intimacy with family members, friends, and boyfriend.

Case example: community intervention

As a coordinator for a community-based outreach project in a large city in the Northeastern part of the U.S., I was asked by an administrator in an urban middle school to help develop psychoeducational group meetings in an afterschool program. The staff and majority of the students at the middle school are African American, and the rest of the students are of Latino, or multiracial backgrounds. The staff at the afterschool program had been increasingly concerned about students' exposure to violence in their neighborhoods. Many of the staff members recognized the stress experienced by the students, particularly a few boys who verbally expressed their anger after witnessing two men mugging a young woman. My colleague, a White American woman, and I arranged a meeting with the staff of the afterschool program.

At this initial meeting with the staff, my colleague and I learned that this type of incident was a relatively common experience for many students, and that traumatic experiences were typically not talked about in the family or at school. The staff hoped to find ways to address students' exposure to violence at a weekly discussion group focused on health topics (physical and emotional) which the students were required to attend. During our meeting, an African American staff member also expressed concern about the ability of "doctors from a predominantly White institution" to relate to the concerns of the school, students, and community. When I heard this staff member's response, I was moved by her honesty, and at the same time felt as though she hadn't noticed my race or ethnicity. It was as though she was solely responding to my White colleague, who was silent through most of the meeting. I acknowledged to the staff that my institution was predominantly White and asked them to provide more detail about their concerns. A different staff member stated, "We really want to make sure that you all understand the community here, and what our kids go through and what is realistic for them." Other staff members agreed and joined in voicing their concerns about our approach to the after-school program. It was clear that the staff were understandably protective of the students' welfare, and cautious about any negative outside influence that would further stress the students. The staff's concerns reflected previous experiences with health care professionals who had disappointed the school community. One example of this was raised by a staff member who stated, "I'm worried about how many of our boys have the label ADHD, and the parents are just told to give them medicine. Some of these boys just need someone to talk to, not all of these drugs, but this is what the doctors tell them to do." As the staff discussed their concerns, I was aware that many of staff and students had previously experienced institutional racism, and of the cultural mistrust toward me possibly because of a concern that I may have internalized the oppressive culture of these institutions, and toward my colleague who may have been experienced as representing institutions that have discriminated against African Americans and other ethnic minorities. Toward the end of our first meeting, my colleague and I thanked the staff for sharing their concerns, and we requested several more meetings prior to starting the discussion groups with the students in the afterschool program. We felt that this was necessary to establish a collaboration to develop an adequate intervention.

While driving back to our office, I asked my colleague why she had remained silent through this meeting. She shared with me that she felt overwhelmed by a sense of sadness and guilt, and worried that she would enact the situation that the staff and she feared, by "taking over" the meeting by talking. She chose to stay silent to cope with feeling simultaneously like an outsider and oppressor. I told her that interestingly, I felt like an outsider since my race and ethnicity were treated as irrelevant or invisible, and that racial difference had been conceptualized around Black-White lines, as they typically are in mainstream American society. My colleague stated that she felt surprised by my reaction, and that she had seen me as an insider because of my Indian background. Indeed, the consultants had felt "othered," and at the same time we wondered whether we had "othered" the staff in some way. We were also aware of being outside of the comfort zone of our offices, and potentially imposing ourselves at the school. It was clear that my colleague's feelings of White guilt and my feelings of invisibility which were connected with long-standing racial dynamics concerning Black-White lines and the ambivalent position of race and racial identity among Indian Americans (Tummala-Narra, Inman, & Ettigi, 2011), contributing to racial dynamics among professionals from African American, Indian American, White American backgrounds that are typically unexplored.

Toward the end of our second meeting, an African American staff member asked me where I was from. I replied by saying that I was born in India and grew up primarily in the U.S. She then stated that she knew that I wasn't from the U.S. I responded by saying, "I'm Indian American. Where did you grow up?" She then told me that she had been raised in the local area. In the coming weeks, during the periods between our meetings with staff, I wondered if I should interpret what I had repeatedly experienced as being "othered," because of my non-Black and non-White racial status. I also wondered for whom (i.e. staff, me, my colleague) and at what point in time an interpretation of racial dynamics would be experienced as helpful. The insider-outsider dynamic that was apparent from the beginning of our interactions conflicted with my wish to belong and be accepted as a credible professional who could consult effectively in the after-school program. In the third meeting with the staff, we engaged in a discussion about students' self-care in the context of violence exposure. Several staff members reported that they worried about the students' physical health as much as their emotional health. Some students mostly depended on fast food restaurants for their meals, and other students ate only one meal per day, at school. The staff also expressed that many of the students did not have access to annual physical exams, because of parents' work hours or unavailability. A staff member stated, "They (students) are treated sometimes like they are adults, like they are supposed to feed themselves, take care of their bodies, and sometimes nobody there to protect them."

As the discussion progressed, we talked about the possibility of developing discussion groups after school focused on physical stress related to exposure to violence in the neighborhood. Specifically, we planned a discussion with the students about how being exposed to violence can be stressful to the body, and strategies to cope with this stress. My colleague and I asked the staff to tell us about their perceptions of students' attitudes toward nutrition. Most of the staff expressed that the students had little exposure to healthy eating. My colleague suggested that we discuss healthy eating habits with the students. I joined by stating that it may be helpful to provide handouts about healthy meals. When we ended the meeting, I realized that the staff hadn't actually responded explicitly to our suggestions, and that in fact, my colleague and I hadn't considered how this approach would be experienced by the staff or the students. I also recognized that I was disappointed in myself for not thinking through the social contextual implications of the nutrition education. In retrospect, I think that joining with my colleague in simplifying or neglecting the social context of the intervention was in part a reflection of my wish to identify with someone (my colleague) who had been more emotionally accessible to me. Up to this point, I had been unsuccessful in my attempts to connect with the program staff and had perhaps resigned to the idea that my help was not going to be accepted.

With three remaining meetings before the initial student workshop, I asked the staff to talk about their reactions to our suggestions from the previous meeting. While some staff seemed reluctant to share their reactions, others stated that they did not know how the students would be able to relate to a healthy eating plan that assumes that people have adequate resources and access to markets and restaurants that sell or serve healthy foods. One staff member stated, "There is no Subway in this neighborhood—only McDonalds and KFC." I then commented, "You may feel then that our idea of talking about healthy foods raises some important questions, like is this plan realistic, or how might someone who doesn't live in this neighborhood understand what it is like here." Several staff members expressed that they wanted this intervention to be productive for the students, and that providing handouts may not feel relevant to the students. Interestingly, no one explicitly questioned our credibility. After raising our outsider status as a potential barrier to the intervention again, one staff member stated, "I don't want to offend anyone, but it's hard to know if what you suggest would actually be what we need here." Another staff member stated, "I think this is a little hard to talk about, but yes, there is a difference in where we come from." I responded, "Thank you for telling us how you feel. I think that this conversation is really important for us to actually be productive and plan a discussion that will help the kids." My colleague joined me in thanking the group for sharing their thoughts.

Later in the discussion, I revealed to the group that I too had experienced feeling alienated and disempowered in predominantly White institutions, and by people who were not familiar with my Indian ethnicity. Several staff members expressed that they appreciated hearing about my experience and that they had indeed assumed that I would not be able to relate to their context because of my privileged status as a professional. Further, they talked about their interactions with some Indian people whom they experienced as "acting more White than people of color." I responded by sharing that race indeed held an ambivalent position with many Asian Indians and with immigrants more broadly, and that I sometimes feel like I'm searching for a place of belonging and identity since race is often seen along Black-White lines in the U.S.

These moments in the meeting marked an important shift in how my colleague and I connected with the staff. Everyone in the room seemed more relaxed with each other, as though we had all felt a bit safer with each other. I came to realize that not only was this discussion critical for creating a general feeling of safety in the room, but also for moving toward a conversation about exposure to violence in the community, an experience shared by the students and staff. In the last two meetings, the staff began sharing some of their own experiences of witnessing and being victimized by community violence. They talked about how they often felt isolated with few resources to access the help that they need. It became clear that the staff's ability to connect with the students' experiences with community violence would be an important part of the after-school intervention. We talked in depth about how the staff could potentially talk about some of their own experiences early on in the intervention (e.g. discussion groups with students) as a way of helping to validate the students' experiences and to collaborate with the students to develop strategies that are culturally and contextually grounded. The staff and students worked together to develop ways of coping with physical and emotional stress related to violence exposure. We decided to continue meeting once every other week over the next several months to discuss the progress of the after-school intervention and to collaborate on brainstorming any potential conflicts or problems that would arise in the program. The staff expressed several times that they appreciated the guidance with attending to the affective and interpersonal processes in our group meetings and in the meetings with the students.

Revisiting psychoanalytic applications and diversity

The case examples that I have presented reflect ways in which psychoanalysis is relevant across treatment and consultation settings, and how community psychology and multicultural psychology can be integrated to better address sociocultural context with individuals and communities. Since its inception, psychoanalytic theory has been rooted in observations from the clinical encounter. In reflecting on the case examples, it is worth considering how psychoanalytic, community, and multicultural frameworks shaped the interventions, and the questions that racial and cultural dynamics in the different practice settings raise for psychoanalytic theory.

In the psychoanalytic perspective, the practitioner/consultant helps to foster emotional insight, and the uncovering of conscious and unconscious feelings and thoughts, which is central to identifying conflict and promoting change. McWilliams (2003) noted that uncovering feelings can allow for experience to be organized, giving "form to chaos" (p. 251). In my work with Reena and with the after-school program staff, attending to affective experiences was necessary for self-understanding. The difficult interactions in which my client (e.g. Reena, after-school staff) and I were able to talk about our emotional reactions to events both inside and outside the therapy/consultation setting helped to create a real sense of safety. I understood these exchanges as the basis for our collaboration. This collaboration established itself through an examination of the intersubjective space in which affect and enactment were mutually influenced by the client, me, and both of our social contexts (Liang, Tummala-Narra, & West, 2011). This is evident, for example, when Reena wondered if my spouse is Indian, reflecting both her transference toward me as an Indian woman who does what an Indian woman is supposed to do (e.g. marry an Indian man), and her wish to be seen by me as someone who can make choices that diverge from this idealized conception of Indian women, and still remain emotionally connected to me and her Indian heritage.

Psychoanalytic theory emphasizes the therapist's ability to bear witness to the client's past and present life experiences and to hold the client's perspective even when it may sharply contrast with that of the therapist. Psychoanalytic practitioners are well aware of the intrapsychic and interpersonal effects of trauma. Through interpretation of transference and education about the problematic nature of trauma, the therapist attempts to differentiate himself/herself from the perpetrator (McWilliams, 2003). The ability to tolerate and engage with multiple subjectivities in the case of traumatic exposure was clearly important in the after-school intervention. For example, it was important that I understood the staff's ambivalence about engaging with mental health professionals from a predominantly White institution as reflective of previous experiences of trauma, both violence in the community and racial trauma directed against African Americans and other ethnic minorities (e.g. Latino/a American). In honoring the reality and significance of these traumatic experiences, I needed to simultaneously recognize my personal experiences of racial trauma as an Indian American, my feelings of sadness about the staff's and students' experiences of racial trauma, and our shared feelings of "otherness." This attempt to examine multiple subjectivities was critical for addressing the insider-outsider dynamic that characterized the group dynamic throughout our meetings.

In bridging a psychoanalytic perspective with community psychology and multicultural psychology, it is worth noting some areas of common ground across these frameworks. All three perspectives value the enormous challenges posed to individuals in the face of loss and injustice. The validation of the individual's distress under circumstances of trauma and cruelty is an important aspect of all of these frameworks. Community psychology and multicultural psychology, however, attend to larger systemic problems, such as racism and poverty, as sources of emotional distress, and emphasize the role of resilience as a contextually determined phenomenon (Liang, Tummala-Narra, & West, 2011). Psychoanalytic theory, which has historically decontextualized individual psychological distress, has the potential to more closely examine the interaction between systemic, interpersonal, and individual sources of distress and resilience. Specifically, the psychoanalytic emphasis on unconscious processes facilitates a more in-depth understanding of individual and collective meanings of experience. For example, a multicultural psychology perspective allowed for closer attention to the effects of racism on Reena's experiences as an Indian

American, and a psychoanalytic perspective was essential to discovering the unique meanings that Reena's experiences of racism held for her sense of self, her relationships with others, and for the therapeutic alliance. A community psychology perspective was instrumental in helping me to develop a frame for the consultation in the after-school program through its questioning of power, privilege, and expert knowledge which indeed belonged to the staff and students in the program. A multicultural perspective helped me with understanding the importance of social location (e.g. race, immigration) in developing a collaborative intervention. Further, a psychoanalytic perspective allowed for an examination of how best to address the fears and hopes that lay beneath the dynamics of race, power, and privilege for both the staff and the consultants.

Another area of emphasis shared by these three perspectives concerns the issue of self-examination. Over the past decade, community psychologists and multicultural psychologists have described the importance of examining one's values, biases, and social location in the context of community collaboration and psychotherapy, respectively (Goodman, Liang, Helms, Latta, Sparks, & Weintraub, 2004; Liang, Tummala-Narra, & West, 2011). Psychoanalytic scholars have increasingly attended to the influence and use of countertransference and intersubjectivity on the therapeutic relationship (Altman, 2010). The role of self-examination was salient in both case examples. For instance, recognizing my wish to belong and be accepted in my relationships with both Reena and the after-school staff was an important step in understanding power differentials in the treatment/consultation relationship and for creating an interpersonal space where authentic discussions about race and ethnicity were possible.

Bearing in mind the potential of bridging psychoanalytic, community, and multicultural perspectives, it is worth considering some implications of such integration on the identity of psychoanalytic practitioners who work across clinical and community settings. Different theoretical perspectives have privileged certain contexts of individual and social change. For example, community psychology has argued against individual psychotherapy in promoting social change (Albee, 1990), and psychoanalysis has tended to dismiss community-level interventions as superficial or incapable of fostering deep internal change (Kaufmann, 2003; King & Shelley, 2008). Multicultural psychology has historically denounced the use of traditional, especially classical psychoanalytic theory, as this perspective has not integrated an understanding of sociocultural context (Sue, 2001). However, in recent years, practitioners and consultants who work across diverse contexts (e.g. clinical, community) and with clients of diverse racial and cultural backgrounds have increasingly recognized the need to revisit these theoretical assumptions (Altman, 2010; Comas-Diaz, 2006; Leary, 2012; Liang, Tummala-Narra, & West, 2011).

The re-consideration of psychoanalytic theory and practice is important for several reasons, including the ability and competence of practitioners and consultants to provide treatment and consultation that fosters meaningful change to individuals and communities who face social marginalization and lack of access to adequate resources. It is worth noting that the valuing of social justice has always been an inherent part of psychoanalytic history, and yet, social justice has largely remained disconnected from a more complete integration of social context in psychoanalytic practice, research, and training. Attending to diversity as psychoanalytic practitioners, researchers, and educators would potentially mean that we raise new questions and redefine our roles. In particular, we can examine how knowledge about specific racial and cultural contexts can inform both conceptualization and technique, in an effort to move beyond only applying existing psychoanalytic concepts to different practice settings and communities. Psychoanalytic technique, such as the use of interpretation, can be modified based on a deeper knowledge of both sociocultural context and the individual's conscious and unconscious identifications with this context. Psychoanalysis can further integrate knowledge of the impact of racial trauma on the individual's and community's day-to-day life, which shapes the psyche. We can examine how our practice, research, and teaching either influence or neglect socially marginalized communities. For example, what part do we play in the "social mirroring" (Suarez-Orozco, 2000) of individuals and communities? Do we explore the potential meanings of our social location in our interactions with clients in psychotherapy? How do we address "microaggressions" (Pierce, 1995; Sue et al., 2007) directed against our clients and those directed against us? How is psychoanalytic practice experienced differently by minority therapists and clients when compared with majority therapists and clients? What role do we as therapists/analysts play in perpetuating institutional discrimination directed against marginalized communities? How might we consciously or unconsciously either encourage or discourage minority individuals and communities to seek help from us?

These questions require a broadening of psychoanalytic theory and technique such that there is a more active exploration of interaction between sociocultural contexts, communities, and individuals. As such, this is time of great opportunity for psychoanalytic theorists and researchers to expand both the theory and applications of psychoanalysis. Eisold (2003) proposed that psychoanalysis move away from a point of isolation and collaborate with other disciplines in order to expand its relevance to broader society. As pluralism within psychoanalytic theory has produced both tensions and creativity in practice, an integration of frameworks that emphasize social context can help to deepen psychoanalytic approaches to diversity. Psychoanalytic practitioners, researchers, and educators would have to further consider changes within institutions, such as acceptance of multiple theoretical perspectives and a commitment to developing relationships with individuals and communities (e.g. minority populations) that do not typically look to psychoanalytic practitioners, researchers, and educators for help. We would have to listen intently to indigenous conceptualizations of health and pathology that contrast with conceptualizations based on our personal life experience or traditional psychoanalytic training. Researchers would approach psychoanalytic concepts such as attachment and object relations from culturally relevant perspectives, rather than solely rely on Western, Euro-American developmental perspectives.

Such an effort would further involve modifications to training, including broadening skills both within and outside of the psychotherapy setting and educating communities and institutions (service and training) about the benefits of psychoanalytic applications within their contexts. In fact, curricula have been proposed for training as a community psychoanalyst (Twemlow & Parens, 2006). However, training curricula that specifically focus on racial and cultural diversity and psychoanalytic theory and technique have yet to be developed and implemented. Furthermore, the experiences of minority trainees and therapists in psychoanalytically oriented graduate programs or institutes are rarely discussed in the psychoanalytic literature, contributing to the problem of isolation for these individuals and communities. Unfortunately, the experiences of minority trainees, in particular, may be additionally influenced by the "authoritative culture of psychoanalytic education" (Lhulier, 2005, p. 468). It would indeed be helpful for psychoanalytic educators to learn more about the experiences of minority trainees and therapists and utilize this knowledge to modify theory, practice, and education. These changes require a closer look at systemic issues within the psychoanalytic profession, through increased dialogue both within and outside of psychoanalytic circles.

Concluding comments

I chose to present case examples from two distinct contexts as a way to illustrate the potential breadth of psychoanalytic applications and to consider how practice across contexts can inform psychoanalytic understandings of racial and cultural diversity. In both examples, the mutual impact of the therapist and client, and the consultant and the community shapes the experience of the healing relationship and raises questions about how we construct theory from real-world interactions with clients. Our clients' sociocultural histories and their ongoing negotiation of social and political aspects of their identity in contemporary society lie at the root of psychoanalytic theory development. The therapist's/consultant's negotiation of these issues in his/her life is also critical to this process of understanding. The examination of multiple subjectivities and narratives drives a psychoanalysis that attends to social and cultural specifics. It is my hope that psychoanalysis moves in the direction of conceptualizing the specifics of diversity and diverse contexts as essential components that shape the psyche, rather than dismiss these specifics as sociological artifacts. I hope that we can consider imagining ourselves as agents of social change in a broader sense than what we have collectively done in past decades and expand discourse on how psychoanalytic practitioners, consultants, researchers, and educators can integrate multiple perspectives in better attending to the needs of minority individuals and communities. I believe that the future of diversity studies depends on psychoanalysis, and perhaps the future of psychoanalysis depends on better attending to diverse contexts.

References

Ainslie, R.C. (2009). Social class and its reproduction in immigrants' construction of self. *Psychoanalysis, Culture & Society. Special Issue: Immigration, 14(3),* 213–224.

Akhtar, S. (1999). *Immigration and identity: Turmoil, treatment, and transformation.* Northvale, NJ: Jason Aronson.

Akhtar, S. (2011). *Immigration and acculturation: Mourning, adaptation, and the next generation.* Lanham, MD: Jason Aronson.

Akhtar, S., & Tummala-Narra, P. (2005). Psychoanalysis in India. In S. Akhtar (Ed.), *Freud along the Ganges* (pp. 3–28). New York: Other Press.

Albee, G.W. (1990). The futility of psychotherapy. *The Journal of Mind and Behavior, 11*, 369–384.

Altman, N. (2010). *The analyst in the inner city*, 2nd ed. New York: Routledge.

Aron, L. (2004). God's influence on my psychoanalytic vision and values. *Psychoanalytic Psychology, 21(3)*, 442–451.

Bodnar, S. (2004). Remember where you come from: Dissociative process in multicultural individuals. *Psychoanalytic Dialogues, 14*, 581–603.

Bonovitz, C. (2005). Locating culture in the psychic field: Transference and countertransference as cultural products. *Contemporary Psychoanalysis, 41*, 55–76.

Borg, M.B. (2004). Venturing beyond the consulting room: Psychoanalysis in community crisis intervention. *Contemporary Psychoanalysis, 40*, 147–174.

Comas-Diaz, L. (2006). Latino healing: The integration of ethnic psychology into psychotherapy. *Psychotherapy: Theory, Research, Practice, Training, 43,* 436–453.

Danto, E.A. (2005). *Freud's free clinics: Psychoanalysis and social justice, 1918–1938.* New York: Columbia University Press.

Darwin, J.L., & Reich, K.I. (2006). Reaching out to the families of those who serve: The SOFAR project. *Professional Psychology: Research and Practice, 37(5),* 481–484.

Drescher, J. (2007). Homosexuality and its vicissitudes. In J.C. Muran (Ed.), *Dialogues on difference: Studies of diversity in the therapeutic relationship* (pp. 85–97). Washington, DC: American Psychological Association.

Eisold, K. (2003). The profession of psychoanalysis: Past failures and future possibilities. *Contemporary Psychoanalysis, 39*, 557–582.

Eng, D., & Han, S. (2000). A dialogue on racial melancholia. *Psychoanalytic Dialogues, 10,* 667–700.

Flores, J. (2007). Social conflict and subjectivity: The analyst's involvement. *International Forum of Psychoanalysis, 16,* 254–258.

Foster, R.P. (2003). Considering a multicultural perspective for psychoanalysis. In A. Roland, B. Ulanov, & C. Barbre (Eds.), *Creative dissent: Psychoanalysis in evolution* (pp. 173–185). Westport, CT: Praeger Publishers.

Freud, S. (1910). 'Wild' Psycho-Analysis. *The Standard Edition of the Complete Psychological Works of Sigmund Freud, Volume XI (1910): Five Lectures on Psycho-Analysis, Leonardo da Vinci and Other Works*, pp. 219–228.

Goodman, L.A., Liang, B., Helms, J.E., Latta, R.E., Sparks, E., & Weintraub, S. (2004). Major contribution: Training counseling psychologists as social justice agents: Feminist and multicultural theories in action. *The Counseling Psychologist, 32,* 793–837.

Granatir, W.L. (2004). A retired psychoanalyst volunteers to promote school-based mental health. In B. Sklarew, S.W. Twemlow, & S.M. Wilkinson (Eds.), *Analysts in the trenches: Streets, schools, war zones* (pp. 137–167). Hillsdale, NJ: Analytic Press.

Greene, B. (2007). How difference makes a difference. In J.C. Muran (Ed.), *Dialogues on difference: Studies of diversity in the therapeutic relationship* (pp. 47–63). Washington, DC: American Psychological Association.

Kaufmann, W. (2003). *Freud, Adler, and Jung: Discovering the mind* (Vol. 3). London: Transaction Publishers.

King, R.A., & Shelley, C.A. (2008). Community feeling and social interest: Adlerian parallels, synergy and differences with the field of community psychology. *Journal of Community and Applied Social Psychology, 18,* 96–107.

Leary, K. (2006). In the eye of the storm. *The Psychoanalytic Quarterly, 75(1),* 345–363.

Leary, K. (2012). Race as an adaptive challenge: Working with diversity in the clinical consulting room. *Psychoanalytic Psychology, 29(3),* 271–291.

Lhulier, J. (2005). Learning in an increasingly multitheoretical psychoanalytic culture: Impact on the development of analytic identity. *Psychoanalytic Psychology, 22(4),* 459–472.

Liang, B., Tummala-Narra, P., & West, J. (2011). Revisiting community work from a psychodynamic perspective. *Professional Psychology: Research and Practice, 42(5),* 398–404.

McWilliams, N. (2003). The educative aspects of psychoanalysis. *Psychoanalytic Psychology, 20(2),* 245–260.

Miller, I.S. (2008). Brief communication preparation for psychodynamic consultation following community trauma: Learning from the "Firehouse Project." *International Journal of Applied Psychoanalytic Studies, 5(1),* 68–79.

Mitchell, S.A. (1988). *Relational concepts in psychoanalysis: An integration.* Cambridge, MA: Harvard University Press.

Pierce, C. (1995). Stress analogs of racism and sexism: Terrorism, torture, and disaster. In C. Willie, P. Rieker, B. Kramer, & B. Brown (Eds.), *Mental health, racism, and sexism* (pp. 277–293). Pittsburgh: University of Pittsburgh Press.

Roland, A. (2005). Between civilizations: Psychoanalytic therapy with Asian North Americans. *Counselling Psychology Quarterly, 18*(4), 287–293. doi:10.1080/09515070500469830.

Shedler, J. (2010). The efficacy of psychodynamic psychotherapy. *American Psychologist, 65(2),* 98–109.

Smith, H.F. (2006). Invisible racism. *The Psychoanalytic Quarterly, 75(1),* 3–19.

Stolorow, R.D. (1988). Transference and the therapeutic process. *Psychoanalytic Review, 75(2),* 245–254.

Suarez-Orozco, C. (2000). Identities under siege: Immigration stress and social mirroring among the children of immigrants. In A.C.G.M. Robben & M.M. Suarez-Orozco (Eds.), *Cultures under siege: Collective violence and trauma* (pp. 194–226). New York: Cambridge University Press.

Suchet, M. (2011). Crossing over. *Psychoanalytic Dialogues, 21(2),* 172–191.

Sue, D.W. (2001). Multidimensional facets of cultural competence. *The Counseling Psychologist, 29(6),* 790–821.

Sue, D.W., Bucceri, J., Lin, A.I., Nadal, K.L., & Torino, G.C. (2007). Racial microaggressionsand the Asian American experience. *Cultural Diversity and Ethnic Minority Psychology, 13(1)*, 72–81.
Tang, N.M., & Smith, B.L. (1996). The eternal triangle across cultures: Oedipus, Hsueh, and Ganesa. *Psychoanalytic Study of the Child, 51,* 562–579.
Tummala-Narra, P. (2007). Skin color and the therapeutic relationship. *Psychoanalytic Psychology, 24(2),* 255–270.
Tummala-Narra, P. (2009a). The immigrant's real and imagined return home. *Psychoanalysis, Culture & Society. Special Issue: Immigration, 14(3),* 237–252.
Tummala-Narra, P. (2009b). The relevance of a psychoanalytic perspective in exploring religious and spiritual identity in psychotherapy. *Psychoanalytic Psychology, 26(1),* 83–95.
Tummala-Narra, P., Inman, A.G., & Ettigi, S. (2011). Asian Indians' Responses to Discrimination: A mixed-method examination of identity, coping, and self-esteem. *Asian American Journal of Psychology, 2(3),* 205–218.
Twemlow, S.W., & Parens, H. (2006). Might Freud's legacy lie beyond the couch? *Psychoanalytic Psychology, 23(2),* 430–451.
Twemlow, S.W., Fonagy, P., Sacco, F.C., Vernberg, E., & Malcolm, J.M. (2011). Reducing violence and prejudice in a Jamaican all age school using attachment and mentalization theory. *Psychoanalytic Psychology, 28(4),*497–511.
Vasquez, M.J.T. (2007). Cultural difference and the therapeutic alliance: An evidence-based analysis. *American Psychologist, 62(8),* 878–885.
Volkan, V.D. (2001). Psychoanalysis and diplomacy: Potentials for and obstacles against collaboration. In D.E. Scharff (Ed.), *The psychoanalytic century: Freud's legacy for the future* (pp. 279–295). New York: Other Press.
Yi, K.Y. (1998). Transference and race: An intersubjective conceptualization. *Psychoanalytic Psychology, 15(2)*, 245–261.

14

The rights of children

Erika Schmidt

The United Nations Convention on the Rights of the Child, a human rights treaty set forth in 1989, contains

> a profound idea: that children are not just objects who belong to their parents and for whom decisions are made, or adults in training. Rather, they are human beings and individuals with their own rights... [Childhood] is a special, protected time, in which children must be allowed to grow, learn, play, develop and flourish with dignity. ("What is the Convention on the Rights of the Child," 2020).

The guiding principles of the Convention include

> non-discrimination; the best interests of the child as a primary consideration in all actions concerning children; the child's inherent right to life... and survival and development; and the child's right to express views freely in all matters affecting the child. ("Frequently Asked Questions on the Convention on the Rights of the Child," 2020)

In its 54 articles, the Convention protects the rights of children; affirms rights to care, developmental support, mental health services and fair processes when families cannot provide for a child; and prohibits abusive actions against vulnerable children.[1] These rights are summarized as the three Ps as they fall into three categories: provision, protection and participation.[2]

Clearly, the Convention is an aspirational document. The tagline reads, "for every child, every right." In the 30 plus years since its enactment, significant improvements have been achieved across the globe.[3] For example, child mortality has decreased significantly, as have the rates of child marriage. A primary school education is more widely available to all, and girls have improved access to schooling. Yet, children who live in poverty remain acutely vulnerable, and are especially so in the face of global pressures such as climate change that impact all children's futures. When examining the treaty, one easily recognizes the impossibility of finding the financial, logistical and resource commitments

DOI: 10.4324/9781003325512-18

necessary to meet the foundational rights outlined in it. Add to this the systemic problems that anchor poverty, racism, unequal access to health care and all forms of social injustice.

Looking deeply, looking psychoanalytically, we can also observe the universal embedded ambivalence elders have toward children that makes it complicated to achieve, or even adopt, the ideals inscribed in the Convention. If all relationships contain ambivalence, the challenge is for the positive attitudes to outweigh the negative and for the adults responsible for children to be able to promote the forward development of children in their care. Children's dependence on parents and caregivers does not obviate their status, as the Convention states, as people in their own right. How is this basic human right enacted within the family, or by the State if the family is deemed unable to provide for the children? And how is it enacted in the implementation of social policy, including the crucial social issue of access to mental health care? On the social level, ambivalence toward children makes for tragic headlines of the immigration crisis and for the quieter but critical problems in providing quality schooling. And on the psychological level, this ambivalence often manifests as a failure to provide adequate interventions, including those intensive therapies of depth, insight and relationship that can remediate the underlying emotional problems children suffer when the ambivalence toward them causes depression or anxiety and the multiple symptoms and behaviors that reflect these root problems.

In this chapter, I will explore the love and the hate of children that allow us at once to mythologize childhood and at the same time to obstruct responses to their legitimate developmental needs. As psychotherapists committed to treatments of depth, insight and relationship, we see this obstruction and its effects upon the individual lives of many of the children who are in therapy or analysis. We also witness it on a social, cultural and global scale where a psychoanalytic perspective can usefully be brought to bear on the phenomenon. I will begin with an exploration of attitudes toward children, including Elisabeth Young-Bruehl's concept of "childism," that is, the prejudice against children, akin to sexism, racism, classism or ageism, that is built into the social fabric. Then I will turn to two areas in which we can vividly see how these prejudices operate and their impact on the lives of children as well as the impact on our social surround. Using Valeria Luiselli's (2019) remarkable book, *Lost Children Archive*, along with recent events and current headlines, I will look at the way immigration has too often become a tragedy for children and their families, supported by social policy. Then I will look at education, using the example of what happened in an urban neighborhood when schools were closed for political purposes as described in the poet-sociologist Eve Ewing's book *Ghosts in the Schoolyard*. Writing this chapter in the midst of the pandemic further highlights the challenges of finding the love that outweighs the inevitable hate toward children. Framing this discussion with the powerful statements about the rights of children in the Convention allows us to keep our ideals in mind as we advocate on behalf of children.

About childism

> Article 2.1. States Parties shall respect and ensure the rights set forth in the present Convention to each child within their jurisdiction without discrimination of any kind, irrespective of the child's or his or her parent's or legal guardian's race, colour, sex, language, religion, political or other opinion, national, ethnic or social origin, property, disability, birth or other status. ("Convention on the Rights of the Child," 2020)

The Convention on the Rights of the Child has been ratified by all member states of the United Nations, save one: the United States. The United States has signed but has not ratified this treaty because no president, including Barack Obama, who campaigned with a promise to do so, has been willing to bring it to Congress. The political cost is apparently too high, given conservative opposition based on the primacy of the authority of the family and religion. In her book, *Childism: Confronting Prejudice against Children*, Elisabeth Young-Bruehl traces the social trends and the anti-child politics and policies that have dominated the United States since the 1970s. The failure to ratify the Convention is one symptom of the childism that Young-Bruehl discusses in her book.

Aligning childism with other prejudices against target groups that are defined by shared characteristics, Young-Bruehl describes the system of thoughts and assumptions that rationalize harm to children and the failure to meet their basic needs. She argues that childism relies on an underlying set of beliefs about children as "immature beings produced and owned by adults who use /them/ to serve their own needs and fantasies...[this] reverses the biological and psychological order of nature in which adults are responsible for meeting the irreducible needs of children" (Young-Bruehl, 2012, p. 36). Note the contrast with the assumption of the Convention that children are individuals with human rights that come as a birthright.

It is important to recognize that ambivalence toward children, which captures feelings of both love and hate, is part of all human experience. Winnicott (1949) suggests that it originates in the hate the mother feels at times toward the infant at a time when the infant cannot yet experience their own hate. He lists a number of reasons for maternal hate. Among others:

> He [the baby] is suspicious, refuses her good food, and makes her doubt herself, but eats well with his aunt. After an awful morning with him, she goes out and he smiles at a stranger, who says: 'Isn't he sweet?' If she fails him at the start she knows he will pay her out for ever. (ibid, p. 74)

In Winnicott's schema, the baby's psychological move from part object to whole object status means that the hate he could only evoke in the mother now can be integrated into the self. This is a complex, ongoing process as children internalize and identify with the significant people in their lives and live amidst the unconscious currents and family secrets that they must sort out. In the course of development, successful integration means that hate will be tempered by love.

The forms that childism takes on a societal level express collective distortions or failures of the integration of hate with love. Without using the concept of childism explicitly, Rosenblitt (2009), in a short, powerful article, highlights the hate of adults for children, which he knows well as a child analyst. Here he explores the way "our ambivalent social policies simply mirror our collective ambivalent inner attitudes" (p. 214). Rosenblitt documents how these inner attitudes find expression in fables and operas, which have a timeless quality, illustrating the persistence and universality of attitudes that are then enacted through social policies or practices. For example, Young-Bruehl cites the rates of incarceration of children and adolescents as an example, as if incarceration could possibly address the problems evidenced by a young person's delinquent misbehavior. In another example, Rosenblitt cites the pharmacological and insurance industries' promotion of medication for children which benefits the industries' bottom line and leads to the gross over-medication of children, often enough with one or more antipsychotic drugs (p. 203). Such social practices as the incarceration of youth and the indiscriminate use of medication for children can be understood through a psychoanalytic lens as the way the unconscious attitudes of adults toward children play out through the use and misuse of findings from the science of child development that are then expressed in national policies, whether conservative, progressive, regressive or liberal. Young-Bruehl provides a good example of this in her extensive case study of the "discovery" of child abuse and neglect and how acutely personal and interpersonal attacks on vulnerable children become national policy and then play out in the sociocultural realm.

Lost children

> Article 22.1. States Parties shall take appropriate measures to ensure that a child who is seeking refugee status or who is considered a refugee...shall, whether accompanied by his or her parents...receive appropriate protection and humanitarian assistance in the enjoyment of applicable rights set forth in the present Convention. ("Convention on the Rights of the Child," 2020)

Do all children have the right to a childhood? Just asking the question points to the obvious answer. This is the question that Parul Sehgal (2019) provocatively asks in her incisive review of Valeria Luiselli's 2019 novel, *Lost Children Archive*. The heartbreaking answer to this question is, "Not every child," as is so horrifyingly evident in recent newspaper headlines of children separated from their parents after crossing the border into the United States seeking refuge. Luiselli tells the story of a road trip undertaken by a blended family coming apart, while simultaneously children desperate to reunite with their families undertake journeys to a treacherous border where the lucky ones are detained and the unlucky ones die trying to get there. The family in the book—Mama, Papa, the boy and the girl—travel to the southwest, each parent on a mission. Papa, a sound documentarian, is headed to Apacheria, the land of Geronimo and the Apaches, hoping to record the echoes of their lives. The story of Native Americans, deported through the Indian Removal Act, converges with the story of families from Central America who are frequently deported from the place they hope will provide refuge and a home. Mama, the narrator, is searching for the two daughters of a friend who are traveling from Guatemala to try to reach their mother. Mama muses how they have come to refer to these girls as "lost children" rather than refugees. "And in a way, I guess, they are lost children. They have lost the right to a childhood" (p. 75).

The narrator's goal is to give voice to these children even as she questions her right to do so and also wonders whether this effort can accomplish anything. As the family travels southwest, their trip is intertwined with the tale of the Central American "lost" children traveling north on the roof of a train they call La Bestia, with its resonances of the Orphan Train movement of the late 1800s to the early 1900s which is also referenced in the book. The narrator ponders her own children's experience, wondering how they take in their parents' pre-occupation with the stories of the lost children and the stories of the Apaches who lost their homeland. What the boy and the girl do is to create their fantasy of being lost children themselves which they play out in the back seat of the car. In this game, they enact the primal fear of losing the needed and beloved parent, as they know the two daughters of their mother's friend had lost their mother. As Freud (1920) theorized from watching his grandson play the fort da game, children use play in an effort to master their anxieties.

As the trip progresses and the boy becomes aware of just how frayed the family bonds have become, he devises a secret plan that he hopes will reengage his parents and prompt them to repair their marriage. He and the girl set out on their own to search for the two lost daughters, thus becoming lost children themselves, and, whether they find the two daughters or not, they will walk to Echo Canyon, the mystical place their father has told them about where the echoes of the Apaches who lost their home can be heard. He predicts their mother will search for them instead of her friend's daughters and their father will listen to them instead of to the echoes of the Apaches. "And here's the most important part," he says to himself, "if we too were lost children, we would have to be found again. Ma and Pa would have to find us" (Luiselli, 2019, p. 238). Here the private psychological drama of the boy and the girl parallels the international immigration drama and the family crisis of the two daughters. The boy adds, "They would find us, I knew that" (ibid, p. 238). Only a child who unconsciously knows he has a right to a childhood could set out on a journey like this with the confidence of being found.

The imaginative journey of *Lost Children Archive* is based on Luiselli's experience as a volunteer translator for children in immigration court in New York which she describes in her 2017 book *Tell Me How It Ends: An Essay in Forty Questions*. It was her task to go through the questionnaire with these children as a first step in obtaining legal representation for them. She recognizes that "few narratives have made the effort to turn things around and understand the [immigration] crisis from the point of view of the children involved" (Luiselli, 2017, p. 44). The consequence of this is a dehumanization of the children. Among the questions she must ask the children are: "Do you feel safe? Are you happy here?" Luiselli points to the absurdity of such questions for children who have fled their homes because of poverty or threats of violence, murder and sexual assault. "In the media and much of the official political discourse, the word 'illegal' prevails over 'undocumented' and the term 'immigrant' over 'refugee.' How would anyone who is stigmatized as an 'illegal immigrant' feel 'safe' and 'happy'?" (ibid, p. 44).

The situation only worsened under the Trump administration with policies that rationalized the separation of children from their parents at the border, treatment so egregious that the head of the American Academy of Pediatrics called it "government-sanctioned child abuse" and the head of Physicians for Human Rights referred to it as "torture" (Szalai, 2020). Public and professional protests forced officials to change this policy, but not before much damage to family ties and mental health was perpetrated on children. And even when forced to end such brutal treatment, it went on. In the fall of 2020, a court case revealed that the US government could not locate the parents of 545 of the children who had been separated at the border because of poor record-keeping, surely a sign of the failure to value the lives of these children and with utter disregard of the meaning of the profound disruption of their emotional bonds. Then news reports revealed that children from Central America were being sent to Mexico, where they know no one, furthering the severing from their families, on the pretext of protecting the United States from the coronavirus. In November, 2020, a court ruling stopped the government from turning children away without an opportunity to apply for asylum (Kanno-Youngs, 2020). Article 21 of the Convention states that children considered refugees, whether accompanied or unaccompanied, are entitled to "appropriate protection and humanitarian assistance" (Convention on the Rights of the Child, 2020).

Education in the life of a child

Article 28.1. States Parties recognize the right of the child to education.

Article 29.1. States Parties agree that the education of the child shall be directed to: (a) the development of the child's personality, talents and mental and physical abilities to their fullest potential; (b) the development of respect for human rights and fundamental freedoms…; (c) the development of respect for the child's parents, his or her own cultural identity, language and values, for the national values of the country in which the child is living, the country from which he or she may originate, and for civilizations

> different from his or her own; (d) the preparation of the child for responsible life in a free society, in the spirit of understanding, peace, tolerance, equality of sexes, and friendship among all peoples, ethnic, national and religious groups and persons of indigenous origin; (e) the development of respect for the natural environment. ("Convention on the Rights of the Child," 2020)

In early spring of 2013, the CEO of the Chicago Public Schools, Barbara Byrd-Bennett decided that the way to solve the budgetary pressures on the school system was to close many public schools, at first a list of over 200, eventually pared down to 53. In May the School Board, all appointed by Mayor Rahm Emanuel, voted to close 49 of these public schools, the most schools ever closed in one fell swoop in the United States (Van Roekel 2013). In fact, school closings have taken place frequently in Chicago and elsewhere as a matter of policy, just not so many at once. The language used by CPS and the media referred to these schools as "underutilized," "under-resourced," "poorly performing" and "failing." CPS promised that the students from closed schools would attend "welcoming" schools that had higher test scores and more "resources" and, to combat fears that children would have to cross gang boundaries to get to their new schools, "safe passage" routes for protection. In her statement to the School Board, Byrd-Bennett declared: "For too long, children in certain parts of our city have been cheated out of the resources they need to succeed in the classroom because they are trapped in underutilized schools. These underutilized schools are also under-resourced" (quoted in Ewing p 55). She went on to emphatically deny that racism played any part in the decision of which schools to close.

In 2011, when Emanuel became mayor, 404,000 students were enrolled in the Chicago public schools. Of these, 42% were Black, 44% were Latino and 9% were white (Karp 2019). Of the 49 schools to be closed, 90% had a majority of Black students, 88% of the students in these schools were Black and 71% of the schools had primarily Black teachers. Students in these schools are some of the most vulnerable in the city in that more were from low-income families, more moved homes frequently, more had repeated a grade and more received special education services (Ewing, 2018b). While CPS argued that enrollment figures, poor outcomes on standardized testing and inefficient use of resources necessitated this drastic step, critics challenged this assessment. They cited the move toward privatization of schooling through reliance on charter schools, essentially to advance a neoliberal agenda. They also identified racism as a motive, insidious, systemic racism that disregarded the voices in the community, students as well as parents, and that led to the so-called under-resourcing and underutilization in the first place (see, for example, Ewing, 2018a; Kristof, 2020; Lipman, 2011; Winslow 2013). On the policy level, CPS justified its actions through fudging the numbers (of student enrollment, class size, budget projections) which opened opportunities for charter schools and activated an expression of systemic racism by virtue of the schools and students affected by this decision. The communities where these schools were located responded with days and days of organized protests and demonstrations.

"Why do people care so much about schools that the world has deemed to be 'failing'? If these institutions are supposedly so worthless, why do people fight to save them," asks Ewing (2018a, p. 6) in her study of these closures. Answering this question requires attention to the voices within the community, the students, parents and neighbors who live with the schools and to the meaning that community members invest in their schools. The New York Times quoted parents speaking against the closings and contradicting the claims of the school board at a hearing: "These parents and these teachers are not dollar signs...They are people with feelings and lives" and another parent protester who said, "We have what you say my baby needs" (Yaccino, 2013). The 1 billion dollar deficit, underutilization and poor performance provided an official rationale for closing the schools. Yet school closings rarely have the promised outcome of improved educational opportunities (Gordon et al., 2018). A researcher who studies school closings summarizes, "In addition to not improving the educational experience for displaced students, it can actually have a damaging effect. 'We know every time you move a child from one school to another it has a destabilizing effect on their education'" (quoted in Webley, 2013).

So what about the feelings and lives of the parents and teachers and the needs of a child? The outrage, frustration and anger expressed at the hearings and during the many protests demonstrated how strongly parents, teachers and students felt about their schools. As an alderman speaking for residents she represented said, "Closing a school is akin to closing a community" (Ahmed-Ullah et al., 2013). Many speakers referred to the school and its personnel as "family." In a discussion of a later school closing in Chicago, 36 students filed a civil rights complaint alleging racial discrimination. After describing the decimation of school resources they had witnessed as students, they concluded, "This history of neglect impacts us—it sends us the message that the Board does not think we are worthy of investment and that our education is somehow less important than the education of our peers around the city" (quoted in Ewing, 2018a, p. 26). They continue, "The closings are traumatic. Dyett [School] has served as a stable institution in our lives" (quoted in Ewing, 2018a, p. 27). Over and over, community members and school personnel describe the school in terms of the community, its place as a home, its participants as family and, importantly, the school as a source of stability. Ewing quotes a student who spoke at the 2013 closure hearings to protest the closing of his school. "Cause the school is like my home. And the teacher is like my, um, mother. And...the students like my brothers and sisters and my cousins" (Ewing, 2018a, p. 107). She elaborates the powerful meaning of the family metaphor. "It's more than a metaphor, given the importance of fictive kinship in African American social life. In African American social networks fictive kin often share the same rights, status and intensity of relational bonds as biological kin" (Ewing, 2018a,

p. 107). Disrupting the social fabric traumatizes the adults and children involved and does violence to the vitality of the community life they have created.

The Chicago Psychoanalytic Institute began the City Project in 2007 to provide group counseling services to children in south side schools, children who had been exposed to violence (Schmidt, Schloerb & Cohler, 2013). As it happened, when we began working in the first school, CPS announced this school was to be closed in an earlier wave of closings from the one that made the headlines. The principal described her school as a "refuge and safe haven" for her students and wondered how they would react to losing this place of safety. It is perhaps not surprising to note how often schools are described as "safe havens." Five years later, several City Project schools were some of the 49 slated to be closed. When the final decision of the School Board was announced, the students had only weeks to prepare themselves, to grieve the loss and to consider the new reality. This was confounded because there was so little specific information from CPS. Students had many questions that could not be answered, and the uncertainty was felt everywhere. In groups, the students spoke of their attachment to the school, their anxiety about moving to a new school and concerns about what they would encounter, even as they acknowledged the violence that had plagued their school and neighborhood. In an era before cell phones, we planned a photography project, giving each child an instant camera to take pictures around the school and of the people who mattered to them. The photos were put into an album as a keepsake. Their ability to mourn the loss of their school helped with the transition to the new school (Schmidt, 2009). The theme of mourning comes up repeatedly in responses to the school closings.

> What happens after the transition from a closed school to a welcoming school? Lipman and colleagues interviewed parents a year after the closings after their children moved to new schools. They found, "(1) Parents believe school closings had a negative impact on their children, and most believe their new schools are not better; (2) Closed schools had deep meanings for children, parents and communities. Closings were a great loss." (Lipman et al., 2014). The UChicago Consortium on School Research studied the outcome of the school closings and published their report in 2019. They found some negative impact on academic functioning at first, but this was mediated with time and the overall academic impact was basically neutral (p 5), despite improved academic opportunity being a rationale for the closings. One of their key findings highlights the mourning and adaptation process necessitated by the profound disruption. When schools closed, it severed the longstanding social connections that families and staff had with their schools and with one another, resulting in a period of mourning. Those impacted by school closures expressed feelings of grief in multiple ways, often referring to their closed school peers and colleagues as 'like a family'. (p. 4)

Ewing focuses on the mourning of the institution that is more than mourning for the institution itself. She comments on remembering that happens "with love."

> In institutional mourning this doesn't just mean love for a school or for the people in it. It can also mean love for *ourselves* within the school. In losing a school one loses a version of oneself—a self understood to be a member of a community, living and learning in relation to other community members. Without the school to act as a hub, that membership is gone. (Ewing, 2018a, p. 131)

As the experience with school closures vividly demonstrates, social policies enact embedded, often unconscious, beliefs about social status, race, class and opportunity and enforce systemic prejudice.

The Covid-19 pandemic has forced upon us a new form of school closures with all the attendant feelings of loss. Though schools closed for everyone, some children are more vulnerable to its impact than others. Ten months into the pandemic, The New York Times issued a special report on schooling. They concluded that the impact of interrupted school-based education affected some students more than others. Those affected are disproportionately non-white and poor. For many of these students, schools are a safe haven, where they have access to food and other supplies as well as adults who recognize signs of emotional distress and trauma and can intervene in helping ways (Taylor, 2021, pp. 4, 5). The problems are many: children whose parents are essential workers may not have the support they need for remote learning; many families do not have adequate access to the technology and some do not have the privacy necessary for concentration on schoolwork; some children require special services because of their individual circumstances; and so on. A New York Times headline—"Virus Closed Schools, and World's Poorest Children Went to Work" (Gettleman & Raj, 2020)—is a reminder that for these children, the basic right to an education, set forth in the Convention on the Rights of the Child, is not available to these children. As the pandemic has stretched out, concern has arisen about the implications of being deprived of social contact with peers and non-family adults, particularly for younger children. The pandemic also points out the ways in which schools function as institutions far beyond their educational purpose as they offer meals, health care and social connectedness. From the middle of the pandemic and in the midst of a presidential transition, it is impossible to assess the long-term impact on children, their development, their education and their sense of the future. Next to family, schools are the most important institution in the lives of children. The sense of uncertainty and confusion about if, when and how to reopen schools is a public health issue. And yet a New York Times op-ed, written during the summer of 2020, raises questions about our social policy priorities. Bars, restaurants and gyms were allowed to reopen even though public health experts claimed that such sites posed a high risk for transmitting the virus. Safety requirements for reopening schools were not given the same level of concern as these primarily social high-risk gathering spots (Nuzzo & Sharfstein, 2020). How effectively this will be managed under a new administration remains to be seen.

Children as individuals in their own right and the right to mental health care

> Article 27 1. States Parties recognize the right of every child to a standard of living adequate for the child's physical, mental, spiritual, moral and social development. ("Convention on the Rights of the Child," 2020)

Interestingly, the Convention does not single out a right to mental health care, though there are several places where mental health needs are acknowledged secondary to the focus of the Article. For example, Article 17 recognizes the importance of the role of mass media and ensures a child's access to it, especially media that promote "social, spiritual and moral well-being and physical and mental health" (Convention). Article 39 addresses children who are victims of neglect, abuse, torture or other "cruel, inhuman or degrading treatment" and states, "States Parties shall take all appropriate measures to promote physical and psychological recovery and social reintegration" of child victims. But nowhere does the Convention assert the primacy of the rights of children to services that meet their mental health needs. This stands in stark contrast to its upholding of the rights of children to a name and identity, to education, to freedom of expression, to safety from abduction, to physical health and so on. It is a curious omission in a document that upholds the status of children as "individuals in their own right" and it leads back to the issue of ambivalence and hatred toward children. Even in a document as well-intentioned and pro-child as the Convention, these "childist" assumptions that deemphasize the mental health needs of children are implicitly built into the text.

In his now classic paper originally written in 1932, "Confusion of Tongues Between the Adults and the Child," (1949), Ferenczi described the analyst's "professional hypocrisy" of behaving politely toward a patient while harboring countertransference feelings of hatred that remain unspoken yet felt by both. He goes on to describe a similar denial by parents who refuse to recognize or acknowledge, much less talk about, a child's traumatic experiences. Children are inevitably harmed by traumatic experiences which, as Ferenczi points out, can be repaired by a parent's empathic response to the child's subjective distress or later by an analyst's empathic understanding. It is the failure to repair that is most harmful. Where are the resources for repair for children?

Some children may be lucky enough to find resources within their environment. A significant adult who intervenes when children are distressed, like a teacher or coach or pediatrician, often promotes a child's development in addition to providing a "facilitating environment" (Winnicott). Social institutions, especially schools but also programing designed to provide such support, can also be facilitating environments when they offer a child a stable community that represents forward development and the future along with the needed responsiveness that allows for progressive development. These "natural" institutions are profoundly important resources that, when disrupted as in politically motivated school closings or pandemic enforced school closings, can mean the difference between forward movement or not for a child. There are many therapeutic experiences that are not therapy per se. They may not provide the benefits of direct mental health services but for children who cannot access mental health care they can mean the difference between psychological life and death.

But the most important resources for children are mental health services that are specific to a child's psychological difficulties. Mental Health America, which tracks both youth and adult mental health statistics and trends, reports a critical situation for youth. Their report states: "Youth mental health is worsening. 9.7% of youth in the U.S. have severe major depression compared to 9.2% in last year's dataset. This rate was highest among youth who identify as more than one race, at 12.4%." Not surprisingly, the statistics are worse for those most vulnerable because of pre-existing problems but also because of the impact of systemic social injustice. The report goes on to cite the unmet need for treatment: "Even in states with the greatest access [to care], over 38% [of youth with major depression] are not receiving the mental health services they need…only 27.3% received consistent treatment [for severe depression]." The pandemic has only highlighted the mental health needs of children during this time of heightened loss and stress as well as the paucity of accessible resources for needed services. The Center for Disease Control reported a significant increase in the number of emergency room visits for mental health crises increased by 24% for children ages 5–11 and 31% for those between ages 12 and 17 from April to October of 2020 compared to 2019. The increase, the CDC suggests, can be attributed both to the stress of the pandemic which may exacerbate pre-existing conditions and cause pandemic-related mental health concerns as well as the mitigation efforts that mean children could not access the usual resources of clinics, community agencies and schools for where their mental health needs are attended to. One of the 1/24/21 headlines in *The New York Times* reads "Surge of Student Suicides Pushes Las Vegas Schools to Reopen" (Green, 2021). They recorded 18 suicides, twice as many as the previous year. Though suicide is a complex phenomenon to explain, the refrain from those quoted in the article about these deaths is hopelessness, disconnection, lack of control and isolation. For other children, the pandemic-associated restrictions and fear have led to problems such as nightmares and aggressive or withdrawn behavior. For children living in communities where systemic racism, poverty and violence are prevalent, the coronavirus is a trauma upon these other traumas or, as psychologist Alicia Lieberman put it, the virus becomes "one more source of uncontrollable danger" (quoted in Levin).

There are too-powerful currents in the contemporary mental health scope of services for children that over-emphasize the use of medication, that focus on alleviation of observable symptoms, that focus on the management of behavior rather than the meaning of behavior, that substitute technological contact for human contact, that promote corporatized forms of pseudo-therapy via phone or text and that falsely proclaim certain therapies as "evidence-based" and others as "unscientific." While any of these interventions may provide some help for children, often enough they fail to address the underlying issues that give rise to the mental health difficulties that interfere with forward development. Development, we know, occurs in the context of relationships, and effective psychotherapy is a developmental process that takes place in the context of development. The Psychotherapy Action Network advocates for therapies of "depth, insight and relationship," as important for children as for adults. Like immigration policies that enforce separation of children from parents and like school closings that ignore the meaning of the school within the community, the inadequacy of mental health services for children that affirm the Convention's foundation that children are individuals in their own right is another version of childism.

If the pandemic has been an object lesson in the importance of mental health care, we should inscribe the following: a child has a right to a sound developmental trajectory and, if that trajectory is derailed for any reason, a child has a right to mental health services that help them to get back on the rails, to acquire psychological resources and emotional well-being. The pandemic, the killing of people of color and the protests in response, and the political binary landscape underscore the multiple systemic problems within contemporary culture. These cultural attitudes are reflected in the headlines and media stories as events unfold. When examining the immigration crisis, school closures, the failure to provide adequate mental health services and the pandemic-enforced constraints on public life, it is possible to see the way in which attitudes toward children can be marked by ambivalence and childism and then become enshrined in social policies that profoundly affect the individual lives of all children. In a newspaper article about two teenage Balinese sisters who have tackled the trash crisis in their country, one of them is quoted as saying, "Us kids may be only 25% of the world's population, but we are 100% of the future" (Paddock, 2020). Children need support to create their own future and to contribute as citizens to their communities, first in the family and expanding to school, neighborhood and the larger world. We need social policies and social justice that support children, and the resources to support individual children when their mental health needs interfere with development. As we recognize the values set forth in the Convention on the Rights of the Child for provision, protection and participation, we must also work to mitigate the ways in which ambivalence and even hatred toward children–childism–manifest in under-resourcing fully adequate mental health services.

Notes

1 For example, the child has the "inherent right to life" and the "right to a name." It also "ensures that a child shall not be separated from his or her parents against their will except when competent authorities…determine such separation is necessary for the best interests of the child." The parties to the treaty "shall take measures to combat the illicit transfer and non-return of children abroad." For full reading of the treaty, see https://www.unicef.org/child-rights-convention/convention-text.

2 The matter of participation by children, in concert with their age-related evolving abilities, is a civil rights issue that remains controversial in the United States. See Mason (2005) for a discussion of this.

3 The full text of the 30-year progress report is available at https://www.unicef.org/media/62371/file/Convention-rights-child-at-crossroads-2019.pdf.

References

Ahmed-Ullah, N., Chase, J. and Secter, B. (2013). CPS Approves Largest School Closure in Chicago's History. *Chicago Tribune* (11/23/13).

Center for Disease Control. (2020). Mental Health-Related Emergency Department Visits Among Children Aged less than 18 Years During the COVID-19 Pandemic—United States, January 1-October 17, 2020. Retrieved from https://www.cdc.gov/mmwr/volumes/69/wr/mm6945a3.htm

Convention on the Rights of the Child. (2020, November 14). Retrieved from https://www.ohchr.org/en/professionalinterest/pages/crc.aspx

Ewing, E. (2018a). *Ghosts in the Schoolyard: Racism and School Closings on Chicago's South Side*. Chicago: University of Chicago Press.

Ewing, E. (2018b). What Led Chicago to Shutter Dozens of Majority-Black Schools? Racism. The Guardian.org (12/6/18).

https://www.theguardian.com/us-news/2018/dec/06/chicago-public-schools-closures-racism-ghosts-in-the-schoolyard-extract retrieved 11/28/20.

Ferenczi, S. (1949). Confusion of Tongues Between the Adults and the Child—The Language of Tenderness and of Passion. *International Journal of Psychoanalysis* 30: 225–230.

Frequently Asked Questions on the Convention on the Rights of the Child. (2020, October 23). Retrieved from https://www.unicef.org/child-rights-convention/frequently-asked-questions

Freud, S. (1920). *Beyond the Pleasure Principle*, The standard edition of the complete psychological works of Sigmund Freud (Vol. 18, pp. 14–17). London: Hogarth Press.

Gettleman, J. and Raj, S. (2020). Virus Closed Schools, and World's Poorest Children Went to Work. *The New York Times* (9/28/20). https://consortium.uchicago.edu/publications/school-closings-chicago-staff-and-student-experiences-and-academic-outcomes retrieved 11/28/20.

Gordon, M., de la Torre, M., Cowhy, J., Moore, P., Saretain, L. and Knight, D. (2018). Research Report School Closings in Chicago: Staff and Student Experiences and Academic Outcomes. Chicago: UChicago Consortium on School Research.

Green, E. (2021). Surge of Student Suicides Pushes Las Vegas Schools to Reopen. *The New York Times* 1/24/21. Retrieved from https://www.nytimes.com/2021/01/24/us/politics/student-suicides-nevada-coronavirus.html?action=click&module=Top%20Stories&pgtype=Homepage

Kanno-Youngs, Z. (2020). 'Public Health' Expulsions of Children Halted. *The New York Times* (11/19/20).

Karp, S. (2019). Grading Mayor Rahm Emanuel's Education Legacy. WBEZ Chicago. (5/16/19). https://www.npr.org/local/309/2019/05/16/723743727/grading-mayor-ahm-emanuel-s-education-legacy retrieved 11/28/20

Lipman, P. (2011). Contesting the city: Neoliberal urbanism and the cultural politics of education reform in Chicago. *Discourse: Studies in the Cultural Politics of Education* 32(2):217–234. DOI: 10.1080/01596306.2011.562887.

Lipman, P., Vaughan, K. and Gutierrez, R. (2014). Root Shock: Parents' Perspectives on School Closings in Chicago. Chicago: Collaborative for Equity and Justice in Education. http://ceje.uic.edu/wp-content/uploads/2014/06/Root-Shock-Report-Compressed.pdf retrieved 11/29/20.

Luiselli, V. (2017). Tell me how it ends: An essay in 40 questions. Coffee House Press.

Luiselli, Valeria. (2019). Lost Children Archive. New York: Knopf Doubleday Publishing Group.

Kristof, N. (2020). We Interrupt This Gloom to Offer…Hope. *The New York Times* (7/19/20).

Mason, M.A. (2005). The U.S. and the International Children's Right Crusade: Leader or Laggard? *Journal of Social History* 38:955–963.

Mental Health America. (n.d.). The State of Mental Health in America. https://mhanational.org/issues/state-mental-health-america#Key

Nuzzo, J. and Sharfstein, J. (2020). America Has Its Priorities All Wrong. *The New York Times* (7/2/20).

Paddock, R. (2020). Teenage Sisters Focus on Bali's Trash Crisis. *The New York Times* (7/4/20).

Rosenblitt, D. (2008–2009). Where Do You Want the Killing Done? An Exploration of Hatred of Children. *Annual of Psychoanalysis* 36, 37:203–215.

Schmidt, E. (2009). City Project. Unpublished document. Chicago Psychoanalytic Institute.

Schmidt, E., Schloerb, A. and Cohler, B. (2013). Growth groups for kids: A school-based psychoanalytic groups intervention project for children exposed to violence. In M. O'Laughlin (ed.), *The uses of psychoanalysis in working with children's emotional lives* (pp. 135–150). NY: Aronson.

Sehgal, P. (2019, Feb 11). Valeria Luiselli's Latest Novel Is a Mold-Breaking New Classic. The New York Times. Retrieved from https://www.nytimes.com/2019/02/11/books/review-lost-children-archive-valeria-luiselli.html

Szalai, J (2020). Your Tired? Your Poor? Forget About It. *The New York Times* (8/6/20).

Taylor, K (2021). What Does it Mean to Go to Public School in the United States During the Pandemic? *The New York Times* (Special Report 1–22-21, pp. 4, 5).

Unicef The Convention on the Rights of the Child. (n.d.). https://www.unicef.org/child-rights-convention/convention-text# retrieved 11/29/20. https://www.unicef.org/child-rights-convention/what-is-the-convention retrieved 10/23/20. https://www.unicef.org/child-rights-convention/frequently-asked-questions retrieved 10/23/20.

Van Roekel, D. (2013). Chicago's Students Deserve Acts of Heroism. *Huffington Post* (5/23/2013).

Webley, K. (2013). Are School Closings Discriminatory? *Time Magazine* (5/11/13). https://nation.time.com/2013/05/23/are-school-closings-discriminatory/ retrieved 11/29/20.

What is the Convention on the Rights of the Child. (2020, October 23). Retrieved from https://www.unicef.org/child-rights-convention/what-is-the-convention
Winnicott, D.W. (1949). Hate in the counter-transference. *International Journal of Psycho-Analysis* 30:69–74.
Winslow, S. (2013). Chicago School Closings Spark 'Wildfire' of Protest. *Labor Notes* 3/27/13. https://www.labornotes.org/2013/03/chicago-school-closings-spark-wildfire-protest retrieved 11/28/20.
Yaccino, S. (2013). Protests Fail to Deter Chicago From Closing 49 Schools. *The New York Times* (5/22/13). https://www.nytimes.com/2013/05/23/education/despite-protests-chicago-closing-schools.html retrieved 11/29/20.
Young-Bruehl, E. (2012). *Childism: Confronting Prejudice Against Children*. New Haven: Yale University Press.

15

Long-term treatment in the rearview mirror

William S. Meyer

It is intriguing for me to reread my paper, "In Defense of Long-Term Treatment" now 26 years old, which included my assessment and interactions with Sue, some seven years into our work together. I suggested in the article that treatment was likely to continue for an indeterminate period. I could not have been more prescient, in that our work together was to continue for a total of 30 years. While Sue generally did what she could to put on her best game face – and when she was on, she had a terrific sense of humor – there were stretches when Sue suffered from unremitting depression and deep feelings of hopelessness.

I will soon return to discussing my work with Sue, even though she was not the primary inspiration for me to write that paper. While I make no mention of it in the article, what prompted me, at that time, to write defending long-term treatment was a suicidal crisis involving a patient of mine, John, a depressed, Duke college freshman. My experience with John was too fresh and too raw to write about at the time and I was too emotionally vulnerable to expose myself.

John

I don't remember much about John, a depressed college freshman at Duke, first time away from home, because his time in treatment with me was so brief. What I do remember is that it was during a time when managed care was pervading the mental health field and all practitioners could feel its presence. There it was, lurking over our shoulders, assessing every diagnosis, every treatment decision, every clinical appointment, and every treatment plan.

It was not that I was unsympathetic to why managed care entered the mental health marketplace. I had worked on inpatient psychiatric units and knew that abuse of the system was common. I had seen long-term hospitalizations provided for people who could have done just as well in outpatient treatment – adults with chronic personality disturbances and teenagers whose problems were no more serious than getting caught smoking marijuana – hospitalized for weeks and months at a time, provided the patients had multi-million-dollar

DOI: 10.4324/9781003325512-19

mental health insurance policies. As a consequence, there was a proliferation of newly built private psychiatric hospitals, which served little purpose other than to drain such funds from insurance companies. A common scenario: Patients would be kept in the hospital because they were deemed too ill for discharge. When their insurance ran out, however, and they could no longer remain in private institutional care, the patients would be transferred to the local state hospital which provided care for the most ill patients in much less plush surroundings than private hospitals could provide. Miraculously, most of these patients, within weeks, days, or even hours, were suddenly well enough to go home, and they and their families would be clamoring for immediate discharge.

When hospitals were monetarily incentivized to keep patients as long as possible, *managed care was necessary* to provide oversight to determine when longer term psychiatric hospitalizations were medically necessary. Unfortunately, this oversight became overarching in all aspects of mental health care, even outpatient care, in all psychiatric clinics, including our own at Duke. The expectation of working quickly and briefly and the frenetic atmosphere it created was becoming pervasive in psychiatry departments and mental health clinics throughout the US. The message was clear: treatments were to be short-term – the quicker, the better. As I mentioned in the original article, managed care was having a "sentinel effect." It was a battle for the mind of the therapist, in which therapists would internalize a hostile sentinel guarding against and thwarting any inclination toward longer-term treatments.

The effect this had on clinicians was profound, and the needs of the patient were replaced by whatever the insurance covered. Clinicians, especially those newer to the field, were inclined to mistrust themselves and trust the communications from the insurance companies. Clinical training in every mental health profession was altered to promote brief treatments. Frequently, programs justified this type of training by saying "we need to prepare the clinician of tomorrow by teaching them the clinical skills that insurance companies will pay for." It cannot be overstated how thoroughly and long-lasting an influence this had on clinical thinking.

With John, I felt pressure to hurry my assessment, rush my treatment, accompanied by the pressure to bring treatment to its quickest possible conclusion. Managed care was omnipresent in our clinic and it affected everything I was doing, not only with John, but with everyone I was seeing at the time. Prior to that time, I was told by supervisors to slow down, take my time, get to know the patient, not to rush to judgment either about diagnosis or treatment.

After the very few sessions that John and I met, during which time I was hurriedly trying to get him to be less symptomatic, I received a call from an administrative dean informing me that John had slit his wrists and would be taking medical leave from the school. Perhaps only a practicing psychotherapist can fully imagine how devastating it is to receive such a call. I was horrified and guilt-ridden, convinced that my departure from my usual, gradual way of getting to know a new patient contributed substantively to this sad outcome.

Long-term treatment? For whom?

In my original article, I used the clinical example of my seven years of work with Sue, not anticipating that my work with her would last so long. I had chosen the case because she had suffered childhood abuse in the extreme, and my rationale was that no one would argue against long-term care for someone who had been subjected to such severe maltreatment. At the time, I thought it necessary to use such an extreme case to bolster my argument that people who had such horrific backgrounds, often required long periods of time in treatment. What I didn't appreciate at the time, due to my relative inexperience, was just how varied are the patients who need or are helped by long-term care.

To be clear, not everyone I see wants or needs long-term therapy. In my practice, some people want to be seen only a few sessions, some for months, others for years, and still others indeterminately. After formal therapy concludes, some stay in touch with me via e-mail and others still may wish to come in on occasion. Moreover, at one time, it was assumed that a geographical move on the part of the patient or therapist automatically ended the therapy. Now, with the increased use of video conferencing, this opens an opportunity for therapeutic work to continue long-distance.

Dr. S.

Dr. S., a prominent physician, who is gay, entered therapy when he was in his 30s. Although his parents, both physicians, cared for him, his life became bleak when, at age six, he was sent for 18 months to a boarding school. The school was run by a sadistic headmaster. Beatings were commonplace and bullying and cruelty by the other boys was an everyday occurrence.

Although he had long considered himself to be his mother's favorite, when at the age of 18 he came out to her, she said, "You are an abomination. I wish you had never been born." At the age of 28, he fell in love with a male roommate and enjoyed a deep friendship that was intimate, but not sexual. When Dr. S. ultimately confessed to his roommate his more amorous feelings, the roommate hastily moved out.

Dr. S. felt lonely and rejected and turned to drugs to compensate. For the next four years, he was hooked on amphetamines. By the time he was 32, he was taking huge doses every day, and at night, chloral hydrate, a hypnotic, to sleep. He began calling in sick at work, sometimes for days at a time, and lost nearly 80 pounds in three months. Nearly one year later, almost always under the influence of some substance, he presented himself for treatment to a male psychiatrist/psychoanalyst, who was approximately his same age. He wrote of that experience,

> I was suspicious ... he was so young ... What experience of life, what therapeutic power, I thought could I find in someone scarcely older than myself? I soon realized that this was someone of exceptional character ... someone who felt I could tolerate and profit from intensive analysis ...

But the psychiatrist insisted that for treatment to continue, Dr. S. must give up drugs, whose use, he said, made success in treatment impossible. Dr. S. never took amphetamines again and wrote that treatment had saved his life many times over. Neither he nor his friends thought he would make it past his mid-thirties. Dr. S. saw his psychiatrist twice a week for nearly five decades!

While the psychiatrist, Leonard Shengold, is known mostly in psychoanalytic circles, particularly for his work and books on "Soul Murder" (1989, 1999), the patient is the beloved, world-renowned author and neurologist, the late Oliver Sacks. The story above is detailed in two books in particular, (Sacks, 2001, 2015); the second memoir, written when Sacks was past 80.

Of note, shortly after Sacks' 75th birthday, he met a man named "Billy." To quote Sacks, "Timid and inhibited all my life, I let a friendship and intimacy grow between us ..." Shortly thereafter, Billy told Sacks, "I have conceived a deep love for you." Sacks writes,

> I had conceived a deep love for him too – and my eyes filled with tears ... It was a new experience for me to lie quietly in someone's arms and talk, or listen to music, or be silent together ... We have a tranquil, many-dimensional sharing of our lives – a great and unexpected gift in my old age, after a lifetime of keeping at a distance.

Who can say which persons can benefit from long-term treatment and how long such treatment should take?

Long-term treatment or brief? If an individual was on a psychotropic medicine that provided symptom relief, would anyone suggest that the person stop taking it? If anything, patients are generally discouraged, and usually strongly so, from tampering with a drug regimen that has demonstrated efficacy. How ironic then, that if it is a human relationship that helps someone feel better, most individuals who have influence in the mental health field (supervisors, insurance companies, mental health agencies) press to know when the date for will be for, of all words, *termination*. Victor Bloom (1997) remarked that he had a patient say, "I don't want to get well; if I did, I wouldn't be able to see you anymore." In reality, Bloom notes, the therapy was the most gratifying situation in the patient's life. For the patient, it was worth every penny, because in the session, the therapist's attention, ameliorating the patient's yearning to be loved and understood, was being gratified, albeit not completely. Why should a patient fear that getting well will necessarily result in the loss of a therapist? As Bergmann (1997) has noted, for many patients, the therapeutic relationship is the best love relationship they have ever experienced.

Sue

While nearly all of my clinical work is standard psychotherapy, built on the convention of the 50-minute, office-based hour, I have always allowed for an unconventional approach to therapy, tailoring what I do to the unique needs of any individual patient. Sue was very special to me. I had been impacted not only by the severity and chronicity of the many traumas in her life, but how, despite such suffering, she maintained her perseverance, dignity, and warm humor. Our work together evolved into a deep, mutually rewarding and intimate collaboration that was anything but conventional.

How unconventional? In the early work of our treatment, Sue found meeting in my hospital-based office too confining, and we had our sessions strolling through the hospital grounds. Sue was a chronic smoker, and once, I told her I would take her to a local baseball game of the famous Durham Bulls, if she would even consider stopping smoking. She knew I would not in any way shame her for trying and that my offer was one of caring for her well-being. We went to the ball game, and while the smoking abated for a time, she resumed within weeks. I took her out to lunch once a year for her birthday and accompanied her to her first visit to a senior citizen's center in the hopes of helping her be more social. Despite this unconventional approach, I took care that no professional ethical boundary would ever be crossed.

Throughout my career within Duke's Department of Psychiatry, I have been involved in training psychiatric residents. Once each year, I would arrange for Sue to give a lecture to them about what it is that helps patients. She would use her clinical relationship with me as a case example. Her favorite admonition was to remind them that they should never talk to patients like they were "reading from a textbook," a trait of mine that she brought up with me with some frequency during the early years of our work. Many psychiatry trainees told me how meaningful their interchange with Sue was, and I know that for her it was an annual event that brought her great joy, as she, with only a high school diploma, was "teaching" the psychiatrists of the future.

Sue's final days

When I met Sue, she was still residing with her mother, having never lived on her own. Ultimately, I worked with Sue for over three decades, seeing her in our early years through several psychiatric hospitalizations, through the death of her mother with whom she lived, then through several moves.

While our counseling sessions allowed Sue the opportunity to tell her story, our most important therapeutic goal was for Sue to get to know how she truly felt and to enable true self-expression with those around her. Although the majority of our time was spent in my listening to and providing psychotherapy for Sue, I, as perhaps only a clinical social worker would, provided concrete help in many ways as well. I supported and helped her through several relocations, from an apartment to a trailer, then to housing for the disabled. Later, when she developed crippling medical problems, I helped her move to a nursing home, where I visited her intermittently. While I did not participate in the actual moves themselves, I arranged for someone to deliver some used furniture from my family to hers and I was able to procure for her a computer from which through e-mail she would update me about her personal life. Usually, however, she would simply send me cartoons and witty postings that she found amusing. I wanted very much for her to have as full a life as possible and did whatever I could to encourage her in that direction, while also providing some of that fullness when I could.

Once, in an e-mail, she wrote me this:

> *Any time I am with you I feel like a weight has been taken off me. I get to smile and laugh with you. There is so much beauty in this world. Sometimes it falls in your lap, other times you have to look hard to see it. Just thank you again for everything you had given me, for my mind and for fun. A song that is in my top 5 is "winter summer or fall, you will be there when I call." Every word is what you mean to me and so much more. All I can work on now is getting well at this time.*
>
> *It has been near 30 years. I am so happy we are still friends. My heart just feels so warm when I think about you, and your caring for me. You have such a big heart, thank you for putting up with me during all that has gone on in my life for so long.*
>
> *I will never forget one thing.*
>
> *Always your friend, Sue*

Much of our treatment involved helping her with life's challenges and helping her to remain out of the hospital, which she succeeded in doing for at least the last 25 years of our collaborative work. She knew how hard I tried for her and the depth of my sympathy for all that she had been through in this life. The type of work I'd done with her contained elements of "supportive psychotherapy" (Werman, 1984), case management (Kanter, 2000) and even palliative psychotherapy. In a brief essay on the latter topic, Kahn (2011) wrote that it is therapy whose goal it is to make another's existence "a little less lonely and painful."

A couple of years ago, I got a call from one of Sue's relatives, informing me that Sue had suffered a severe stroke, had been rushed to a nearby hospital, and was lying comatose. The call came during a weekend and I was able to make it to the hospital and plant a kiss on my dear friend's cheek, the day before she died.

To illustrate one small element of our work, there came a time when we focused primarily on the need for her to stand up for herself to family and friends. I tapped into her sense of humor at the end of one session by saying, "Now this week, don't take no shit off nobody." Sue loved that line and for years we would say this to each other at the end of every session. During this period, she told me about a television program she had just seen. I was so moved that I wrote a poem about it and gave it to her as a holiday gift. In the poem, I mention a patient encounter I had in the high-risk obstetrics clinic, where, in addition to my psychotherapy practice, I have now worked for the past 20 years.

She had the poem framed and kept it at her bedside:

FOR SUE,
AND THE VANQUISHED SOULS OF BABY ELEPHANTS
"I just saw a TV show about an elephant," you told me.
"I used to be just like him.
When he was a baby they chained his ankle.
He squealed and squirmed until there was no more fight left in him. He was just too puny to pull away.
Now he has a chain around his mind.
His baby memories run so deep he doesn't realize that now he is grown and powerful.
Why he could pull that chain out of the ground any old time he wants to. He just doesn't know it. So all he does is stand there.
I used to be just like him."

I remembered how our weeks of therapy turned into months turned into years.
You couldn't trust me at first. No wonder, given the nightmare that was your childhood.
Over time, our therapy became infused with love.
You brought me your pain, your courage, your integrity, your warmth, and your humor.
Once at the end of a session I looked you square-in-the-eye and said,
"Now this week, don't take no shit off nobody!" You laughed.
At the end of the next session, you looked me square-in-the-eye and said,
"Now don't you take no shit off nobody!" We both laughed.
And so it went. Every week we would end the session with a square-in-the-eye-look and say, "Now don't take no shit off nobody!"
It was a good way to end our sessions.
Link by link your long chain fell away.

Yesterday, in clinic, I saw a wisp of a woman who had a pregnant belly and a blackened eye.
She had come to her appointment with HIM. HE had dark glasses and stank of alcohol.

"I bumped my head on a door," she lied to me.
I looked through her medical chart. An emergency room visit, and Another, and ANOTHER.
she had been hit, Punched, PUSHed and KICKED.
I dug back through her chart to when she was a child.
abuse, abUSE, ABUSE. bad parents, Foster Care, MORE FOSTER CARE.
"I can help you," I told her.
"I can get you in a shelter that will keep you safe. Just don't leave here with HIM."
HE had already started down the hallway. HE looked back with a dagger-eyed glare.
First at me, then at her. What HE expected was clear.
She walked – toward HIM, paused, turned around and – for one eternal moment – fixed her eyes upon mine.
I pleaded with my look. As hard as I possibly could.
But she lifted her chin, did a half-pirouette, and flashed her sad smile – at HIM.
Arms entangled, they departed.
All I could do was stand there. And watch them get smaller in the distance.

Perhaps one day, like you, she will find the land where the elephants all run free.

References

Bergmann, M.S. (1997). Termination: The Achilles heel of psychoanalytic technique. *Psychoanalytic Psychology*, *14*, 163–174.

Bloom, V. (1997). Interminable analysis? *Journal of the American Academy of Psychoanalysis and Dynamic Psychaitry*, *25*(2), 313–316.

Kahn, M.W. (2011). Palliative psychotherapy. *American Journal of Psychiatry*, *168*(9), 888–889.

Kanter, J. (2000). Beyond psychotherapy: Therapeutic relationships in community care. *Smith College Studies in Social Work*, *70*(3), 397–426.

Sacks, O. (2001). *Uncle Tungsten: Memories of a chemical boyhood*. New York, NY: Vintage Books.

Sacks, O. (2015). *On the move: A life*. New York, NY: Alfred A. Knopf.

Shengold, L. (1989). *Soul murder: The effects of childhood abuse and deprivation*. New York, NY: Ballantine Books.

Shengold, L. (1999). *Soul murder revisited: Thoughts about therapy, hate, love and memory*. New Haven, CT: Yale University Press.

Werman, D.S. (1984). *The practice of supportive psychotherapy*. New York, NY: Brunner/Mazel.

Stepping toward the future

PsiAN's vision

Linda L. Michaels, Janice R. Muhr and Nancy Burke

Psychotherapy of depth, insight and relationship has an essential and vital role to play in the much-needed healing of the world. This epilogue, written by the three founding co-chairs of the Psychotherapy Action Network (PsiAN), revisits some of the central themes from this special issue and considers both the reasons for hope and the threats to the overarching vision captured in this special issue.Psychotherapy of depth, insight and relationship sits at a nodal point, embedded between psyche and social life, between the inner and the outer of our most personal experiences, between the obstacles we face and the opportunities we create. It's not called "the impossible profession" for nothing; in our rich and broken world, it evokes many roles at once – parent, interpreter, doctor, shaman, scientist, judge, teacher, sociologist, priest, alchemist and poet – but perhaps most central is its function as container of the most difficult and profound aspects of human suffering and healing. Admittedly a tall order, and yet we see possibilities that are as incomplete as they are invaluable. In short, psychotherapy of depth, insight and relationship has an essential and vital role to play in the much-needed healing of the world.

We three founding co-chairs of the Psychotherapy Action Network (PsiAN) for the last five years, and we hope that the essays in this volume have given voice to the significance of therapies of depth, insight and relationship. These therapies have not only transformed individual lives but have rippled out to affect family, friends, vocation and culture, acting, at their best, as both a force and a forum for social justice. Personal and social embedded tiers of healing are inextricably linked and we need to attend to both as we stand up for the rights of people to be treated as subjects rather than as objects, and protect arenas in which relationships based on recognition, rather than on reductionism or exploitation, can flourish. These broad, lofty goals are enacted concretely step by step, session by session, in consulting rooms around the world, but they also increasingly inform the efforts of organizations and institutions to stretch themselves to encounter more directly the communities, events, systems and ideologies in which they are embedded.

If therapies of depth, insight and relationship share an overlapping vision and stand with other social movements that aim to protect human rights and

DOI: 10.4324/9781003325512-20

cultivate respect for difference, they also face parallel threats, as the first series of essays in the **Social, Political and Economic Context** describe. Psychotherapists cannot be blind to the steady encroachments into the fields of psychology, psychiatry, social work and related disciplines of quantification, capitalism, fundamentalism, authoritarianism, reductionism, scientism and so many of the other "-isms" of modernity. The study and practice of mental healthcare writ large have been vulnerable to corruption since its inception by social currents and economic demands that not only have bent its methods to bolster dangerous social programs, but also have argued against the legitimacy of fundamental ideas of internal life, and with them, therapies of depth, insight and relationship. Clearly, psychotherapy cannot do its part in helping people to appreciate the values and meanings of both the internal and external aspects of their lives if we allow our field to be guided, either unconsciously or uncritically, by forces that devalue both.

While the movement toward so-called evidence-based treatment has gone a long way toward dismissing these therapies as unscientific and without sufficient data to support them, there is, in fact, an abundance of evidence – quantitative, qualitative, experiential – to establish their essential value. Depth therapies have been found to offer significant, long-lasting, global results, not merely in remediating symptoms but in changing lives. For all of this, we call them "therapies that stick" (Michaels, 2020). They are highly cost-effective, particularly when viewed in the larger context of long-term social benefit. In our advocacy, we must find clear and compelling ways to communicate this strong and growing evidence base to multiple audiences including policy makers, legislators, mental health professionals and the general public. Meeting this challenge will be crucial if we are to sustain the relevance of therapies of depth, insight and relationship in a social climate and mental health milieu that tends toward reductionism, a misapplied understanding of scientific method, and quick fixes, and away from the healing nature of relationship.

It is often the *experiential* evidence, patients' and practitioners' day-to-day witnessing together of change and growth, that is most compelling to those who encounter it. While this form of evidence isn't as easily studied in randomized controlled trials and is unlikely by itself to impress lab-based researchers, insurers, and policy makers who often make decisions without the benefit of personal knowledge of what therapy can do, it speaks for itself to students, practitioners and patients alike. When other types of interventions have disappointed them, those who haven't given up have been able to locate the failure in the intervention – not in themselves. They have turned to deeper treatments, and then often stuck with them because they know the investment they've made in the process and, more importantly, in themselves is worth it.

Thus, in the second series of essays, **Therapies of Depth, Insight and Relationship**, we hope you have found compelling descriptions, not only of these therapies, but of the hope they hold. Central to the contribution made by psychotherapies of depth, insight and relationship is their view of human problems not as pathologies to be excised, but as personal expressions of distress which are meaningful and can be understood and appreciated. Depth psychotherapies have developed a multitude of vocabularies for describing emotional suffering, and they take as their starting point the question, "What happened to you and how have your reactions to those experiences shaped you over time?" in stark contrast to interventions that begin with the question, "What's wrong with you?" These therapies encounter symptoms not by seeing them as less but as more, as messages whose translation leads to letting go of, rather than cutting off or dissociating, troublesome patterns of thought and action. This refusal to pathologize and reject parts of the self-offers not only a crucial tool for the resolution of internal fragmentation and conflict in our patients, but a prototype for comprehending and addressing those forms of prejudice that often lead to efforts to excise unfamiliar groups on a mass scale.

There is no more important time than the present to support the appreciation and availability of psychotherapies of depth, insight and relationship. We live in an age of social upheaval characterized by widespread experiences of intergenerational, complex trauma, both acute and accumulated. Moreover, there has been a simultaneous erosion of cultural resources that can absorb this outsized need for healing. There are too few social institutions that can rise to meet suffering people where they are, and too many societal and economic influences that increasingly offer superficial options for repeating traumas rather than resolving them. However, rather than protect us from the marketplace demands of better-faster-cheaper-easier-simpler, our educational institutions and professional organizations have too often allied with the economic and ideological forces that feed these pressures. We need professional organizations that place creativity, personal connection, and deeper well-being among the experiences and outcomes most worthy of study. We also need a shift in the foci of clinical education to engender internal, experiential growth and the cultivation of sensitivity, empathy and capacity for connection, as of equal importance with the dissemination of declarative knowledge. In the arenas of education and of practice alike, the PsiAN aims to support those who value intensive treatment, both through advocacy on its behalf and by working to reach a generation of therapists-in-training enlivened by its insights and potential. We are committed to ensuring that in-depth treatments are available not just to those with means, but to those who need them most.

Our last section of essays, **Implications and Future Actions**, holds perspectives on an admittedly incomplete number of compelling contemporary issues, social and technological, that we need to understand and integrate into how we work, in order to utilize the powerful force for healing of both individuals and society that is inherent in our therapies. In our own research with the public, we find that people want to understand the root of their problems and believe this undertaking and growth in self-awareness are worth the time it takes. However, we learned that people do not know what these forms of therapy are called, let alone how to access them. Helping to educate the public, in addition to elevating their expectations for therapy, form a crucial part of our mission. We cannot do this without also grappling with the ways socially induced suffering is lived by our patients and manifest in our work. This means integrating into our sense of professional identity and social responsibility a heightened understanding of the world outside of our offices – how it contributes both to inner suffering and to inadequate mental health systems, and how we need to engage with it to accomplish healing in both arenas.

The work of PsiAN has just begun, but we are confident, five years out, that its path is one of significance and growth. A strong and vibrant advocacy organization that can speak forcefully in defense of psychotherapy stands not merely to preserve its practice for the next generation and beyond, but to contribute to the knowledge base of psychoanalytic, humanistic and other depth and relational perspectives by helping therapists look outside of their offices to become more vividly aware of and engaged with the wider context of systems, populations and communities in which their practices, patients and selves are embedded.

Our ambitions are inescapably large: to create an available vocabulary that is embraced by the public, an educational program that cultivates the relational capacities of students, a sufficient roster of engaged clinicians and an economic system that recognizes the value of personal transformation. It will require the sustained effort of many in what is, in the end, not just a defense of psychotherapy, but of what's human in us and can be expressed humanely in our world. We are grateful that our all-volunteer membership and our advisors, many of whose articles are included in this volume, have already contributed so significantly to PsiAN's efforts. We look forward to the partnership of those who will join us to reclaim a landscape in which therapies of depth, insight and relationship can set roots and flourish, and hope we have convinced you to be among them.

Reference

Michaels, L. (2020, March 24). Why depth therapy is more enduring than a quick fix of CBT. Aeon. Retrieved February 09, 2021, from https://aeon.co/essays/why-depth-therapy-is-more-enduring-than-a-quick-fix-of-cbt

Index

Note: **Bold** page numbers refer to tables and page numbers followed by "n" denote endnotes.

abuse of discretion 69
academics 214; professional organizations and 214; and therapists 170
accountable care organizations 103
Acemoglu, D. 246
Affordable Care Act (ACA) 9, 38, 57, 58; essential health benefits 59, **59**
Akhtar, S. 256
alliance building 122–123
American Psychiatric Association 24
American Psychoanalytic Association 10
American Psychological Association (APA) 86–88, 114, 173
Angell, M. 140
anti-Semitism 85, 86, 93
artificial intelligence (AI) 251
awareness of therapy 226–227

Bakan, D. 84, 85
Beck, A.T. 23, 81, 91
behavioral intentions 221–224
Bellah, R.N. 188
Bendat, M. 3, 46, 48
Benedict, R. 191
Benjamin, B. 116
Bentall, R.P. 140
Bentham, J. 20–21
Bergmann, M.S. 294
Bernstein, R. 183
Bion, W. 155n9
Bloom, V. 293
borderline personality disorder 43, 45
Borg, M.B. 257
Bornstein, R. 178
Boss, M. 192
Brigham, C.C. 85
Broken Brain model 135, 137–138, 141, 142, 146, 151–153
Bugental, J.F.T. 122
Burke, N. 1, 6
Byrd-Bennett, B. 280
Byron, L. 186

Caligor, E. 176
capitalism 100, 101, 114, 116
capitation 103
case formulation 163, 178
Christensen, C. 246
Churchill, S.D. 195
Clark, D. 26
clinical depression 24
cognition 26, 27
cognitive behavioral therapy (CBT) 2, 19, 40, 92, 212; human nature 25–26; neoliberalism and managerialism 24–25; NICE 33; psychiatry and clinical psychology 23–24; psychoanalysis and 227–229; research 28–33; treatment 26–27
Colaizzi, P.F. 195
Community Mental Health Act 57
Cornelius, J.T. 4
Corno, F.D. 178
cost-effectiveness 41–46
COVID-19 14, 211, 283
critical psychiatry 24
cultural identity 221, 262, 279

Dalal, F. 2
Danto, E.A. 83, 255
declarative knowledge 121, 300
Delboy, S. 5
depression 43, 172
diagnosis 162; academia 170–172; cost containment 166–167; legacy of changes 164–166; pharmaceutical corporations 167–170; present-*versus*-absent criteria 173
Diagnostic and Statistical Manual (DSM) 162
dialectical behavior therapy (DBT) 32
Dilthey, W. 184
Duke, D. 92

Edwards, D. 193
Eisold, K. 269
electroconvulsive therapy (ECT) 136, 140
Ellis, A. 3, 81
Emanuel, M.R. 280
empathic immersion 123–125
Employee Retirement Income Security Act of 1974 ("ERISA") 59, 64
Erickson, E.H. 82, 86
Erikson, E. 255
Essig, T. 5
"evidence-based" claims 221
evidence-based practice (EBP) 100; administrative costs 103; dominates 101–102; free market 105; free market economy 103–104; landscape of mental health 111–113; movement 102; neoliberal exploitation 106–108; neoliberal illusion 108–110; pharmaceutical costs 103; reality 102; social forces 101; systemic forces 101
Ewing, E. 275, 281
Eysenck, H.J. 92

Fanon, F. 83
Federal Parity Act 58–60
Ferenczi, S. 284
Fischer, C.T. 195
Flores, J. 257
Foa, E. 173
Fox, G.K. 193, 194, 195
Frank, K.A. 125
Freud, S. 78, 79, 82, 83, 197, 254, 257, 278; "Wild Psychoanalysis" 254
Friborg, O. 102
Friedman, M. 25
Fromm, E. 83, 255

Gazzillo, F. 178
Geisteswissenschaften 184
Gendlin, E. 187, 192
genuine/authentic care 125–127
Gergen, K.J. 199
ghost networks 213
Giorgi, A. 182, 183, 191
Gnaulati, E. 4
Goddard, H.H. 85
Goldacre, B. 28
Goldstein, K. 192
Gordon, R. 178, 179
Granatir, W.L. 258
Greenspan, S. 175, 176, 177

Hall, G.S. 79, 80, 84, 86
Halling, S. 192
Health and Human Services (HHS) 58
Health Insurance Portability and Accountability Act of 1996 (HIPAA) 70
Heidegger, M. 184, 187
Hollander, N.C. 116
Horney, K. 83
Husserl, E. 184, 187

illegal insurance protocols 46–48
Increasing Access to Psychological Therapies (IAPT) 34–35
insurance companies 9, 242
insurance reimbursement 38–40
intensive psychotherapy 42, 81
International Classification of Diseases (ICD) 162

James, W. 3, 79, 80, 81, 184, 191, 192
Johnsen, T.J. 102
Jung, C.G. 131

Kahn, M.W. 295
Kant, I. 21
Kennedy, J.F. 57
Kernberg, O.F. 173, 176, 178
King, R.A. 257, 258
Kirk, S. 24
Klein, M. 255
Kuhn–Popper debate 183
Kutchins, H. 24

Layard, R. 20, 26
Layton, L. 116
Lazar, S.G. 2
Leichsenring, F. 40
Liang, B. 258
Lomas, P. 128
long-term psychodynamic psychotherapy (LTPP) 44, 45, 290–297
Lowen, A. 192
Luiselli, V. 275, 278, 279
Lukoff, D. 193
Luria, A.R. 82, 191

Madsen, R. 188
Malberg, N. 178
Malone, J. 178
managerialism 24–25
Martin, G.B. 27, 28
Marx, K. 85, 86
Maslow, A. 184, 191, 192
Mayes, L. 178
May, R. 184, 192, 197
McCance-Katz, E. 102
McWilliams, N. 4, 266
medical necessity guidelines 38, 39, 46, 65, 66, 67, 71, 104, 213
medications 39, 137, 221; psychiatric 213; psychotropic 43, 136, 153, 155n10; research on psychotherapy *vs.* 169; scientific comparison of 169
Meehl, P.E. 32
mental distress: biasing influence 141; Broken Brain model 135, 137–138; drug manufacturers 139; epidemiologic evidence 139; psychiatric diagnoses 145–146; suicide rates 140; symphonic perspective 135, 146–149
mental health parity: appealing 70–72; applicability laws **60**; clinical considerations 72; cloaking the identities 62; enforcement challenges 63–65, **64**; inadequate access 57; in- and outpatient care 59; “independent” review organizations 65–66; litigation 66–67; prohibitions **63**; proposed solutions 67–69; regulations operationalize 61–62
The Mental Health Parity and Addiction Equity Act (MHPAEA) 9, 38, 39, 57
Messer, S.B. 192
Meyer, W. 6
Michaels, L. 1, 5, 6, 11, 241
Midgley, N. 178
Miller, I.S. 258
Miller, M. 193, 195
mindfulness-based cognitive therapy (MBCT) 31, 32
Moyers, B. 200n1
Muhr, J. 1, 6, 11
Mundo, E. 178

Nageotte, J. 178
National Alliance for Mental Illness (NAMI) 155n1
National Association for the Advancement of Psychoanalysis 10
The National Institute for Health and Care Excellence (NICE) 33
National Registry of Evidence-Based Programs and Practices (NREPP) 102
Neem tree 22–23
neo-Kraepelinian diagnosis 162, 164
neoliberalism 24–25
NICE *see* The National Institute for Health and Care Excellence (NICE)
non-quantitative treatment limitations (NQTL) 61
Norcross, J.C. 173

O'Neil, J. 178
Overskeid, G. 91

Parens, H. 258
patient health questionnaire 27–28
personality disorders 42, 45
physical illnesses 163
Plotkin, D. 177, 178
Polkinghorne, D. 183, 191
postmodernist philosophy 183, 198–199
price elasticity 38
PsiAN *see* Psychotherapy Action Network (PsiAN)
psychiatric medications 213
psychiatry 163
psychoanalysis 78; American Psychological Association 86–88; applications 266–271; case study 259–266; and CBT 227–229; community intervention 257–259; critiques and dismissals 82; cultural

fascination 83; dissident force 114, 115; diversity 256–257; exclusion 78, 88–90; formulation 82; history 79–86, 90–92, 100; insights 113–114; late-stage capitalism 114; marginalization 78; neoliberal system 114; political mythology 104–105; time 115
Psychodynamic Diagnostic Manual (PDM) 162, 175–179
psychodynamic therapy: cost-effectiveness 41–46; "evidence-based" research protocols 40–41; illegal insurance protocols 46; insurance reimbursement 38–40; lawsuit 46
psychological wellbeing practitioners (PWP) 34
Psychotherapy Action Network (PsiAN): accessibility 13; activists-from-the-margins 13; committees 12; evidence base 10; extensive qualitative 10; insight and relationship 10; instant-gratification ideology 9; insurance companies 9; marketers 8; multi-faceted advocacy organization 14; organizational structure 12; principles 11; quantitative market research 10; space and time 8; tremendous value 10; vision 298–301
psychotropic medications 43, 136, 153, 155n10
Public Health Service Act (PHSA) 59

qualitative research 215–216
quantitative research 216–219

racial identity 221, 236, 261, 262, 264
racism 93, 115, 263, 267–268, 280; systemic 280–281, 285
Rand Health Experiment 39
randomized control trials 190, 212
Rayner, R. 80
Reich, W. 192
relational healing: alliance building 122–123; empathic immersion 123–125; genuine/authentic care 125–127; humanistic revamping 127–130
relationship 121; insight and 10
remote treatment 247
remote *vs.* in-person therapy 221
Rennie, D.L. 195
Restrepo, P. 246
rights of children: about childism 276–277; education 279–284; lost children 277–279; mental health care 284–286; principles 274
Rogers, C. 184, 192
romanticism 5; benefits 191–192; complementary value 192–198; origins and nature 183–184; postmodern challenge 198–199; price of discarding 189–191; psychology 186–189; threats 184–186
Rosenberg, L. 178
Rosenblitt, D. 277
Rosner, R.I. 91
Rushton, J.P. 92
Russell. G.I. 244

Sacks, O. 293
Sampson, E.E. 199
Sartre, J.P. 127, 187
Sass, L. 186
Scheel, K.R. 32
Schmidt, E. 6
Schneider, K. 5
Schneider, K.J. 192, 195
Scholom, A. 3
Schore, A.N. 123
Schultz, D.P. 82
Schultz, S.E. 82
scientific validity 142–145
Sehgal, P. 277
self-actualization 191–192
Seligman, M.E. 3, 20, 81, 82, 86
Shedler, J. 33, 41, 42, 102, 176, 178
Shelley, C.A. 258
Shore, K. 188
Skinner, B.F. 3, 81, 86
sleeper effect 43
Smith, H.F. 257
Society for Psychoanalysis and Psychoanalytic Psychology 10
Speranza, A.M. 178
Speranza, M. 178
Spitzer, R.L. 23
Stein, D.B. 127
Steinert, C. 40
Stevick, E.L. 195
Stricker, G. 163
Sullivan, H.S. 83
Sullivan, W.M. 188
symphonic perspective 4; beginning treatment and deprescribing 151–152; costs 152–154; emotions

147; listening, context and dialogue 149–151; modern psychoanalytic theory 147; mood complaint 147; priority 146
systemic racism 280–281, 285

Tipton, S.M. 188
treatment-resistant depression 28, 44
Trump, D. 101
Tummala-Narra, P. 6, 258
Turkle, S. 244
Turner, E. 29
Twemlow, S.W. 258
Twenge, J.M. 32

United Behavioral Health (UBH) 213; conflicts of interest 46–47; guidelines 47–48; Wit *vs.* 49
U.S. health care system 104
U.S. Substance Abuse and Mental Health Services Administration (SAMHSA) 102

Valle, R. 192
valuable aspects of therapy 224–225
Van Deurzen, E. 130
the Vienna Circle 21–22
volkenpsychologie 182
vulnerability 80, 105, 109, 114, 220

Waldron, S. 178
Walker, E. 91
Wallerstein, S. 176
Wampold, B.E. 173
Watson, J.B. 3, 23, 79, 80, 81, 84, 86, 91
Web 2.0 250
Wertheimer, M. 191
Wertz, F.J. 192, 195
Westen, D. 33, 176
West, J. 258
"Wild Psychoanalysis" (Freud) 254
Winnicott, D.W. 155n9, 276
Wittgenstein, L. 162
Wolpe, J. 81, 82, 87
World Health Organization 43
Wundt, W. 182

Yakushko, O. 3
Yerkes, R.M. 84
Yin, R.K. 194, 195
Young-Bruehl, E. 276